Douglas H. Ruben, PhD

Publicity for Mental Health Clinicians: Using TV, Radio, and Print Media to Enhance Your Public Image

Pre-publication REVIEWS, COMMENTARIES, EVALUATIONS . . .

"**T**he book *Publicity for Mental Health Clinicians* by Dr. Douglas H. Ruben provides a well-thought-out and unusual approach to unique problems experienced by mental health professionals. Dr. Ruben's book clearly provides avenues for public awareness that are much needed in the field of mental health."

Nancy R. Macciomei, EdD
*Area Coordinator
of Exceptional Children's Programs,
Charlotte-Mecklenburg Schools,
Charlotte, North Carolina*

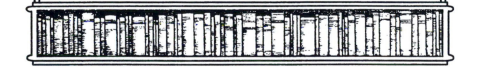

"**D**r. Ruben's latest book, *Publicity for Mental Health Clinicians*, is a must for all private practitioners in the mental health field who are attempting to survive the catacylsmic changes that have occurred in the last few years.

Dr. Ruben's book provides an excellent and very efficient way of continuing to develop the referral source for the private practitioner. His suggestions of building a referral base by using local public radio and TV has been extremely important for me in my practice. Because I am a licensed psychologist who happens to be blind as well, it is more difficult for me to contact physicians, teachers, and clergy who can refer to me. Radio or TV exposure may facilitate my efforts in this area.

I feel that this book is an absolute must for anyone trying to survive in the current jungle of health care delivery."

Winfred J. Smith, PhD
Hope Counseling Center,
Lansing, Michigan

"**M**anaged care, increased competition, and other market forces have led to an even greater need for mental health professionals to be able to ethically and effectively promote their services. Dr. Ruben's newest book serves as a helpful guide on how to achieve this.

This book is filled with creative ideas, not the tired standards that less innovative works repackage. The style of this book makes it readily accessible and useable by the reader. Dr. Ruben explains all the aspects of these marketing methods. His samples are remarkably helpful and are primarily ones he has successfully used.

Dr. Ruben is an expert in this area, and he lets readers in on many of his successful secrets. His book benefits readers with his skills and expertise as fully as if he were providing a complete marketing how-to consultation. Novices and professionals alike will gain much from this valuable work."

Chris E. Stout, PsyD
Chief of Psychology
and Associate Administrator,
Forest Health Systems,
Des Plaines, Illinois

The Haworth Press, Inc.

Publicity for Mental Health Clinicians

Using TV, Radio, and Print Media to Enhance Your Public Image

HAWORTH Marketing Resources
Innovations in Practice & Professional Services
William J. Winston, Senior Editor

New, Recent, and Forthcoming Titles:

Publicity for Mental Health Clinicians

Using TV, Radio, and Print Media to Enhance Your Public Image

Douglas H. Ruben, PhD

The Haworth Press
New York • London

The Haworth Press, Inc., 10 Alice Street, Binghamton, NY 13904-1580

Library of Congress Cataloging-in-Publication Data

Ruben, Douglas H.
    Publicity for mental health clinicians : using TV, radio, and print media to enhance your public image / Douglas H. Ruben.
        p.   cm.
    Includes bibliographical references and index.
    ISBN 1-56024-953-6
    1. Mass media in mental health education. 2. Mental health services–Marketing. 3. Radio in publicity. 4. Television in publicity. I. Title.
RA790.87.R83 1995
362.2′068′8–dc20   95-6249

CONTENTS

ABOUT THE AUTHOR

Douglas H. Ruben, PhD, is host of a locally syndicated cable show called *Recovery Shop*, a producer of television shows, and president of Best Impressions International Inc., a speaker's bureau. He is a clinical psychologist specializing in family and addiction who has within the last 6 years turned media consultant in various disciplines. He appears regularly on television and radio talk shows from coast to coast and is currently touring for his book *No More Guilt*. The author and co-author of more than 31 books and professional articles, Dr. Ruben's popular and scholarly books have covered topics ranging from family issues and psychotherapy to addiction and behavioral psychology.

Foreword

Some years ago, well-known artist Andy Warhol made the often-quoted statement "In . . . the future, everyone will be famous for 15 minutes." Having been in the public's eye for the last three decades, I would like to add, "But you're only as good as your last 30 seconds. And not unless someone knows about it."

Suppose somebody builds a mousetrap. It's good, but you can do better. Maybe you have already built the better mousetrap (probably computerized). The question is, "How does that deed alone guarantee the world will beat a path to your doorstep?" There seems to be a step missing–that of letting the world know you have that better mousetrap, and, more important, *why they need it.*

The following is *not a fairy tale–*

Once upon a time, there was a very good hypnotherapist who was successfully helping people to stop smoking and to lose weight. This was years ago, in the days before it was commonplace and accepted. In fact, today he chuckles, "Then, if I told anyone I was a hypnotist, their responses would invariably be–you do what?" Today people know what that is.

This hypnotist was the first, and for many years, the only one to do group sessions for habit control. In 24 years, hundreds of thousands attended his sessions from coast to coast and not one penny was spent in advertising. Lucky? Maybe. But there was definitely a method.

First of all, he had learned his craft well. Starting in a seminary studying for the priesthood, he was introduced into the world of the subconscious by his philosophy professor who, at the time, was working on his doctorate in psychology. His dissertation was on experimental hypnosis. After leaving the seminary (he discovered girls), he continued his quest into psychology in college. He was fortunate to have as his mentor Dr. Milton Erickson who was considered the world's leading medical hypnotist in his day. Not bad, huh? But there's more to this tale.

After leaving college, the yen for "show-biz" got the best of him and he spent 14 years in radio and television and did hypnotherapy in his spare moments. Finally he became so busy with the sessions that he left broadcasting to pursue hypnosis full time.

One day, a friend from his broadcast days called. This friend was Bill Baker, who later became President of Westinghouse Broadcasting. At the time, Bill Baker was producer of the *Allan Douglas Show,* a well-listened to radio talk show in Cleveland. Bill wanted to know if he would be a guest on the show to discuss hypnosis and its uses. They would fly him in, put him up in a hotel and maybe he could even pick up a few clients while in town. This sounded like a good idea, so he accepted.

The first half hour or so of the show ran smoothly with our fellow entertainingly answering questions and generally having a good time. The host of the show (Allan) just casually mentioned that the hypnotist could be reached at his hotel later if anyone had further questions. And then it happened!

An emergency phone call came for our friend, the guest, off the air. It was the manager of the hotel calling from across the street. He was as mad as the proverbial "wet hen" and threatened to call the police. Instead of the few expected phone calls, it seemed that the switchboard was jammed and on the verge of burning out.

After pacifying the hotel manager, the fellow agreed to hiring, at his own expense, three telephone operators to handle the flood of calls for many days. Lesson learned! The power of the media was rather forcefully demonstrated then and there.

Drawing on his broadcast and show business knowledge and experience, our friend created a companion career to parallel his chosen field of therapy. This was well before the days of Dr. Joyce Brothers. He laughingly calls himself a "professional guest" for talk shows.

To date he has appeared on *Johnny Carson's Tonight Show, The Merv Griffin Show, Mike Douglas Show, Oprah, Jenny Jones Show, Sally Jesse Raphael* (more times than anyone else–17), *ABC's 20/20, Larry King Show, CNN,* and *Entertainment Tonight.* He also was the subject of a nationally aired infomercial and has been a guest on virtually every major radio talk show in the country. In fact, after appearing numerous times on *Regis & Kathie Lee,* Regis calls him "The finest hypnotist in the country today–amazing."

In addition to numerous newspaper stories around the country, he has been written about in *Time* magazine, *US* magazine, *USA Today, Woman* magazine, *Cosmopolitan, Playgirl, The National Enquirer,* and *The New York Times.*

Did any of these shows or publications come looking for him? Did someone say, "You're what these shows or magazines are looking for. Let me book you." In a word–no! He used many of the methods and ideas you'll find here in the following pages. Not only has it been successful, he'll be the first to tell you that he has had a *ball!*

By the way, I know for sure that this story is true. That fellow is me–Damon Reinbold.

Think about it. Your skill is of little use to you or anyone else if nobody knows about it. Yes, you can advertise and get referrals. But in this age of the information glut, your public image is what really counts. If it's on radio, TV, or in the papers, it must be good, *right?*

The media certainly is the way to reach the marketplace and make your valuable talent, which you already have spent considerable time and effort developing, available to those who can most benefit from it. Doesn't it make sense to spend just a little more effort to explore the public arena?

And the media is continuing to expand. There are many more opportunities today than there ever were when I started decades ago, and every day more are being added. Whether you would like a national, regional, or local reputation, all the resources are here for you. If nothing else, it can get you out of the humdrum office routine and as I said, it can be fun and exciting.

The results can be surprising too. You never know who you are reaching or what the outcome will be. For me, it has gotten me into places and situations that otherwise would probably have not happened. I have experienced everything from doing a session in the White House, another session on death row of a maximum security prison, to spending a Fourth of July weekend as a guest in a movie mega-star's home. Those experiences and many others would never have happened without the public image I had established in the media.

Now for the good news. There is no real luck and there certainly is no magic to any of this. With the proper guidance, anyone can do it.

When I first read Dr. Doug Ruben's manuscript, I thought, "My God, he's been following me around for most of my adult life. It's all here—and then some!" And that is the truth of the matter. It *is all here and more.*

Doug Ruben knows whereof he speaks. This book is no pipe dream and it's not just a bunch of theories that sound good but aren't practical. Unfortunately, many books are like that these days. But not so here.

As I have in my way, Doug Ruben in his way has lived and developed and used everything he describes. He was bitten by the "bug" and since that time has been on countless shows including the *Phil Donahue Show*—all without an agent or public relations firm. He did it himself.

I am more than proud to count Doug Ruben among my few close friends and colleagues. His knowledge and enthusiasm is most inspiring and it sure is catchy.

Doug reminds me a great deal of the Wizard in *The Wizard of Oz.* The wonderment and real magic is in his common sense, keen insight, and oftentimes unusual viewpoint that works. In his unique style, he has jumped into the wacky world of the media and he not only has survived—he has prospered. He now generously shares it with you—all of you—in detail.

You too can "follow the Yellow Brick Road" to success. It is all here in these pages you now hold in your hands. And some day soon I hope to run into you in some talk show's "green room" (which is never green). Be sure to say, "Hi!"

Now, it's *magic time.* Take a deep breath, turn the page, and be prepared for one heck of a trip into the wonderful universe of the media. There's none other like it.

I envy your experience.

Damon Reinbold

Preface

Showbiz is everywhere. It's foolish to think that years of formal academic training robbed you of the dream to walk down the aisle in the Dorothy Chandler Pavilion for an Oscar award. It certainly beats walking down the aisle to receive your diploma. But that's about the closest most of us have come to stardom. Venturing out of the insulated boundaries of academia or a private practice is no simple thing. Forget for the moment the time and energy involved in even getting started. How about the real issue–how *frightening it is*. You have to be somewhat crazy, don't you? Why would you write a book, appear on radio, or worse yet, let millions of viewers watch you scratch your nose on television? We're talking *millions of viewers*. Local shows may be picked up by cable, syndication, satellite, microwave, even by scanners. Everybody and his brother can know *you appeared on the air.* And all for what?

To build your public image. It's a fast, competitive clinical practice out there, and even under the protective shields of academia the vultures lurk to devour you. Nothing is forever safe and secure in the business of mental health. For example, once upon a time psychologists and psychiatrists ruled the nests on service provision. But many state laws have changed this landscape. Now social workers have insurance reimbursement status, and forging ahead are school counselors, rehabilitation counselors, family and marriage counselors, substance abuse counselors, and the list of certified and credentialed providers goes on ad infinitum. More eager hands are grabbing a piece of the clinical pie, putting up their own shingles, and are determined to succeed. All providers differ in training, in orientation, in preferred clientele, and in running their businesses. These differences are obvious.

What's less obvious is another difference. Most practitioners are perfectly content in private or academic life following the daily routines of a patient load. Ambitions beyond an expanded clinical practice are minimal. Some providers, for example, undertake administrative duties or enlarge their services to include mental health management. This is a good beginning; it means charting new territory outside the norm of clinical training. But once administrative duties involve *the media,* that is, appearing on television, radio, or being interviewed in the newspaper, providers get cold feet. "I'm not an actor," they say. "I wouldn't know what to do!" And so the fears abound. The less chances taken, the safer a practice remains. And so life continues in the Norman Rockwell tradition of a happy, secure existence. Forget the risks, forget becoming another Michael Douglas. Public image, you feel, is for those idealistic "wanna-be's" who are impulsive and looking to make an extra buck.

But not so. Those extra-buck media seekers are not professional actors. They're trained mental health experts turned TV and radio personalities after they realized the enormous volume of business and personal respect that public media generated for them. Sure, on high ladders of media success are Dr. Joyce Brothers (syndicated columnist, TV guest), Dr. Sonya Friedman (TV host), and Dr. Barbara DeAngelis (TV host), to name only a few. But these folks are the exception, not the rule. Even authors of best-selling self-help books such as John Bradshaw, Wayne Dwyer, Claudia Black, among others, are not natural media experts. Time, effort, and plenty of personally spent money went into building their public images.

So how did they get that way? What did they know that most professionals never know? How did they get that extra boost to experiment with the public media? All of these professionals started at the same base: "Nobody naturally taught me to do this, so I'll have to do it myself." Wayne Dwyer, for example, toured his first book around the nation by loading up an inventory in his station wagon and making the bookstore-signing rounds. That's perseverance. Most writers, academic and self-help, believe once the published book hits the library or bookstore, it will sell itself–that intuitively readers will spot its value and spread the gospel. But nobody buys books. *People buy people.* Readers buy books written by authors they know.

"Who wrote this? Stephen King? Fine, I'll buy it."

The same is true for TV and radio. If Dr. Joyce Brothers says it, it must be true. Experts are believable and sell their books, their ideas and their promises all because the power of media transforms people into persuasive giants. Consumers agree: "If they got on TV, they must be somebody special." Does that mean any Tom, Dick, or Harry can "be somebody special?" Absolutely. That is how info-mercial gurus such as Anthony Robbins can corner the market on success-building tapes. He appeals to a basic human instinct: self-esteem. And so, all public media moguls like Anthony Robbins tap the inner core of human emotions: greed, vanity, success, and pow-er. Is it wrong? Are they exploiting the gullible public with lies, deceptions, and unfulfilled dreams? No, they're not. They're selling a product exactly like yours. They have a book, a tape, or a video. You have a clinical practice *and also maybe a book, tape, or video.* You are one-up on the self-help heavyweights because you have what many of them never received but wish they did: a formal clinical training.

Never underestimate the *power of your credibility.* It goes beyond using it to set up a business. It goes beyond the diplomas, the edito-rial boards, and the memberships to organizations. Clinical expertise makes you a scarce commodity because media industries want hon-est, legitimate advice on down-to-earth issues. Whether on a local show, or touring the big-time with *Oprah Winfrey, Sally Jessy Ra-phael, Regis and Kathie Lee, Donahue,* and *Jenny Jones*, producers will seize your valuable expertise. Actors and people with life expe-rience give the raw data. But you personify that raw data with a glow of interpretation and insight. Insight that directly relates to everybody listening to and watching your show. Why? Because you're talking about real things: *human behavior.* The public knows your topics: fears, panic attacks, drug abuse, sexual abuse, physical abuse, anger, love, marriage, divorce–and on and on. Every word you speak, every suggestion you give, every idea about human behavior has a com-mon language. Your advice always is relevant.

When your product is that saleable, why not try to sell it? That's why you should use your public image in clinical practice. This book offers a guide through the steps of media-building and skill development needed in TV, radio, and print markets. Chapters de-scribe planning materials, how to make contacts, prerequisites and roadblocks, and troubleshooting those roadblocks so you don't trip over your own feet. Remember, you're not alone. Except for the few professionals having acting experience, most academically trained providers did not take "Acting 101" in their master's and doctoral programs–not even as an elective. So, here's your chance to a get a condensed 16-week course in a short manual. It's easier. And it's a faster reference for hard-to-answer questions that might pop up. Read this guide as you would a roadmap, not in one sitting. You don't need to. Just flip to one of the four parts with corresponding chapters to get your bearings.

But here's the best part. Unlike many media handbooks, *Publicity for Mental Health Clinicians* should remain fairly accurate despite ups and downs in the media business. Studio buy-outs, shows that come and go, and shifts in personnel should not change your promotions approach. Technology may enlarge, so plan on expanding your arsenal of computer and electronic media communications. Otherwise, basic strategies for developing a media image will hopefully endure the passage of time.

What *will* change is your "mind." Don't be fooled by competition, the seemingly endless rejections producers send you, or because nobody replied to your inquiries. That's normal. And it is also normal to be booked, promised, and prepared for a show that cancels you at the last minute. Media opportunities do not guarantee media appearance. That's why your own perseverance is important. Stick with your plans on using a new avenue for exposure no matter how discouraged you initially feel. You're not trying to win the lottery. Odds of winning the media lotto are far greater, more predictable, and increase your probability of repeating that same media market in the future.

Of course, insider information on media business is hard to come by and doesn't just land on your doorstep. In my case, I owe many debts of appreciation to TV, radio, and print industry people who enlarged my vocabulary, awareness, and appetite for showbiz all at once. They also got me to step back and realize there needs to be a road map for inexperienced media seekers. They are indispensable contributors to this book: for instance, the distinguished and nationally syndicated hypnotist Damon Reinbold. For 20-odd years Damon's habit-control workshops and TV appearances from *Carson* to *20/20* have been the exemplar of "do-it-yourself" in public image. Damon's friendship and insights breathe through every page of this book. Second, I personally thank the publishers of my books, both academic and self-help, for tolerating my stupid questions and insane propositions that always got answered as: "Are you serious?" Fortunately, they explained what I really wanted to know and how I could get that knowledge.

Damon's son, Jay Reinbold, may not realize it but what he told me in two days during the shooting of an Infomercial was equivalent to a bachelor's degree in "studio production." His talents and knowledge are extraordinary. But there's only one person whose support beats any media expert: my wife Marilyn. Her confidence to see me try new things in the media is inspirational. So are her snappy questions such as "Are you flying with a plane that has one propeller or two?" "Are you sure you're not staying at the Bates Motel?" "Do you *really think they care about your books?*" Well, hopefully somebody does. And you'll find there are plenty of eager listeners and viewers immediately impressed by your opinions. They're there. And your job is to tap that audience before somebody else does.

D. H. R.
Okemos, Michigan

PART I.
LOCAL HOLLYWOOD: GETTING ON TV

Nothing is as easy as it first appears. Talk show hosts make life in front of a camera look simple, such as teaching a class or talking to friends. Even their guests look comfortable, polished, and attractive. Surely they must all have natural talent. But not really. A behind-the-scenes look at TV hosts and guests reveals untold truths that most of them are afraid of the camera. It took many rehearsals, nicotine, caffeine, alcohol, or other relaxants to subdue anxieties about goofing up a live broadcast. Fear is natural and is worse when there are studio audiences. You have no idea exactly how audiences will behave. So, no matter how talented or experienced a TV personality, guest, or expert seems, every show holds new surprises and jets the adrenaline as if it were the first show they ever did.

Why, then, should mental health providers suffer hours of fear appearing on TV? Here's why: TV is the most powerful media tool directly affecting the mass public. More powerful than radio and print media, TV is watched by one out of three people in America. With cable capacities, accessibility and variety of TV has tripled in the last 20 years to become the nation's leading influential information source, watched by all age groups at all hours of the day. From 24-hour news to 24-hour religion, TV shows broadcast entertainment, business, weather, sports, and consumer interest topics. TV focuses in on nearly every aspect of human behavior, shaping society both nationally and internationally. Household reception of TV is so easy on cable that family meals and gatherings revolve around TV as the prime instrument for recreation.

TV information not only is plentiful, it is consumed rapidly. People tune in to weather and traffic reports, watch news events, and Hollywood gossip, all while they are doing something else.

Periodically they look at the television screen, but not always. TV offers background noise while dressing in the morning, cleaning the house, preparing and eating meals, and doing homework. Activities while the TV is on allow viewers to keep busy, and from time to time see who is on the tube. The reason? Television generates multiple sensory stimuli enabling persons to perceive, identify, and comprehend what's going on without their undivided attention. When TV (like videos, or slide shows) has sound and sight, information is consumed with very little effort.

Because TV is so powerful, there is a premium to use it. Advertisers pay high fees for air time. News and entertainment shows go through extensive test marketing before running on network or nonnetwork time. Calculated efforts go into planning, selecting, programming, and revamping shows. Ratings predict their survival. A show rated high during "sweeps" week lives another month, possibly is renewed for another year. Low ratings may kill a show or require extensive rewriting, rehosting, or involve such major facial reconstruction that it looks and sounds totally different when it reappears. The demand for viewer ratings is competitive and highly depends on finding the right resource, at the right time, with the right message. That's where the mental health professional comes in.

Chapters 1, 2, and 3 invite you to be a part of the TV world and promote your public image. There are calculated ways to do it and beat the red tape and fears involved. Marketing your public image does not involve paying for advertisement. At least not in this book. Paid advertisement is a viable, but expensive, route you can take. But disadvantages are many, primarily because the viewer does not know who you are except for what your paid advertisement claims. Claims are impressive but insubstantial unless backed by viewers who used your advice. Advice *sells your product. And your product is your expertise, your practice, or some other accomplishment (book, film, etc.).* So, sit back and enjoy the many ways TV can become your public relations friend.

Chapter 1

Guest Appearances
and Resident Expert on TV

Most people know what a guest appearance is. *CBS This Morning* has several segments devoted to medical and family health. Frequently a physician or psychologist offers opinion on a controversial news story or health condition. For instance, medical ethicists commented on Dr. Kevorkian's suicide machine. Rape experts took sides during the young Kennedy trial and again when boxer Mike Tyson was accused and later convicted of sexual assault. Scores of experts commented on racial oppression following the Rodney King verdict and Los Angeles riots. And spin doctors from all sides of the fence speculated on O.J. Simpson's tragic fate. How do these experts get air time? How do they beat other experts to the punch?

It's simple. Experts who offer these opinions either are invited or solicit their expertise to appear on the show. Experts are authors who promote their latest book, nationally known specialists, or *resident experts*. A resident expert is a professional repeatedly appearing and trusted by the show's producer for his reliable information and presentable style. Resident experts may or may not be under studio contract, but are frequently consulted for news stories or commentary on controversial issues.

Steps to become a one-time or regular guest on TV are not hard. Initially the effort is sending a letter or making a phone call to the producer, introducing yourself, and making a pitch. The *pitch* is significant because it represents a succinct description of your product; namely, that you have some expertise beneficial to the TV show. Let's take a closer look at other preliminary steps for moving into local Hollywood.

HOW TO GET STARTED

Computer, Desk-Top Publishing

Preparing inquiry letters, press releases, and all other correspondence require professional stationery and the flexibility of databases to make changes on your copy. One option is to use a word-processing program on computer. The diversity and complexity of word-processing software depends on individual taste. IBM and IBM-compatible users are accustomed to several writing programs from *WordStar* and *Professional Writer*, to *Microsoft Word*. Macintosh users generally are happy with *MacWrite, Microsoft Word*, or *PageMaker*. But, whether an IBM or MAC enthusiast, you're in luck. Nowadays, advancing efforts to marry IBM and MAC have resulted in computers accepting software from both computer types. Plus, with *Windows* on the scene, the landscape of an IBM looks more like a Macintosh every day. Add to this hybrid a fierce computer price war lowering costs of IBM and IBM-compatible hardware and software, while Macintosh prices remain relentlessly high, and you'll find it pays to think twice before investing in only MAC supplies.

Just another note for you DOS-lovers resisting conversion to *Windows*. Clinics and companies who make that reluctant leap to *Windows* now enjoy multiple programs open at one time and find *Windows* software easier to learn and use. DOS-based software can operate in the *Windows* environment, but there are many limitations. If you have thought about converting to *Windows*, look first at your hardware. *Windows* programs use more memory and require a faster computer. An optimal level machine would be a 486 DX/33 with 8 megs of RAM, but expect the need for more memory and faster computers to increase in the future. But be prepared for magic. *Windows* products are simply unmatched in the DOS world for ease of use, power, and functionality.

Pricing out software and hardware is only half the reason for program flexibility. Another reason for program flexibility is so that you can alter names, addresses, and text easily, rapidly, and efficiently without messing with a labyrinth of commands. *Microsoft Word* (IBM and Macintosh), for example, is a desk-top publishing program combined with a word processor that allows for text and graphics. You can edit pages, use many different type styles ("fonts") at any size ("point"), and organize the page to look like a publisher laid it out.

Printing the copy is also important. A neat, professional-looking inquiry letter, press release, and correspondence is an eye-catcher for busy producers. They have very little time to wade through towering piles of over-the-transom mail. Letters printed from a letter-quality typewriter or high density dot matrix (DPI-75 to DPI-1200) are safe to moderately acceptable. Ideally, the letter should be printed from a postscript laser printer or Ink-Jet printer (e.g., Apple LaserWriter IINT, Personal LaserWriter, Canon Bubble Jet Printers, Hewlett-Packer Ink-Jet printers). Laser and Ink-Jet printers deliver sharp text with smooth, dramatic grays or eye-catching color. Many printers have resolution enhancement for printing on plain paper, glossy or special papers, transparencies, and envelopes. Printers with higher DPI's (600 DPI to 1200 DPI) produce exceptionally professional-looking output that adds instant credibility and readability of the letter so that producers believe your material comes from a public relations agency.

Inquiry Letter, Fax, or Phone Call

Inquiry letters and faxes are advisable over cold telephone calls. This is a product pitch, but you need not be a salesman. Telephone calls directed to the senior producer or producer's assistant are ineffective initially, because the listener relies entirely on your words. Since telephone discussions are brief, details describing your product, your background and expertise, and relevance to their show all are lost unless the producer asks the right questions or you know ahead of time precisely the facts they need.

Depending on your media, inquiry letters may focus on radio or TV. On TV, letters may differ according to local talk shows, regional and nationally syndicated shows, and news shows. Figure 1.1 is a letter to a regional talk show. Open the letter with a reminder of who you are, if previously appearing on the show, and the high ratings it enjoyed. Otherwise, grab readers with a tabloid-like heading such as "A new diet to relieve fear," or "Fear-relief in minutes!" Next, briefly describe how you can deliver your product or message consistent with the talk show format. In the third paragraph, one or two

FIGURE 1.1. Pitch letter to regional TV talk show

BEST IMPRESSIONS INTERNATIONAL INCORPORATED

4211 OKEMOS ROAD, SUITE 22, OKEMOS, MICHIGAN 48864, U.S.A.
TELEPHONE: 517-347-0944 or 517-347-1811

December 24, 1992

Ms. Lisa Fisco, Executive Producer
Kelly & Co
WXYZ Television
29777 W. 10 Mile Road
Southfield, MI 48037

Dear Ms. Fisco:

You may recall I appeared on your show a year ago discussing parenting and my book *Bratbusters: Say Goodbye to Tantrums and Disobedience.* The show scored high in ratings and re-ran several times. You invited me to contact you following release of my new book, ***Avoidance Syndrome: Doing Things Out of Fear.***

Avoidance Syndrome is a nationally released anti-fear manual that I can discuss on upcoming segments of KELLY & CO. A perfect title for fighting the holiday blues or seasonal depression. It gets to the heart of why people hate doing things. Imagine a panel or point counterpoint on "Why do I procrastinate?" "Why do I hate conflict?" and "Why do I hold feelings inside?" From fears and phobias to having bad moods–let's tell your viewers firsthand why it happens and what they can do about it.

For myself, I've now authored over 30 books on families and habits and appeared on local and regional TV talk shows. Last year I appeared on *Kelly & Co* (WXYZ-Detroit, MI), *Morning Exchange* (WEWS-Cleveland), *Good Company* (KSTP-St. Paul, MN), *A.M. Northwest* (KATU-TV, Portland), *Top of the Morning* (Birmingham, AL), and *Conversation with Ed Clancy* (New Orleans), to name a few.

Enclosed, for starters, is a press release. I would be happy to forward a copy of the book and additional information upon your request. I look forward to your thoughts and hopefully working together on KELLY & CO.

Please feel free to call me at the phone numbers above.

Very sincerely,

Douglas H. Ruben, PhD

sentences should introduce your credentials. The final paragraph tells about the press release and invites the producer to ask for more information, and a copy of your product (if you have one). Don't send your product right away. Just offer it in the press release. This will save mailing costs, the number of products in your inventory, and will minimize the producer's review time. Figure 1.2 is a slight variation of the first letter, on a different topic, and focused on late night talk shows.

Figure 1.3 is a fax to a regional talk show. Shoot the reader between the eyes with a boldly typed, large-printed heading followed by shocking statistics that only you and your expertise can explain. Of course, research your statistics and be prepared to support the data if asked–and you will be asked. Create a need for newsworthy commentary by relating your facts to high-profile headliners such as "Was O. J. Simpson HRV-Positive? (high risk to violence)," "Tonya Harding's Secre Wweapons–Fear and Aggression" or "Why Paula Johnson Isn't Lying about the President." Although sounding alarmist, curiosity is instantly stimulated in the minds of viewer-conscious producers looking to spice up news stories before the other networks do. The last paragraph briefly identifies your credentials and precisely how your expertise or product *will save the day.*

The note at the bottom of the fax is a great incentive for rapid communication. Sure, fax is fine; but toll-free numbers are better. Media-ambitious practitioners frequently use 1-800 numbers, answered by a multiple voice-mail system. Top-dollar digital answering machines are one approach, many now even have two or three mail boxes built in for easier information routing. On advanced levels, for computer literates, is a fabulous *Windows*-based communications program called TyIN 2000 (National Semiconductor). This program operates as a full-function digital answering machine which can record telephone messages in a highly compressed form into the hard disk. You can create multiple mail boxes, use different greetings, record memos, and essentially replace secretarial support with the many voice-mail features.

When do you send the inquiry letters? Planning ahead is always best. Booking dates usually run three weeks to one month in advance. Producers may need lead time to consult production staff or

FIGURE 1.2. Pitch letter for night show

BEST IMPRESSIONS INTERNATIONAL INCORPORATED

4211 OKEMOS ROAD, SUITE 22, OKEMOS, MICHIGAN 48864, U.S.A.
TELEPHONE: 517-347-0944

February 29, 1992

Executive Producer
RON REAGAN SHOW
FOX Broadcasting Company
PO BOX 900
Los Angeles, CA 90213

Dear Producer:

ARE YOU A PARENT? DID YOU KNOW LATE NIGHT VIEWERS ARE ALMOST ALL PARENTS? So, why not treat them to stuff they can use the next day. Like–**Bratbusters: Say Goodbye to Tantrums and Disobedience** (Skidmore-Roth, Publishers).

Bratbusters is a nationally released parenting book that I can discuss on upcoming segments of the RON REAGAN SHOW. Why a night show? Because that's when today's parents *really* watch TV. Life begins after dark.

Viewers want direct no-nonsense answers on how to handle tantrums and children who don't "mind." And they want it to be entertaining. That's why **Bratbusters** is a great segment piece. Excite your viewing audience with questions and answers on stopping temper tantrums, lying, stealing, not following instructions, and overachieving.

For myself, I've authored some 28 books on families, kids, and parenting, hosted a cable show, and appeared on local and regional TV talk shows. I have recently appeared on *Kelly & Co.* (WXYZ-Detroit), *Morning Exchange* (WEWS-Cleveland) and *Top O' the Morning* (WVTM-Birmingham, AL).

Enclosed, for starters, is a press release. I would be happy to forward a copy of the book. I look forward to your thoughts and hopefully working together on the RON REAGAN SHOW.

Please feel free to call me at the phone number above.

Very sincerely,

Douglas H. Ruben, PhD

FIGURE 1.3. Fax of pitch letter with clenching headline

BEST IMPRESSIONS INTERNATIONAL INCORPORATED

4211 OKEMOS ROAD, SUITE 22, OKEMOS, MICHIGAN 48864, U.S.A.
TELEPHONE or FAX: 517-347-0944, or 1-800-595-BEST

FAX COVER SHEET

DATE: 6-6-94

ATTENTION: Maria Garcia, WLNS

FAX NUMBER: 374 7610

FROM: Paul Smith, Best Impressions International Inc

NOTES: Here's something your viewers will definitely tune in for–

Was O.J. Simpson HRV-Positive?

That's High Risk to Violence (HRV-positive)– the social virus linked to teen violence. It's because–

- 80% of youth watch violence
- 60% of adolescents are thrill-seekers
- 40% of parents encourage aggression

Anti-violence expert Dr. Ruben will explain what to do about it.

National anti-violence expert and family psychologist Dr. Ruben puts answers at your fingertips–a first-aid kit on protecting kids from violence. Dr. Ruben currently is touring his workshop on "Youth Survival Skills Against Violence and HRV." Workshops are in public schools, outreach programs. Author of over 31 books, Dr. Ruben will identify five reasons why aggressive violence occurs at home and school and five solutions for it.

For info, booking segments/shows, call 1-800-595-BEST

remote camera crew, or to round up a panel of guests or audience members for the show. If your letter arrives in mid-March, plan on scheduling early to mid-April dates. Exceptions, however, do occur. Booked guests do cancel, opening up a segment for your interview.

The urgency of your expertise following a crisis or headline story also takes precedence. For example, suppose you're booked to speak on post-traumatic syndrome in one month, but today another hostage crisis emerges, turning the nation's eyes to the dangers of Americans in captivity. The producer may ask you to be available on the spot for commentary. Naturally, TV appearances during significant life events receive high audience exposure and carry your expertise or product to many more consumers.

Because scheduling can be so impulsive, certain implicit rules may help guide your inquiry process. First, always send your letters so that they arrive on a *Monday or Friday*. Why these days? On Monday, producers arrive earlier to work, weed through correspondences from the week prior and over the weekend, and rush to make decisions before starting the week full of meetings and last-minute show arrangements. By Friday, after the last talk show of the week ends, clean-up work begins. Piles of week-long correspondence are reviewed, decisions are made without time pressures, and producers plan ahead for forthcoming weeks. In other words, expect few decisions made from Tuesday through Thursday, during the height of production.

Another way experts find they combat this Tuesday to Thursday busy time is, again, by sending a fax correspondence. Faxing has many advantages. First, rapidly transmitted information alerts producers of your availability, especially pertaining to local or national events in headline news. Second, faxes reduce the waiting period between mailing your inquiry and a reply from the studio. However, fax correspondences can be piled up along with other mail unread by the producer until Friday. So, reserve the faxing approach for two situations. First, fax materials immediately that are requested by the producer or those that are likely to determine a decision to book you on the television show. Second, fax materials that are brief (two to four pages), supplementary, or that notify producers of critical scheduling changes and additional facts for the hosts or are needed by the TV crew. For example, at the "11th hour," one producer left a message asking what my product (book) was about. I faxed her a list of questions for the host to incorporate into the interview.

Besides the cover letter, facsimiles additionally can include two other pages. One is a graphic page with your picture on it that embellishes your product and expertise (see Figure 1.4). A second page is less neon and more explanatory, following a Question and Answer (Q & A) format on why your product or expertise promises high viewer interest (see Figure 1.5). Both pages efficiently convey your topic as simple, digestible, and directly valuable to that station's stake in reputable news coverage. But showing your picture is always more marketable. Here's why. First, personalizing the pitch with a photo looks like you're saying the words on the page. Second, producers can instantly determine if you are photogenic and will appear honest, casual, and professional.

Be aware, however, of two problems. On some fax machines, transmission of illustrations and pictures may be imperfect. Blurred, smudged, or blackened discolorations will ruin received pages, unless the sending machine can be set on "Picture quality." Second, federal regulators recently have stiffened rules against sending unsolicited multiple faxes for direct sales marketing. Does this apply to your faxing strategies?

It could, but not if you protect your credibility by following basic and smart rules when faxing materials. First, identify the exact person's name to whom the fax is sent. Second, relate your product or expertise to recent programming or current events on that station or TV show (e.g., Normandy Anniversary). Third, directly point out your goal is educational, not financial. Pitch materials that clearly and convincingly promise free information and meet four consumer-related goals. These include: *satisfy a need, solve a problem, search for truth,* and *Simple Simon.*

Satisfy a Need

Satisfy a craving for humorously hot and controversial news by offering proof, speculation, and explanation on what's going on. "Why are Rosanne and Tom Arnold *finally splitting?*" "How is Don Johnson's boozing a typical price for Hollywood slumps?" Stay away from perpetuating myths or riding the coattails of high-

FIGURE 1.4. Fax of pitch letter with picture and brief biography

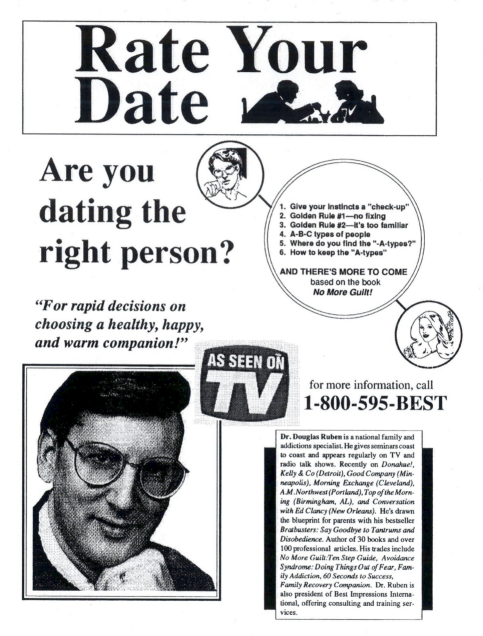

FIGURE 1.5. Fax of explanatory pitch letter and offer to coordinate the show

BEST IMPRESSIONS INTERNATIONAL INCORPORATED

4211 OKEMOS ROAD, SUITE 22, OKEMOS, MICHIGAN 48864, U.S.A.
TELEPHONE: 1-800-595-BEST; FAX or PHONE:517-347-0944

Believe it or not–

- 3 out of 5 men hate to argue.
- 60% of single men say they'd like to but never marry "nice girls."
- 90% of married men today will cry and admit feelings to their wives.

Men don't naturally do these things, do they?

Dr. Ruben says they do. He's author of *"No more shame: 10-step guide to a shame-free life."* Interview him alone or with a panel and get the facts firsthand. He'll explain: men are "approval-junkies." They're afraid to be mean. They feel too guilty when they hurt some-body's feelings. So, they become wife-pleasers. Forget this macho-stuff. They're the opposite of it.

That's not what most women think.

So let's set the record straight. Hear a panel of 2-3 men in abusive relationships tell your viewers the way it is. They suffer pain, panic, and punishment just as many women claim to–but men keep it hid-den. They won't talk about it–until now. On your show.

Psychologist and author Dr. Ruben has appeared from coast to coast on TV and radio talk shows–*Donahue, Good Company, A.M. North-west, Morning Exchange, Kelly & Co.,* among others. Ruben is author of over 30 books including self-helpers *Bratbusters: Say Goodbye to Tantrums & Disobedience, Avoidance Syndrome: Doing Things Out of Fear, 60 Seconds to Success, Family Recovery Companion,* and *One-Minute Secrets to Feeling Great.*

He'll arrange the panel and help plan the show.

This will be one of your easiest shows to put together. Just let him know when you want the show and what you need. For more informa-tion, booking, or sample of *No More Guilt*, give us a call at:

1-800-595-BEST.

profile celebrity-watch syndicates such as *Entertainment Tonight, E! News, Inside Edition, Hard Copy, A Current Affair,* or even from leaks of inflated gossip from such nationally circulated tabloids such as *The Inquirer* and *The National Examiner.* By contrast, use articles featured in *Variety,* which reputably reports up-to-date, fast-paced changes in the entertainment industry impacting all segments of the media.

Solve a Problem

Offer a solution for some nerve-racking problem affecting millions of viewers. "How to cure sleepless nights." "How to relieve migraine headaches in the heat of day."

Search for Truth

"Do UFO's really exist?" "Is Bigfoot a hoax?" "Are adult children of alcoholics really psychic?" Search the hidden scientific truth underlying mysterious phenomena, either by exposing fraudulence or by verifying claims of unusual events. Investigate your own personal "X-Files" with riveting discoveries on why, for example, "UFO abductees all share similar psychological profiles before they're abducted." Really? Is it true? Yes, and you'll explain why.

Simple Simon

Put ideas into simple-to-remember acronyms. "Say goodbye to anxiety with NBD (no-big-deal)"; "Are you suffering from PBS (Post-Birth Syndrome)?" In a recent antiviolence promotion (see Figure 1.3), we faxed TV and radio stations to announce the epidemic of HRV-virus (High Risk to Violence virus). Acronyms instantly act as mental-minders of vitally personal information and the person delivering this information.

Pitch. Can you rattle off a 10-second abstract of your product or expertise without saying too many "Uhmms?" The pitch is really the art of brevity. Briefly, explain in your letter or later on the telephone exactly who you are, what you have or do, and why this specialty is entertaining or relevant to the talk show viewers. Remember the underlying human emotions of greed, vanity, success and power. Also, satisfy those four consumer goals. How your product appeals to any one of these guidelines can compel producers to seriously consider you on a segment.

Be flexible, as well. Brainstorming new ideas may generate off-the-wall possibilities that seem tangential to your topic. If pitching parenting skills, imagine the new topic of "Are mothers over 40 better parents?" It seems a far cry from the original methods to handle tantrums and disobedience but then, *what sells?* A producer already may have booked 20 child psychologists and family specialists that year; the topic of parenting may be boring or saturated, or the hosts dislike it. Any reason for rejecting your first concept is possible, none of which may deal with *your ability or inability to present the material.* Thus a good lesson from pitching sessions is: never take it personally. Just be creative and come up with new angles.

Press Release. Cover letters frequently replace the old standby of press releases. Producers are less technical about what they receive, as long as it piques their interest and contains follow-up information. However, much trial and error goes into composing successful pitch letters and usually what gets you over the frustration and writer's block are press releases. The press release is an announcement of your product, with key details naming what it is, who you are, and where they can get the product or more information on it (see Figure 1.6).

Most press releases are double-spaced, originally started as a courtesy to newspaper editors who could edit the copy before printing it. Press releases can follow several publicity guidelines. First, state in bold letters at the top FOR IMMEDIATE RELEASE. Second, hook the reader into a catchy phrase or idea (Figure 1.7). This allows editors to lift the text verbatim as part of a news story. Alternatively, describe exactly what the product is. Third, briefly state who you are. Fourth, annotate the product's parts or contents. Fifth, indicate who the product is for. Sixth, give the name or names of contact people for product availability or purchases.

Photo. What do you look like? Most TV producers who buy your pitch still have no idea who you are. They realize you're a profes-

FIGURE 1.6. Press release of book for TV

FOR IMMEDIATE RELEASE

NEW PARENTING BOOK

BRATBUSTERS: Say Goodbye to Tantrums and Disobedience

FOR INTERVIEW, CONTACT: DR. RUBEN, 517-347-0944

When times are rough, and kids are tough... Who ya gonna call? **Bratbusters!**

MICHIGAN FAMILY SPECIALIST Dr. Doug Ruben is author of the new parenting book, ***Bratbusters! Say Goodbye to Tantrums and Disobedience,*** published by Skidmore-Roth (paperback, $12.95). **BOOK DISTRIBUTED TO NATIONAL CHAINS.**

This book teaches parents, teachers, and anyone how to be a Bratbuster using simple, ready-to-use methods in each chapter. Methods offer rapid ways to stop temper tantrums and noncompliance (not minding) in a day. Nothing hard. Nothing to memorize. Just basic principles put into easy terms for dealing with everyday child problems.

Readers first learn why kids are bad and good. This involves dispelling myths about children and seeing exactly what goes on with behavior. Second, readers get a picture-perfect idea of why kids have tantrums, and then reasons not to take them so personally. Advice follows with precise methods on stopping tantrums, noncompliance, and parental anger. The last three chapters are especially valuable. "Is There Life After Children?" describes parenting woes and best ways to survive the marriage and family during rearing years. Even how to handle kids after visitations with a divorced spouse. Plus, how to introduce kids to your new partner. Then, on daycare, advice eases fears of sending kids to daycare versus keeping them at home. The last chapter tells it straight: "When is therapy needed?" This will help parents make prudent decisions.

Dr. Douglas Ruben is in private practice in Okemos, Michigan. He is also President of Best Impressions International, a consultant firm. He is author of over 28 books and many professional articles on parenting, family problems, and adult relationships. His workshops on family issues are national. TV and radio appearances are nationwide.

For interviews, contact: Douglas H. Ruben, PhD
Best Impressions International, Inc.
4211 Okemos Road, Suite 22
Okemos, MI 48864 (1-517-347-0944)

FIGURE 1.6. (continued)

For publisher information,

contact: Linda Roth, Publisher

                                    Skidmore-Roth Publishers

                                    1001 Wall Street

                                    El Paso, TX 79915 (1-800-825-3150)

sional, not a model, and physical appearances will vary. But it is an illusion to believe talk shows select experts entirely based on credibility. Physical attractiveness is important. Size and shape may be invalid gauges of competency but can predict viewer appeal and higher ratings. The more popular the show, the greater the value placed on physical stature. Less circulated shows may overlook this criterion. For clarity, then, send an 8″ × 10″ glossy photo, taken at a professional studio.

Photos are "mug shots" for the TV industry and a facsimile of your personality. Be sure the photo is a head shot or from the shoulders. Let your face look humble, friendly, compassionate, and competent. Overly serious, comedic, or academic-looking photos (glasses lowered on edge of nose; pipe in mouth, standing in front of bookcases) will be a turnoff. Let your photogenic face communicate "trust" and "camaraderie" with the general public. Producers already know you are an authority on topics and need not be convinced by the picture. Send the photo after the producers want more information. Never send it with the initial inquiry letter.

Demo. Producers now know what you look like. But can you perform? Can you be animated, speak articulately, handle questions from the studio audience, and essentially charm their viewers? That's why they ask for a demo tape. A demo tape is a five-to eight-minute collection of your best segments or spots from previous TV shows. The way to get this collection started is simple. On your first TV interview, ask the producer, stage manager, or host for a tape of the show. They may only tape your interview alone. Empty

FIGURE 1.7. Press release of book with tabloid-like heading

FOR IMMEDIATE RELEASE

CLOSE ENCOUNTERS WITH PSYCHIC!

Michigan author and syndicated columnist Joyce Hagelthorn finally has done it! She has assembled the best, most compelling stories from her popular column, "I've Never Told Anyone But..." into a book. Stories told to Hagelthorn are from hard-nosed scientists, skeptics, and magicians about some personal psychic experience they had as a child or adult. Stories of the strange and supernatural blend with current psychic research and ARE EXPLAINED!

Contents include dreams, clairvoyance, precognition, going back in time, out of the body, poltergeists, and life after death. Virtually everyone has some experience they cannot explain–Joyce explains it with the help of science.

Follow Joyce Hagelthorn through the mystery and maze of psychic events–finally explored–finally explained, as real "natural events." Now only $11.95. Order from Best Impressions International Inc., 4211 Okemos Road, Suite 22, Okemos, MI 48864.

tapes you provide ahead of time are a nice courtesy. Take a VHS cassette tape or three-quarter-inch BETA cassette tape for them to use. Ideally, a three-quarter-inch tape provides sharper quality for later editing and reproduction.

Once you have two or three shows taped, work with a local video studio on selecting impressive spots and options for splicing them together. Editing costs add up quickly on lengthy demos, lengthy editing time in the studio, or where you insert text in between shows. However, keep the price low by following these steps: (a) figure out the segments ahead of time, (b) sit with the video technician in the studio and direct him or her on where to cut and splice, (c) include the jingle and opening title of the show you're on, (d) at the end of each segment, dissolve the scene to a blackout, and (e) at the end of the demo, have text run for 20 to 30 seconds on who to contact, address, and phone numbers for booking.

A less expensive route is doing the editing yourself using computer-based software connected to the camcorder and VCR. For example, IBM *Windows* runs *VideoDirector* and Macintosh runs *Movie Movie, SuperMac, and VideoSpigot,* among other programs. Video software compiles and sequences video clips for faster editing and allows for storage in a video library for later retrieval. Of course, disadvantages of video software are not to be taken lightly. First, many digital software programs require specific camcorders or VCA brands without which even simple applications are futile. Second, size requirements are very large for computer operations and memory storage to run video software, unless you own a new multi-media machine with built-in sound-boards and expandable memory (MB, RAM-Random Access Memory).

For providers who are illiterate in computers, can't afford fancy multimedia hardware or who would rather be "equipment junkies," your boat has arrived. Put together a home-editing studio using remarkably advanced equipment put out by several firms such as Videonics. They supply several devices on mixing sound effects, inserting special effects, editing, and title-making that customize segments into high-resolution broadcast quality.

Follow-up letters, product sample, and phone calls. Replies to inquiries are usually made by phone. Producers do not have time to draft letters. This is not a corporation on Wall Street. Formality is spared in the interest of efficiency. Impulsively, producers may use the telephone and fax materials. The first call in reply to your inquiry may request a demo tape or product sample. The product sample is the book, audiotape, or other accomplishment. Finally it might happen: All the promotional materials you prepared are in the producer's hands.

What's next? Frequently the producer consults with her writers, staff, and hosts about how to work in your product or expertise. Brainstorming of ideas goes beyond the problem solving you did with the producer. The question now is, *will it play?* Once decided it will play, the producer calls you back to book a date.

So, how long is this wait? Is the wait as long as journal editors take to accept or reject your professional manuscript? That takes three to five months, sometimes six months before you hear a reply. The answer is: Never that long. TV is like all of Hollywood. It is impulsive and decisions made today revolve around headlines made yesterday. Tomorrow the headlines may be gone and so will the potential high ratings. Producers usually act within two days after receiving your demo and product, *if they want you.* If they do not want you, that does not mean your appearance is dead in the water. There is the possibility that your material (a) got routed to the wrong person, or (b) got lost in the mail shuffle. Syndicated shows such as *Maury Povich, Donahue,* and *Jerry Springer* are difficult for nonsolicited experts to appear on unless their product and sales pitch are strongly enticing or involve celebrities. Biographies of Elvis Presley or J. F. Kennedy instantly get the author a fair shake, not because the author is well known, but because the topic is a household word.

When the waiting game is two weeks old, call the producer again and ask about the status of your material. He or she may politely tell you that the material is under review or "We'll get back to you if we want you." Accept their answer for now.

Interview questions. Impulsivity seems to be the name of the game in the television industry. But that's usually behind the scenes, where producers and stage crews rush around to make a show look perfect on the air. By air time, guests, hosts, cameramen, director, and all key players of the broadcast generally know exactly what to do and how to do it. They have a production script to follow. One type of script you can provide to the producer ahead of time is a list of interview questions that elicit key facts about your expertise or product. Questions are brief, in simple words, or in vernacular (slang) and should spotlight your unique insights, concepts, and strategies (see Figure 1.8).

Questions also relieve the host or anchorperson who may or may not be familiar with your product ahead of the interview. Frequently, last-minute additions and deletions of copy can be frazzling and TV personalities may use the TelePrompTer because they can't remember everything. Your questions make their job easier since they rely on *you as the expert to reply rapidly and get them through the segment.*

However, bear in mind that not every anchorperson or show host wants your interview questions. Reactions vary from open arms to feeling insulted. Most producers are open to receiving the questions in preparing *sound bites, bumpers,* and series of interview hooks. Sound bites are key words or phrases used as cliffhangers thrown out to the viewers to entice their patience. Bumpers are statements or facts appearing across the screen during the break before a commercial begins. On the screen the viewer may read "Children who are tired have more temper tantrums—more on this when *Top of the Morning* returns."

While your questions provide strong material for preparation, some TV personalities believe questions are too contrived and violate good journalistic practice. They believe spontaneity and letting the interview "just flow" is more natural and entertaining to the viewing audience. They maintain that questions stiffen up the dialogue and make it look too rehearsed. Instead, they rely on your press release, the product (book, etc.), and some background credentials. But what is good for the goose may not be good for the gander. In effect, they are "winging-it." Not knowing what to expect may be journalistic but it is very uncomfortable and can cause stage fright. Unless you're good at improvisation, ask the host to stick with some semblance of questions or topic area to ease your fears.

Contacts. The adage that "It isn't what you know, but who you know" is the prophecy of TV. Contacts in the TV industry are as crucial as having a credit history when applying for a loan. And like

FIGURE 1.8. Interview questions from TV show

QUESTIONS FOR INTERVIEW

ABOUT THE BOOK IN GENERAL

1. BRATBUSTERS? Are kids really brats?
2. Why do parents need a parenting book?

ABOUT TANTRUMS

1. Let's get down to some specifics. Most parents know what tantrums are. Why do children have tantrums?
2. Your book warns parents not to take tantrums personally. What does that mean?
3. You say there are four steps to stop tantrums. What's the first step?
4. Won't parents think kids are controlling them when behavior gets worse?
5. What are the other three steps?

ABOUT "MINDING"

1. I don't know what's worse, tantrums or not minding. Why do kids not mind their parents?
2. What should parents do to get their kids to listen to them?
3. Sounds easy, but how do kids react to step two, taking something away?
4. How do you know when these steps work? Is it because kids mind their parents better–is there more?

credit, few newcomers to TV already have contacts, so they must build those contacts slowly. But not too slowly. The way to find somebody *who knows somebody* is actually easier and faster if you follow certain guidelines. First, contact your local TV studio and set up an appointment with the anchor person. Introduce yourself and ideas, while asking if they can direct you to talk to show producers. Most major local stations are network affiliates, which means they carry shows from CBS, NBC, ABC, or FOX. They are also privy to the politics of major networks. Chances are, that anchor person himself or herself is looking to advance professionally and may have insider information beneficial to both of you. Second, contact a colleague, friend, or respected professional who recently appeared on the talk show you want to appear on. Ask this person which producer he or she worked with, what the hooks were, and whether you may use this person's name as a reference. Figure 1.9 announces this connection right at the beginning of the letter. Create the impression in the producer's mind that you are *part of the show's inner family and naturally should be invited to dinner.*

Marketing rep and agent. Time is always scarce. Like most practitioners, you probably are on a tight schedule of clients, teaching, and raising a family. Research and writing activities further devour valuable hours in the day and limit campaign efforts to promote yourself on TV. Or, you may perceive yourself as the nonaggressive marketing type, more capable of performing and less capable of planning. Whatever the reason, you may consider hiring a public relations agent to get booking dates. There are many obvious advantages of agent representation, primarily that somebody else can sweat through contacts, rejections, and booking complications. In fact, many larger publishing houses already have in-house marketing agents (publicists) who do everything from booking shows to arranging lodging, meals, and transportation. All you do is go through the motions. This is a luxury that is more uncommon than common. For first-time authors or newcomers to TV, rarely is there a paid tour scheduled.

Agents can rescue you from TV phobia but they are expensive, unpredictable, sometimes unreliable, and not always looking out for your best interests. Costs range from advanced fees of $500 to $3,000 just to retain the agent, to $5,000 after the entire booking

FIGURE 1.9. Letter to TV producer showing connection with a previous guest

BEST IMPRESSIONS INTERNATIONAL INCORPORATED

4211 OKEMOS ROAD, SUITE 22, OKEMOS, MICHIGAN 48864, U.S.A.
TELEPHONE: 517-347-0944

April 24, 1992

Mr. Burt Dubrow, Executive Producer
SALLY JESSY RAPHAEL
Multimedia Entertainment
75 Rockefeller Plaza, 22nd Floor
New York, NY 10019

Dear Mr. Dubrow:

Your frequent guest and good friend of mine, Damon Reinbold, suggested I contact you about my book, ***Bratbusters: Say Goodbye to Tantrums and Disobedience*** (Skidmore-Roth, Publishers).

Bratbusters is a nationally released parenting book that I can discuss on upcoming segments of SALLY JESSY RAPHAEL. A perfect title for interview, panel, or point-counterpoint on "Why do children have bad behavior?" and "Parenting: the right way and wrong way." And especially controversial is "Does your child have ADD–Attention Deficit Disorder?"

Viewers want direct no-nonsense answers on how to handle tantrums and children who don't "mind." Let's show them how. First by talking, then by demonstration. Excite your viewing audience with questions and answers on stopping temper tantrums, lying, stealing, not following instructions, and overachieving.

For myself, I've authored some 28 books on families, kids, and parenting, hosted a cable show, and appeared on local and regional TV talk shows. Recently, I appeared on *Kelly & Co.* (WXYZ-Detroit, MI), *Morning Exchange* (WEWS-Cleveland), *Good Company* (KSTP-St. Paul, MN), and *A. M. Northwest* (KATU-TV, Portland, OR).

Enclosed, for starters, is a press release. I would be happy to forward a copy of the book. I look forward to your thoughts and hopefully working together on SALLY JESSY RAPHAEL.

Very sincerely,

Douglas H. Ruben, PhD

schedule is ready and other services are rendered. What other services? Consider one publicity agency's plan. They try appealing to novice media buffs by offering an introductory test package that includes:

Local Radio Talk Show	$ 275
National Radio Talk Show	$ 550
Local TV Talk Show	$ 550
National TV Talk Show	$1,100
Local Article Mention	$ 550
Local Feature Article	$1,100
National Article Mention	$1,100
National Feature Article	<u>$2,200</u>
Any combination of the above totally	$2,750
+	
Media Kit Charge	<u>$ 275</u>
TOTAL AMOUNT	$3,025

Now that's a sizable hunk of change for promises. And this represents a retainer's fee payable immediately upon signing the contract, even before you step inside a television studio. Is this expense really worth it? Maybe. That is, if you do some price shopping and realize that their regularly priced show packages start from $5,500 (for 20 TV/radio shows) and go up as high as $27,500 (for 100 TV/radio shows). And that's with quantity discounts.

Plus you must work through your agent each time the producer has a question, schedule change, or problem. If agent representation is for legal purposes, protect your "rights" by asking a good lawyer friend or one you frequently do business with to handle any unforeseen issues. However, there is nothing to legally protect and very little paperwork before appearing on TV. The only paperwork involves standard consent forms and waivers that indicate there is no remuneration for your appearance and that you indemnify the TV studio for all claims made. Negotiating different language in these forms is a waste of time, money, and probably will reflect negatively on your cooperation with the producers.

Media resources. Who do you contact? How do you get the names of producers, studios, and the shows they run? Your academic training no doubt makes you familiar with reference-hunting skills. Most college libraries carry directories, indices, and other compendia listing TV and radio shows nationwide; some even include names of talk shows and personalities. In entertainment cities, such as Los Angeles, specialty bookstores (e.g., Samuel French bookstore) carry an extensive inventory of publicist trade handbooks and periodicals. Annual trades also put out their own collection of principal contacts in the entertainment field. So there are many places to choose from. The best resources, updated annually, for network and cable TV (and radio) that give you names, addresses, telephone numbers, and shows follow:

Bacon's Directory of TV and Radio Stations,
  and Programming Contacts
Bacon Information Inc.
332 South Michigan Avenue
Chicago, IL 60604

Gale Directory of Publications and Broadcast Media
Gale Research, Inc.
Book Tower
Detroit, MI 48226

Hollywood Creative Directory
3000 Olympic Blvd.
Santa Monica, CA 90404

The Producer's Masterguide
330 W. 42nd Street
New York, NY 10036-6994

Studio Blu-Book Directory
The Hollywood Reporter
PO Box 1431
Hollywood, CA 90078

MEDIA COMMITTEES

Endeavoring in TV need not be a gamble. Before launching your career, consider working alongside seasoned media experts in the mental health or allied health and science fields. Many of your colleagues sit on community, local, and national *media committees.*

Committees vary from those which announce fund-raisers and other public services, to committees that advocate political and social positions. The ACLU media watch committees are outspoken on civil and human rights infringements. The Jewish Federation media watch committees alert the public to anti-Semitism. In mental health, for example, the media watch committee for the Association for Advancement of Behavior Therapy (AABT) looks for misrepresentations of behavior modification in TV, radio, and print, corrects those mistakes, and promotes a humane perspective. Media watchdog groups act as public relation agents spreading a positive image about their organization (e.g., *the product*). They use members to volunteer as spokespersons, doing PSA's (public service announcements). This is a simple and professional avenue to gain media experience.

CABLE SHOWS

Most people think of news and talk shows on the big stations such as ABC, NBC, CBS, and FOX. But there is a new world of networks transmitted nationwide gaining viewer attention by the millions. Think about it: Whose news did you watch during the Persian Gulf War? CBS? Maybe NBC? Probably not. Nielson ratings strongly indicated that CNN monopolized daytime and prime time viewing. And how about sports? TNT and ESPN now cover major national playoffs, from college to professional tournaments. Still, did you ever watch the Comedy Channel, the Travel Channel, the Family Channel, USA Channel, and Lifetime? Of course you have. These cable stations globally compete with major networks by running news, talk shows, sports, and other entertainment. Since most households in rural and urban America have cable, alternative stations reach a heterogeneous audience ready and willing to consume your product and expertise.

Take QVC–the cable home-shopping giant who lures high-paying customers on a regular basis. QVC's viewership reaches multi-millions and will gain a wider radius after possibly merging with TCI. On QVC, discounted products sell when celebrity stars or authors promote the product, providing live testimonials on its benefits. Recently, comedienne Joan Rivers attempted a bonanza on her QVC selling success rate by hosting the show *Can We Shop?* Unfortunately, the hour-long grocery-store plus interview show fared poorly in ratings and QVC canceled it.

Think of it. If QVC or another home-shopping network can turn off a big star on early Nielsen stats, just imagine how quickly it might pull the plug on your own product or selling efforts. In fact, getting your product considered for the QVC showcase is fiercely competitive. David Whiteford (1994) recently warned eager product developers of the tedious steps involved in TV catalog sales including *QVC, Valuevision, TSM,* and *HSN* shows. Frequently the show has an "open-vendor" day on which marketing agents vie for the few slots of product reviews. Marketing agents may or may not succeed at pushing your product, considering that five out of 200 products submitted receive a viewing.

That makes cable home shopping, for the time being, out of the beginner's league. Unlike, say, Multimedia Entertainment's proposed advertiser-supported *Talk Channel,* a 24-hour cable network. This show will focus on topics issues in its 16 hours of daily live programming, mostly drawn from headlines or trends–a potentially great marketplace for your expertise. And that's only one example. Cable's ever-changing landscape from 50 channels to over 500 channels comprising the information superhighway, known as *Info-pike,* is blasting open doors for career and product-promotion opportunities. The direction is twofold. First, look for multiple TV cable channels offering a range of entertainment, education, and sports. Second, look for interactive television using advanced computer technology. With over five million current subscribers to on-line services such as *America-on-Line, Internet, CompuServe,* and *Prodigy,* TV companies are planning to sell their myriad of services (movies, shopping, banking, videogames, etc.) through computer screens. The two-way pipeline of computers allows viewers to receive and send messages at a high rate, churning out sales rapidly. Responses to talk shows, which currently rely on traditional telephone lines, will be sent through a full-functioned keyboard and mouse, making it easier to interact with a computer than a TV. It might not be too long before the entire family gathers together for a night of watching the computer.

And that's why you want to be there when it happens. The first step is to send inquiries to shows appearing on cable and the super-stations (WWOR, WGN, WTBS, WPIX) just as you would inquiries to regular network shows. For example, contact producers of *Sonya Live (CNN), Real Personal (CNBC), Best Talk in Town (WPIX), Point of View (KTVT), Arlene Hersen Show (CTN), Your Family Matters (Lifetime),* or *Healthy Kids (The Family Channel)* Cable shows are personable, offer product exposure, and help pre-pare you for major network shows.

NEWS SEGMENTS

Every urban and rural city nationwide has a news program. Small stations with limited programming even have live news broadcasts or simulcasts with other local programs. On each show, news coverage follows a routine format of (a) headlines of national and international news, (b) local news, (c) sports, (d) weather, and (e) community interest stories. Stories about local events range from celebrities in town to seasonal or holiday themes. Around Christmas, remote cameras are out looking for the fanciest decorated house. On New Year's Eve, reporters crash a bourbon-bouncing party in progress. Or, anchors may run a special report or series on a socially prevailing problem such as infant mortality, safety of airline travel, or grocery coupon wars.

Topics frequently take a mental health perspective, such as "Minding your manners" (about children's misbehavior), "Drugging ADHD (attention-deficit and hyperactivity disorder) children," and "Dating without fear of AIDS." Human interest stories also tie in with significant world and local events. For instance, troops returning from the Persian Gulf War brought interest in post-traumatic stress syndrome. So did the release of the American hostages from the Middle East. Attacks on Dow Corning's leaking breast implants raised interest in body image distortion and inter-personal relationships. And the O. J. Simpson saga brought out victims of domestic violence. So, be patient. Ultimately your area of expertise will come up.

Be ahead of the game by following news developments and contacting local news stations to offer your expert commentary or consult on a multiple-part series. Live interviews may last one to two minutes, or may be taped earlier and edited down to 30 seconds, but that is plenty of time for your message or product to reach consumers.

Believe it or not, a newer trend in local news is starting the show a half-hour or hour earlier, devoted to live interviews with call-in questions. Some morning news shows actually have changed their names, changed their format, and now are a mixture of standard journalism, entertainment, and talk show. They've become "Oprahtized." *Top O' the Morning* in Birmingham, Alabama is one of these. The weatherman and news anchorwoman still play their traditional roles but are talk show hosts to a wide variety of guests. They feature fashion designers, veterinarians, book authors, and take cameras on the road to capture unusual happenings about town. Because local news shows want top billing, they will experiment with live studio audiences, call-in questions, and invite unusual guests or controversial topics. Authors who can entertain and enlighten with solid advice are top priority. News programs consequently are open markets for talented experts who can entertain and sell their products.

LOCAL TALK SHOWS

Celebrity hosts become a household name when they first appear on the local circuit. That's how Phil Donahue got started, airing live out of studios in Ohio. Then, after building a reputation and moving upward into national shows, their reputation doubles in impact. The same is true for your reputation. Booking on local and regional shows may seem inferior to booking on the Cadillacs of nationally syndicated talk shows, but nothing could be farther from the truth. First, what is a local and regional talk show? This is a talk show run just like *Bertice Berry, Geraldo*, or *Regis & Kathie Lee*, except that it transmits on a frequency covering only the state it is in, unless picked up by cable. Shows start in the morning, around 8 a.m. or 9 a.m., last one to two hours, and feature several talents, from sports, authors, entertainers, cooks, to local personalities. Segments are three to five minutes long, usually interspersed with call-in questions, a live studio audience, and product demonstrations.

Some shows have been on TV for many years and gained loyal viewers and respectability. Cleveland's *Morning Exchange* leads the national pack, celebrating its twentieth year of broadcasting and regarded as powerfully influential in product sales. Shows with live studio audiences such as Detroit's *Company*, Minneapolis' *Good Company,* and Portland's *A.M. Northwest* draw high ratings for their polished mixture of humor, business, and audience participation. Appearing live with a studio audience also enhances your credibility, because viewers see you humbly explain to everyday people why your product works. All you need is one audience participant to say, "I agree with the doctor," and you just sold your product or idea to millions of home viewers who vicariously agree.

NATIONALLY SYNDICATED TALK SHOWS

Now you've made it. Nationally syndicated shows offer mass publicity to viewers who hunger for controversy, gossip, and stripping the taboos off of every national headline. Underlying each show is a need for explicit *exposure. Geraldo* perhaps ranks highest in this compulsive desire to unleash deep secrets and get to the facts. He, personally, and his shows come under frequent attack for being too crude, zealous, and undermining the integrity of solid journalism. But in defense of *Geraldo*, that's the purpose of his show, and every talk show does this who competes for high Nielson ratings. The way in which they sneak in or disguise their crude topics is the magic of the industry.

Watch, too, as the talk show industry undergoes many face-lifts as bright new hopefuls gamble for a piece of television stardom. This past year alone witnessed the sharp rise and fall of motivational mogul Les Brown *(Les Brown Show)*, Carol Burnett's sidekick Vicki Lawrence *(Vicki!)*, comedy actor Chevy Chase *(The Chevy Chase Show)*, and nightlife stimulant Arsenio Hall *(The Arsenio Hall Show)*. Say goodbye, also, to NBC's *Jane Whitney Show*, replaced by ordained minister, psychologist-comedian Dr. Will Miller's *The Other Side*. Rising with Nielsen fever was talker *Rolonda*, and actress Ricki Lake *(The Ricki Lake Show)*. Low ratings naturally worry station affiliates who buy daytime and nighttime talk shows and ultimately determine the show's win-loss record.

Viewer ratings from television and the box office equally influence choice of talk show host; newly acquired *The Gordon Elliott Show*, for example, will fill gaps in the daytime TV schedule around the soap operas.

Of the leaders, from *Oprah* and *Sally Jessy Raphael* and *Donahue* to *Montel Williams*, every show books ahead one to two months with exceptions to guests who are part of a breaking news story. Segments vary from five minutes to the entire hour. Frequently, executive producers already have planned themes for which they need experts. Your specialty or product may fit in perfectly. Other times, you must pitch your idea and possibly do much of the footwork before it sells to production staff. Footwork involves proposing the hook, assembling and videotaping testimonials, and any other steps that spare the producer of background research. The more you can research and prepare details under their "supervision," the faster a confidence develops with production staff who perceive you as a healthy risk for the show.

Figuring that one person in every household watches at least one talk show a week, and a higher number tune into the same show daily, the chances of product visibility remain quite optimistic. Suppose you book the show and are there discussing your book. Hosts who enthusiastically praise the book's value and call it compulsory reading are a publisher's dream. For example, when *Oprah* talks, people listen. *Donahue, Sally Jessy, Rush Limbaugh,* and many high profile talk stars who put their seal on a product will propel sales into overnight bestsellers. This happened when *Oprah* told the world she'd already bought 1,000 copies of Marianne Williamson's book *A Return to Love*, and was giving one to all her friends and all the people in her Chicago studio audience. Convinced viewers took her advice verbatim and across the nation 70,000 books were sold immediately. Other books catapulted by Oprah and talk show hosts to No. 1 on the coveted *New York Times* list include Kaye Gibbons' *Charms for the Easy Life*, Deepak Chopra's *Ageless Body, Timeless Mind,* John Gray's *Men Are from Mars, Women Are from Venus,* and Richard and Linda Eyre's *Teaching Your Children Values.*

COMMERCIALS

Catchy commercials are getting harder to find. However, keep an eye on European creativity, where taboo-free ingenuity mixes erotica with product promotion. It doubles marketing success and adds credibility to another branch of cinematography. But in America, advertisers are still cautious about risqué messages and stick with wholesome depictions of "home on the range." Defectors of this tradition such as the garment and cosmetic industries, eagerly strive for a new image–something between pornography and classic romance. Their goal is to *psychologically tap the core emotions of greed, vanity, power, and success.* Your expertise is precisely what they need.

The trend in TV commercials is to hit the viewing audience fast and hard and elicit impulsive actions. Burger King commercials sizzle their giant-size hamburgers on the screen. Pizza Hut commercials heap giant helpings of cheese on a mouth-watering, deep-dish pizza. Why? Because food buyers are gullible to enticing advertisements. If your product or expertise can help marketing and advertising companies construct impulse-eliciting commercials, they want to hear from you. Opportunities for entering this mass media field are competitive for MBAs and public relations experts, but not for media or industrial psychologists. Just as psychologists have entered the courtroom–screening jurors, calming witnesses, and predicting the verdicts–so there is a need for mental health experts in the advertising field.

Begin by contacting a local public relations firm and offer your product or expertise for free. Or, contact advertisers who you know are kicking off a major media campaign, such as a political campaign: how about the Presidential campaign? Economists, political advisors, and other socio-demographic experts already are on board but not the person who *really can assess the motivation and needs of a voting constituency.* That is what you can do.

For instance, imagine calling yourself a behavioral consultant; a specialist in consumer behavior. You're not lying; your training prepared you to predict and judge human behavior. Your expertise can separate fact from emotion, can explain short-term and long-term voter gains, losses, and roadblocks. And you can offer strategy to boost voter confidence, either by redesigning or rewriting the commercial. As behavioral consultant, you give input on conflict resolution, habits of the constituency, speech writing, interpretations of voter motivation, and negotiate options of attack against opponents. In other words, you become an indispensable team member who uses scientific principles of behavior to mobilize political advice. Why *you?* Because most political aides do not know how to do this. Commercials of all types increasingly depend on a fresh perspective of behavior that only mental health experts key into (see Figure 1.10).

INFOMERCIALS

Do you know what this is? Most TV watchers do not. And people who rarely watch TV absolutely have no idea what this is. But learn about them. Study them. Infomercials are becoming one of the nation's hottest product-promoting commodities in history. And the industry is still in its infancy. Infomercials, by definition, are commercials. They are 30-minute commercials that either provide customer leads or sell business opportunities, educational products, or self-improvement programs. One 30-minute show can run 50 to 200 times per week on cable and broadcast television. *Variety* recently compared infomercials to snake-oil salesmen. And here's why. Each half-hour length program looks like and acts like a real program, but unmistakably sells like commercials. They air early in the morning or late at night; these are the cheapest times to buy TV space. Costs for productions vary from $10,000 to $400,000, depending on how fancy they get. *Fancy* means who the spokespeople are, what the set looks like, and other casting and equipment expenses.

Products sold on infomercials range from juice machines and cosmetics, to dog-training manuals and stop-smoking methods. But no matter what the product, one thing is increasingly clear to infomercial producers: millions of dollars are made. Not for every infomercial made, however. In fact, one out of every ten infomercials fails. Even using celebrities such as Cher, Jane Fonda, Farrah Fawcett, Brooke Shields, Ali MacGraw, and Fran Tarkington may not guarantee infomercial success. The reason is that product sales call

FIGURE 1.10. Behavioral Consultant advertisement

Behavioral Consultant

What is a Behavioral Consultant? by DH Ruben, PhD

A *Behavioral Consultant* is a specialist in political and consumer behavior. This specialist uses techniques borrowed from behavioral sciences to identify what kinds of psychological variables have impact on voter decision making. Voters can be individuals or organizations; constituency or cohorts. Behavioral consultants begin by analyzing factors that might precipitate, disrupt, or sabotage innovative bills and lobbying. Once known, carefully chosen tactics build support and convert opponents. All steps from writing to passing a bill require these people to do things for you. Consultants tell you fast ways to make this happen.

> *Carefully chosen tactics build support and convert opponents. . . .Consultants tell you fast ways to make this happen.*

Behavioral consultants have the expertise to use science of human behavior to separate fact from emotion. Facts explain motivation. Facts explain short-term and long-term voter gains, losses, and roadblocks in Congress–things the polls never tell. Consultants trace problems from personal advisors to public appearances. From in-house interviews to outside surveys, solutions restore and boost voter confidence.

WHAT CONSULTANTS WORK ON

Evaluation and selection of staff, communication strategies with advisory and adversarial groups, speech writing, mental health research, converting opponents, negotiations team with business and health agencies, training staff.

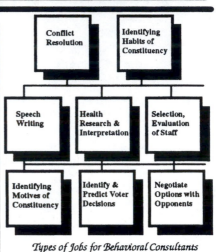

Types of Jobs for Behavioral Consultants

Consultant Helped in House Concurrent Resolution 172

*H*ouse Concurrent Resolution 172 with respect to considering battery as a factor in child custody awards is now law due to elected officials working closely with advocacy groups and behavioral consultants. Resolution protects against awarding child custody to a spouse abuser. Consultants did research legwork, provided profiles of abusers, coached legislators on speaking with abused parents, and helped with language on drafts.

> *Have you or your aide contact:*
> *Douglas Ruben, 517-347-0944*

for a delicate balance between *persuasion* and *honesty*. Winning producers such as Guthy-Renker Corporation, Rock-Solid Productions, Bill Powers, and Jim McNamara all share common insight on unique selling propositions: Products must be needed, consumable, and *valid*. Deceptive products are not tolerated. Valid products appeal to those basic human instincts: Vanity, greed, power, and success. That is why Victoria Jackson's cosmetics, Kathy Smith's fat-burning system, Susan Powter's calorie-cutting program, and Anthony Robbins success-building tapes are blockbuster hits. *Everybody needs them.*

And so, why not investigate whether everybody needs *your product?* The steps to infomercial development and making your first deal with producers involve a series of risks that begin with: *I have nothing to lose by trying.* It's true that Hollywood moguls do not know you or your practice in Sioux Falls, South Dakota, or, in my case, Okemos, Michigan. But they soon will if you try the following strategies.

First, check *Variety, The Hollywood Reporter,* or other entertainment trades for conventions and conferences on infomercials and whether you can attend. If travel and registration costs are prohibitive, find out whether transcripts, videos, or audios will be available after the program. Second, watch at least two infomercials on TV to get the gist of format, sales pitch, and types of products peddled. Third, write to an infomerical producer describing *briefly* who you are and a product proposal. After an opening paragraph or two, here is one way to pitch your product succinctly:

The Power of Parenting

Sales Pitch:	Four steps to teach parents how to manage their children: 1st step–don't take it personally; 2nd step–stay calm; 3rd step–ignore tantrums; 4th step–get kids to mind you.
Program Design:	Interviews, demonstrations, testimonials
Products:	Book-*Bratbusters: Say Goodbye to Tantrums and Disobedience* (Skidmore-Roth Publishers); video–same title (Videowave productions); audio–can be prepared.

Buyer:	Parents, grandparents, teachers, nannies, day-care providers. Appeals to mothers with new-borns, up at all hours. Appeals to their need for power and control.
Testimonials:	Available from ten years of clinical practice and from people who bought the book.
Research:	Proof of its effectiveness shown in experimental and applied studies, and in countless clinical cases.

Let's review this sample:

Sales pitch–tell exactly what you plan to sell.

Program design–name the main ways you believe the product can entice viewers.

Products–identify the existing book, video, or audio ready for packaging and shipping. Available products are a plus because it reduces overhead expenses and months of preparation. Then, too, some producers want to start from scratch so they have more *control*.

Buyer–who wants your product and how do you know they watch TV at those odd hours of the day?

Testimonials–infomercials thrive on real-life, unpaid people who bare their souls on the merits of the product. Where are you getting them? Therapist-authors usually base their self-help treatise on case studies, together with theory and research that round out prescriptions for a healthy lifestyle. On testimony, it's tempting to solicit voluntary help from the anonymously named clients in the book, thinking they would assuredly sing your praises. And, they might. But ethically this practice is "iffy," unless the client is perfectly comfortable emotionally undressing in front of millions of viewers and there are genuine therapeutic gains for the client. Even then, ask yourself if putting the client on public display entirely for personal gain is exceeding your authority as trusted teacher, friend, and confidant. If it is, no pursual of media height is worth losing your professional reputation over ethical violations.

The alternative way to seek authentic testimonials is by running a classified or display advertisement in which you offer to have people use your product (e.g., read your book) for free. Volunteer participants receive an informed consent stating benefits and risks of the product and that they are not under any financial or ancillary obligation to you, the provider. Next is a statement asking their permission to be contacted for live or written testimonial for TV, radio, or print media. By contrast, neutrally acquired testimonials spare you the ethical dilemma of placing your client's troubles on the auction block for public bidding.

Finally, *research*–just the facts. Why is your product valid? Should the producer be interested, and the deal struck, the company's attorneys will investigate the validation issue more thoroughly and ask your expertise on providing journal studies, books, or other corroborative documentation.

The final step in your infomercial gamble is selling your expertise. You can offer to be the expert who endorses the self-help product (as long as you really believe in the product), or the one who does the background research on it. Product development, arranging realistic testimonials, and scripting the commercial are just some of the services you can provide.

EDUCATIONAL/BUSINESS VIDEO

Does your product or expertise appeal to the mass populace? Can it be turned into an impulse purchase or loss leader in a bookstore, grocery store, video-rental store or through direct mail or telephone marketing? If so, what are you waiting for? Why not promote your expertise or product *educationally* using videotape, or consult with a video production studio on their own educational and industrial projects. *United Training Media, Video Arts, Human Resource Development, Dartnell,* and *Cally Curtis Company,* among many others, specialize in videos on labor relations, interpersonal relations, and home and family life. Videos employ unknowns or feature-named actors such as John Cleese or Lilly Tomlin, and directly sell as training and development aides to organizations. More narrowly focused topics, say, on ethics (e.g., *Ethics Resource Center, Inc.*) distribute to a larger business market because of state and federal mandates to clamp down on indiscretions.

Connecting with a video producer for your own product is the next step. There are two ways to approach it. First is subsidy production; the other is attracting investors. Subsidy or self-production means you put up the costs and contract with a video company. They in turn arrange all the steps from studio and equipment rental, hiring actors and crew, post-production, storage of inventory, and setting up distribution channels. How much you participate in each step depends on your time, experience, and cost-saving ambitions. For example, can you write the script? Chapter 11 probes this possibility in more detail. Do you have friends or relatives in theater or who know actors willing to work at nonunion or reduced rates? Cutting corners where you can cheapens the process, but not *necessarily* the outcome.

The second route is interesting investors in your product. Investors such as friends, colleagues, and independents are naturally skeptical about return on their investment with interest. Prove your product can earn profits by test marketing it on a sample population at your expense, using a prototype. Results of that test substantiate initial risks and allow reasonable projections of product growth. For example, suppose you planned a video on dog training. First, put together a prototype home video basically instructing and demonstrating methods, with few testimonials, similar to an infomercial. Use your VCR camera and friends or family as actors. Then take your copy to a local video studio for editing or use your home-based editing equipment; smooth out the transitions in between each scene, creating a simple and flowing video. Make three to six copies of the video. Editing and reproduction costs should be kept low, under $200. Frequently production runs of six or more copies entitle you to a substantial discount. Take advantage of this savings even if you planned on only a few copies. Now take your copies to three or four public libraries in your county area. Invite them to rent this video to their patrons; provide them with a small sign or flyer describing the video. Ask the librarian to keep a tally of daily video rentals and comments made by the viewers. Let the test marketing last about one month.

High numbers of video rentals indicate your product is saleable and will convince investors their money is in good hands. Low rental numbers signify many things, but primarily that it's back to the drawing board before calling an investors meeting.

Finally, put your expertise in human resources to good use by writing local, regional, and national video companies about who you are and why they can benefit from your input. Letters are like inquiries for infomercials: short and sweet. Most financially successful producers already have consultants on board and reject outsiders. That's okay; you *don't know what their responses will be until you send an inquiry letter.*

Chapter 2

Your Own Local Access Cable Show

The recent movie and sequel of *Wayne's World*, the take-off of *Saturday Night Live*'s sketch of two cable TV junkies, has the world taking a new look at cable vision. This mass communication outlet is literally a free opportunity for ambitious, inexperienced TV seekers to get camera time. Access cable provides educational shows using studio equipment, a production crew, and post-production facilities identical to a network TV operation. Cable also is big on individual autonomy. All you need is a show idea, available time slots, and trained production crew, credentialed or approved by the studio manager, and your show becomes reality. For first-time TV exposure, nothing beats it. However, there are specific steps to go through in setting up a show and being programmed into the schedule.

CONTACT A LOCAL ACCESS CABLE COMPANY

These are all around you. Ask yourself, "Who is the company I pay my cable bill to?" That company may have a working studio that telecasts amateur shows on a regular schedule. Call the cable company in your area first, before checking other local cable studios. Ask for the production manager. That person can explain (a) which live or taped shows can be done, (b) the crew requirements (number of, credentials, and where to find them), (c) the type of new shows being considered or preferred, and (d) time slots available for rehearsal and programming.

Ideally, propose a show combining humor such as *David Letterman* with a serious side for discussion of social, medical, mental health, or political issues. Design a simple, 30-minute format of guest interviews or telephone call-in mixed with a barrage of simple tech-effects for variation. Stay away from the "bopping-heads" format of two people sitting across from each other asking and answering questions. While still popular in interview shows, this format is a deadend. Just ask yourself why you do channel surfing on Sunday morning when you see politicians being interviewed. It's not the politicians, it's the sedative-hypnotic trance of the camera rotating headshots. Figure 2.1 describes a different proposal for a show called *The Recovery Shop*. Note how time segments are defined, interspersed with bumpers, and focus is upon controversially charged topics aimed for night viewership.

ASSEMBLE PRODUCTION STAFF

Who runs the show? Is it you? At first, perhaps. You conceive the show idea, do the groundwork for pitching the cable show and gather leads on crew recruitment. But where do you find a crew? Crews consist of three to four trained audio-video specialists ambitiously seeking air time for class credit, credentialing, or because they do it for a hobby. And good thing; most cable crews work for free. Crews include a sound-controller, two floor camera operators, and a director. The director is not like a motion picture director who says "CUT" or visibly appears on the set giving orders and acting tips. Directors instead hide behind a panel of TV monitors and choose which camera is on, at what angle, and coordinate all other crew members. The best place to find crews is at colleges in media and communications departments. Place a notice on the departmental bulletin board or find out from the secretary which students are looking for internships involving practical and direct hands-on experience. Believe me, the secretaries *will know this answer*.

Once recruits volunteer their time, schedule a first meeting together to plan out rehearsal and taping schedules, time commitments, and to solicit their technical input. Crews should be regarded as valuable assets and treated politely and royally. They are, after all, volunteers and only will remain faithful to your project if they feel special, enthusiastic, and see their ideas put to use.

FIGURE 2.1. Proposal for cable show called *The Recovery Shop*

The Recovery Shop
for WELM-TV

Host: Dr. Doug Ruben

Length: 30 mn

Frequency: weekly, night.

Co-producer: Best Impressions International Inc.

Purpose: Consumer awareness of medical and mental health topics and solutions facing today's community. Gives insider secrets on health improvement and pitfalls to watch out for when seeking help.

Guests: Arranged by Best Impressions International Inc, if desired.

Show Topics: Is there such a thing as too much sex? Finding the right sex partner? How much drinking is too much? What's the price of love?

Format: Segments include:

1.	15 sec	Logo—Best Impressions International Inc. presents . . . and title
2.	2-3 mn	intro of topic—cliffhanger, stay tuned
3.	1 mn	pre-taped voice-over/bumper called CAN YOU BELIEVE IT? with facts, figures of illness
4.	10-15 mn	introduce guest and interview on topic, "back with your questions in a minute."
5.	1 mn	CONSUMER BEWARE or REAL LIFE OUCHES prepared ahead of time based on expert's advice with pretaped info, v.o. bumper
6.	5-7 mn	Questions taken from phone or from live audience
7.	1 mn	closing.

ASSEMBLE SPONSORS

Some, not all, of cable show programming requires sponsored advertisement. Educational cable stations refuse advertising and in fact refuse product promotion of any sort, so your show has to remain entirely educational. Titling your show toward commercial ends, such as "The amazing panic-controller device," won't make it; it violates cable regulations for acceptable air time programs. Try instead "The Fear, Phobia, and Personal Health Show." Promise a wide variety of mental health information, among which is your panic-controller device. Other cable companies are open to product sales but ask for minimal assurance of paid advertising time before each weekly telecast. For example, Joyce Hagelthorn, host of a show on the paranormal, enjoyed high weekly ratings and even expanded to a studio audience. But the cable company faced economic realities and asked that all shows be underwritten by paid advertisers. This meant Joyce, herself, had to beat the pavement for interested sponsors, knowing that cable commercials are financial losses. Several months passed before companies agreed to a limited sponsorship contract and allowed her show to re-air.

Sponsored shows can sweep you into the next stage of TV popularity. After you run two to three shows, decide on a simple measure of viewer ratings. For example, using live telephone call-ins, compare the number of questions called in from one show to the next; some shows invite mail-in questions which can act as another gauge of viewer interest. There's no need for rigorous empirical research on your show's success, as long as the ratings system chosen is applied reliably and accurately. Get a little data under your belt and try sorting through easy questions such as–Is the viewer response rate increasing from one show to the next? How about demography? What type of person is calling? Where are they calling from?

Depending on your show's impact, for-profit cable stations managers are always looking for syndicatable material. Don't laugh; your chances of winning the small-time syndication lottery are much higher than winning *Publisher's Clearinghouse*. Why? Because it's a matter of timing and politics. The timing is right if your show pilots a viewpoint or unique style catching on like hotcakes and is locally publicized in community newspapers, radio, or network TV news. It's a political bonanza if your cable studio is owned or operated by a statewide or national cable company through which public access shows can be transmitted, transferred, or bought. Take, for example, TCI, the nation's cable magnate. Locally produced shows under TCI stand a powerful chance of selling to other TCI-owned cable stations in neighboring cities or states. Out-of-state programming may be on different days and time slots and, of course, may mean modifying format, such as no more live telephone call-in. But that's a small price to pay for syndication.

Chapter 3

Prerequisites and Roadblocks for TV

Convinced you're the TV type? You should be; many practitioners or instructors who do clinical therapy are accustomed to talking and improvising in the session. TV allows ready access of these skills and your product to a wider clientele, but through less intimate contact. That's one difference. Differences between therapy, teaching, and TV become more obvious after making blatant mistakes and realizing afterwards what you did. The biggest mistake is not so much what you did wrong, but *what you didn't know to do right*. Below are key roadblocks mental health experts face on live and taped television because they treat this medium the same as giving a lecture, presenting a workshop, or conducting therapy sessions. TV is not these things and the effective guest plans ahead to modify wrong expectations.

SIMPLE AND SLOW LANGUAGE

One of the first lessons taught directly or indirectly in college is that there is a technical vocabulary and talking in this language is your ticket to survival among faculty and peers. Don't say "rewards," say "reinforces." Don't say "the pigeon does it again," say "there is an increased probability of that behavior occurring in the future." Vernacular doesn't die, it goes on "extinction." In graduate school, technical language replaces English. You are no longer bilingual–you can't speak normally and do professional jargon; it becomes 24 hours of thinking, eating, and breathing *only* jargon. And if you forget the words, some other doctoral student vying for your orals date will make sure the faculty knows you slipped up. So, you don't slip up. Even after earning your degree the rewards for jargon are numerous, from journal articles and edited books you publish, to speaking engagements at conventions. You are professionally known by your eloquent, technical speech.

Well, say goodbye to eloquence. TV hates it. Jargon is inappropriate when promoting your product or expertise to the public. College-educated consumers might understand a word or two, but don't count on it. And other viewers, with no education or barely a ninth grade education, certainly will miss the point. Words must be simple, not two-thousand dollar words. Nobody knows what "mastication" means; but you know what they think it will mean. Misunderstood words can ruin your impact and convey a negative image, even if you appear likable on the screen. Even your advanced reputation cannot excuse confusion. For example, most of the public has heard of B. F. Skinner. One talk show about ten years ago featured Skinner being interviewed about child discipline and reasons for a positive approach. Asked why firm discipline was a no-no, he replied that "Punishment was okay on interval schedules but not on continuous schedules." On what? What's an interval schedule? What's a continuous schedule? Or worse, "See, the expert said it was okay to PUNISH my child." Technical words hit the airwaves and completely distorted his message.

Use simple words and speak slowly. Even when words *seem simple*, they may only be simple in comparison to your heavy technical jargon. Suppose you're describing how tantrums get started. Think simple. You start by saying "Kids do attention-seeking behavior and get their parents' reinforcement." Okay, now omit from the sentence any compound or slightly technical words and replace them with *taboo words*. Words you were never supposed to say during college years because it made you look unprofessional. Now the sentence might sound like this: "Kids yell and say bad things and parents want to calm them down; but parents give love and affection for the wrong behavior." That makes sense. Believe me, some god out there will not strike you down for betraying your code of professional obedience.

WATCH BODY LANGUAGE

Be careful to spot where your hands move, and how you sit in front of a camera. Hand gestures are excellent tools for animation but may detract from your words if used too much. Frequently camera shots "crop" you from the waist up, and excessive gestures may actually block your face. If hand motions *help you speak effectively*, restrict the gestures to around your waist, not raising them higher than your chest. Exercise similar caution with sitting. Sit with your legs crossed at the ankle (men), at the ankle tucked inward or to the side (women) or at the kneecap (men and women). Sit erect in the chair, and lean forward during your delivery. Forward leans convey sincerity, humbleness, and compassion.

KNOW YOUR PRODUCT

Surely by the time you start TV you know the product very well. It is second nature to you. That is how you want viewers to understand the product; that using the product or advice is so simple, so commonsensical, that it becomes a fixture in every American living room. Convince the viewers that life is so much easier and personally satisfying using your product and advice. Compel them to impulsively jump on the bandwagon of success and power and give up their bad habits. Persuasion does not have to be evangelical. Charisma is a plus but not essential. Product sales depend on explaining how *something new* eliminates a sensitive problem in every viewer's life. One way of identifying with viewers is to share how *you suffered until you discovered the miracle ways of this product or advice*. For example, recently a habit specialist explained why his stop-smoking tapes worked years ago when he was a two- to three-pack-a-day smoker and needed a safe, effective approach to change his life. That pitch not only was *true*, but it *played well*.

KNOW YOUR AUDIENCE

Who are you speaking to? Certainly not to a college audience. But that much we already know. Consider, then, other factors in the composition of the studio audience or TV audience. Metropolitan audiences out West are different from those in the East, South, and from those of the Midwest. Certain parts of the country have different demographics, family attitudes, and product needs. Certain states have larger ethnic, racial, or religious groups whose customs and practices are worth consideration so you don't offend the viewers. Audience variables also predict your *pitch*. Hard-selling pitches are probably best for the Midwestern and Eastern states. Southern and Western states react better to soft-sell.

MEMORIZE VS. TELEPROMPTER

TV is not an oral dissertation defense. It is not necessary to memorize every detail that can possibly be asked of you about why the product works, who says it works, and what happens if it doesn't work. This only causes panic. Let your creative ideas flow and follow the interviewer's questions. Three- to ten-minute segments go by rapidly and rely on some "stock" answers scripted ahead of time, but the majority of discussion is spontaneous. On longer shows, infomercials, educational videos, or scripted copy require some memorization to assure accuracy of product description and consistency for the filming crew. Hard-to-memorize facts can appear on a TelePrompter, or computer cue card. Full or abbreviated sentences typed at a keyboard project across the lens of the camera where you are looking. You can read the words from line to line without *looking like you're reading anything.* Of course, voice intonations and soft facial expressions also deflect attention from your "reading."

FLEXIBILITY

Remember that television lives or dies on ratings. Scheduled segments survive as long as the TV show exists or is not interrupted by an exclusive news story. Advanced scheduling may instantly change if the show must interview newsmakers or cover a headline event taking priority over your expertise and product. This is not always common, but when it does happen, never take the "eleventh hour" change personally. Be flexible. Producers behind the scenes usually are very happy you showed up and will reschedule an appearance.

A second last-minute change affects not your segment, but what you plan on talking about. Intentions are one thing; *what plays well and generates high ratings is what counts*. Producers booked you, for example, because your product pitch was perfect for an upcoming show. Now you've arrived for the show, but find out that upon "further thinking the segment through," the senior producer wanted a different slant, a more catchy angle, and so do this instead. New angles usually pertain to your product and expertise, but you may have to rewrite your mental script with little time to spare. Last-minute corrections usually are relevant, easy to adopt, and will probably generate higher audience reaction.

IMPROVISATION

How important is it to *let things just happen?* By the time the floor director says "3, 2, –" (points finger to host), your adrenaline already has been pumping wildly and has wiped out everything you memorized. You can't remember a thing you rehearsed except the name of your product and your own name. Seconds later the host introduces you and the promotion begins. Panic never lasts long and is absolutely normal the first couple of times you appear on live or taped television. That is why a good rule to follow is *wait for the cue*. Let the news anchor or show host lead you down the path of questions based on prescripted material and any chats you had before the telecast or in between commercials. Details about *why your product works* or general advice will feel normal when responding to familiar questions. Oddly enough, call-in telephone questions are easier for practitioners than purely being interviewed. This is because the voice of an emotionally distraught person reminds you of clients who you talk with all the time.

Follow the lead of the interviewer even if the direction he moves in goes astray. Suppose you start off talking about obsessive compulsive behaviors. Conversation rapidly drifts to problems of adult children of alcoholics, not exactly your specialty, but also not outside of your competency. *Combine the two*. Find a common link between both topics, for example, "Yes, they both have trouble with perfectionism." Relating the two topics shows your creativity, spontaneity, and capacity to keep the conversation flowing naturally as if you've rehearsed it. The more natural it looks, the more viewers think you're best friends with the host and there is automatic product endorsement.

SERIOUS VS. COMEDY

Academic training is a serious endeavor. Nobody disputes this. From bachelors to doctoral degrees, homework and political appeasement of committee members occupied your wakeful hours. Obstacles to graduating, no matter how few or many, were tedious and took every ounce of concentration. Now, as a practitioner, therapy takes every ounce of serious concentration. If your expertise is a serious one, and your product treats serious problems, why be funny about it? Here's why–because *funny works*. Not comedy, *funny*. Even when you appear on a "medical show," humor integrated into your pitch plays more effectively than dry descriptions. First watch how the show hosts set the tempo. Questions starting with, "Now, seriously, tell me . . ." deserve frank replies without a smile or laughter. If the host laughs or jokes with another host, joke along with them *if it fits*. This is still their show. Let them be the stars of it. But knowing that a lively rapport sells products, it pays to use animated expressions or share humorous examples. Levity used in moderation keeps the conversation upbeat and shows you're *only human.*

A dangerous mistake is forcing people to know this is *not a laughing matter.* On a recent show, an author of a self-help book on depression appeared with her daughter. Every time the show hosts joked about "a depressed child being easier to handle than a hyperactive one," she lit into them with a fierce "Hey, I don't think this is a joking matter." She perceived their comedy as ridiculing her book and discrediting her and her daughter's awful experiences. Consequently the author looked defensive, angry, and at odds with the lovable hosts of this metropolitan town. The mistake? She took it too personally. The outcome? Her book sold poorly in that town. The lesson? Look humble and likable across the airwaves, mixing honesty with soft humor.

MAKE THE HOST(S) LOOK GOOD

You're a guest, so have the common courtesy to make the host look good. On any show, but particularly nationally syndicated shows, hosts ride on their reputation. Oprah Winfrey frequently appears on *The National Inquirer, The Star,* and other tabloids depicting some new crisis in her life. Whether or not crises really exist is less important than her receiving continuous publicity. That public image *starts on the show.* Guests must not compete with her reputation by making her look stupid or ill-informed. Instead, follow her initiative, charm, and respond in agreement with her opinions. Exceptions are when the host completely misses the point or is dead wrong about what the product does. Correct the host gently by flowing one idea with another idea, for example: "That's very true, but another reason for this product is . . . ."

Hosts are not out to get you. Even offensive jabs they take at your product or expertise are entirely for entertainment; they can arouse the live studio audience into anger or frustration by treating you a certain way. But remain calm, answer the questions frankly and warmly, promoting your product as the *remedy* for their anger and frustration. In this sense, upsetting the viewers sets you up as the hero, the rescuer. You only think you look bad or your product failed, if you fall for the oldest trick in the book: good cop, bad cop. Hosts who play devil's advocate on controversial topics afford you a remarkable opportunity to beef up your pitch. Seize it with zeal but make it look natural.

REIMBURSEMENT

As your own publicist, you quickly learn one thing about TV talk shows. They're cheap. They want you but can't pay for you. Expense accounts for local, state, and regional (even Superstation) shows are minuscule and virtually no funds are allocated to reimburse guests unless they are major celebrities. Travel, lodging, food, and related expenses go toward next year's tax deductions as part of gaining experience in media. Paying for your trips seems costly and downright ugly as an incentive for out-of-state shows. That's why initial booking should be on local news, talk shows, or shows within a radius of 100 miles. Let your car build up mileage and make the greatest expense be for gas. But once you've exhausted locality, try booking on shows in neighboring states. The farther you go, the more the costs build up. Some shows are sympathetic, offering to pay one night's lodging. But that's it. It's time to get to know your credit cards.

There are many ways to save money using membership privileges and advanced preparation. First, buy your airline tickets two weeks or more in advance of the show, or try scheduling a flight over a weekend. For example, depart on Sunday night for a show Monday morning; do a show Friday morning and return home Saturday. Check out new fare plans among rival airlines. For example, American Airlines recently unveiled cheaper fares for business travelers. Purchase tickets from a reliable travel agency or on your own using the Prodigy or other computer on-line systems (e.g., EAASY SABRE). Second, build up *frequent flyer miles* on domestic flights during your tour. American Airlines, Delta, Northwest, Continental, among others, all offer mileage awards such as free one-way or round-trip tickets after, for example, earning 20,000 to 80,000 miles. Or, third, take the credit card plunge. Major credit cards (MasterCard, Visa, Discovery, etc.) now offer credit-for-mileage programs, where dollars spent translate into miles flown. On Northwest Airlines' program, for example, $20,000 of credit charged equals 20,000 earned miles and a free round trip in the continental USA, good for two years. Fourth, earn free round-trip tickets by volunteering your seat on overbooked flights.

Fifth, select a hotel or motel discounted by any membership status. For members of the American Psychological Association, for instance, corporate room discounts are available at participating Hyatt Hotels, Holiday Inns, Sheraton properties, and Howard Johnsons. Sixth, arrange ahead of time for the hotel's shuttle to pick you up at and return you to the airport. If car rental is a must, again use your membership discounts. Fourth, eat modestly and rely on meals served on the airplane. By the time you check into the hotel, you're ready for a light dinner. Eat the dinner but plan on missing breakfast the next morning unless you bring your own food or eat a complimentary pastry at the studio before the show. After the show, you're headed back on the airplane and can relax with lunch.

Pay-as-you-go is the principle of talk show tours unless you hit the big time. Compensation is available for travel, lodging, and meals on nationally syndicated shows. You may also receive additional "spending money" for recreation and entertainment. Shows in New York, Chicago, and Los Angeles realize most guests are not natives and probably want to enjoy their brief stay before traveling home. Budgets are discussed as part of booking arrangements, including your flight schedules and lodging accommodations.

So, dare yourself to be a hustler on a small scale. Devise a plan on how to break into local TV using many of the techniques outlined in this chapter. You'll see in no time how easy TV contacts can be, and you'll be surprised how creative you are. Once it happens, you'll say to yourself, "Now, really, was that so hard?"

PART I:
REFERENCES AND SUGGESTED READINGS

Em, M. (1994). The ever-changing story: Writing for the interactive market. *The Journal of the Writer's Guild of America, 7*, pp. 16-21.

Helitzer, M. (1987). *Comedy Writing Secrets*. Cincinnati, OH: Writer's Digest Books.

Minch, S. (1992). *A Life Among Secrets: The Uncommon Life and Adventures of Eddie Fields*. Seattle, WA: Hermetic Press.

Sullivan, J. (1993). Interactive media: Birth of a market. *The Journal of the Writer's Guild of America, 6*, pp. 15-19.

Walters, D. & Walters, L. (1989). *Speak and Grow Rich*. Englewood Cliffs, NJ: Prentice-Hall.

Whiteford, David (1994). "TV or not TV." *INC*. June, pp. 63-66;68.

PART II.
AM, FM, OR PhD?
THE VOICE OF RADIO

Who do you listen to on the radio? DJ's? Sports announcers? Weathermen? Probably all of these people. Consider the facts: Radio is the second oldest form of mass media, reaching millions of listeners. It breaks socioeconomic barriers: white collar, blue collar, rich, poor–almost everybody owns a radio. Radios are tall, small, cheap, portable, pocketable, and follow people wherever they go from bedrooms and bathrooms to the workplace. The *voice of radio* wakes you up, drives you to work, follows you home after work, and keeps you company at night. Everywhere you go, radios can be found.

So, it makes logical sense that radio is the perfect medium to pitch your product and expertise. While TV is clout, radio is popular. Don't count on radio gaining you a status symbol. Radio *does* communicate messages rapidly, repeatedly, and is easier to hook into than TV. News and talk shows always are open to human interest stories, authors, inventors, and expert commentary on prevailing social issues. AM and FM equally provide numerous opportunities for the novice performer to break into showbiz, gain confidence in public speaking, and promote products cheaply while in the convenience of your own office.

Chapters 4, 5, and 6 introduce ways to better maximize radio technology for public relations and ultimately to expand your image-building efforts using another media resource.

Chapter 4

Guest Appearances
and Resident Expert on Radio

Just as with TV, start by selecting radio stations featuring news and talk shows that invite guests and frequently use resident experts. Guest spots on radio usually are longer (10 to 50 minutes), more relaxed, and require far less advanced preparation other than booking a date.

HOW TO GET STARTED

Contact radio stations for interview. Start by asking, "Who do I want to hear me?" Choice of radio stations locally, statewide, or nationally are infinite and easily found in *Bacon's Directory of TV and Radio*. Choose a city and state. Suppose it's your hometown. Now consider what the radio station plays–rock, country, golden oldies, gospel, solid gold, classical, TALKNET, or all news? Music determines listener profiles and this indicates weak and strong potentials for product sales. Adult contemporary talk shows generally attract parents between ages 35 and 50. Rock stations cater to teenage and early adult ages. Talk show varieties run AM (morning hours), PM (afternoon hours), AD (morning drive time), PD (PM drive time), LN (late night), or PT (prime time). Send an inquiry letter to the show's senior producer, pitching your product or expertise, similar to that done for TV. Figure 4.1 is a letter saying that you are "radio-friendly" from past airwave experience. Figure 4.2 is a fax version, appealing to the mass market quick-fix mentality. Incidentally, the term "Shame Doctor" played off of media terminology; at the time listeners were getting a steady diet of "Dr. Death"

(Dr. Jack Kevorkian), and the "Love Doctor" (Dr. Leo Buscalia and his followers).

Use a National Distributor

Direct mail to radio stations can become a financial headache. First, addresses must be correct. Second, bulk mail discounts get confusing and inevitably involve hours of presorting according to a myriad of post office regulations: Thank you, but no thank you. Third, tracking replies, rejections, and stations which require follow up takes reliable record keeping and updated spreadsheets. Computer users may find this labyrinth of paperwork a challenge and an escape from daily monotony. That's fine, but computer illiterates are less ambitious; heavy documentation is a sure way to kill your incentive. This is why many radio-seeking guests use national distributors.

National radio distributors are firms who compile names of politicians, athletes, and celebrities into a monthly newsletter sent nationwide to nearly every talk radio station. The newsletter gives an abstract on each potential interviewee, describing his credentials, why he is newsworthy, and interview hooks. *Newsmaker Interviews* of Los Angeles for example, issues their newsletter only to paid subscribers. Producers interested in an interviewee contact that person directly for a booking. The distributor neither represent the interviewee nor coordinate radio appearances. Their job is exclusively to apprise producers and show hosts of what's out of there.

Media Representative

Volunteering your expertise on local mental health boards and community organizations provides an easy step to radio. Ask to be designated the media correspondent or PR (Public Relations) liaison, speaking to reporters and granting interviews. As spokesperson, you describe current policies and decisions or may articulate one side of a controversial problem. For example, after becoming a trustee on the church board, you make the media rounds updating the church's position on abortion, corporal punishment, and attempts to curb the city's crime wave. News and talk shows offer

FIGURE 4.1. Pitch letter for radio show

BEST IMPRESSIONS INTERNATIONAL INCORPORATED

4211 OKEMOS ROAD, SUITE 22, OKEMOS, MICHIGAN 48864, U.S.A.
TELEPHONE: 517-347-1811, FAX or PHONE: 517-347-0944

April 13, 1993

Mr. Dennis Daly, Producer
AMERICAN MONTAGE
UPI Radio Network
1400 1 St, NW
Washington, DC 20005

Dear Mr. Daly:

A year ago I appeared on national radio talk shows discussing parenting and my book, *Bratbusters: Say Goodbye to Tantrums and Disobedience.* But now adults have a tougher problem–they "avoid things too much." That has prompted ***Avoidance Syndrome: Doing Things Out of Fear.***

Avoidance Syndrome is a nationally released anti-fear manual that I can discuss on upcoming segments of AMERICAN MONTAGE. A perfect title for call-in questions, ***Avoidance*** gets to the heart of why people hate doing things. Get answers to "Why do I procrastinate?" "Why do I hate conflict?" and "Why do I hold feelings inside?" From fears and phobias to having bad moods–let's tell your listeners firsthand why it happens and what they can do about it.

For myself, I've now authored over 30 books on families and habits and appeared on radio shows coast to coast. Recently I appeared on JP McCarthy's *The Focus Show* (WJR-Detroit), the *Bob Cudmore Show* (WGY-Schenectady, NY), and booked nationwide through *Newsmaker Interviews*.

Enclosed, for starters, is a press release. I would be happy to forward a copy of the book and additional information upon your request. Telephone or in-studio interviews arranged. I look forward to your thoughts and hopefully to working together on AMERICAN MONTAGE.

Please feel free to call me at the PHONE or FAX numbers above.

Very sincerely,

Douglas H. Ruben, PhD

FIGURE 4.2. Fax pitch letter for radio show

BEST IMPRESSIONS INTERNATIONAL INCORPORATED

4211 OKEMOS ROAD, SUITE 22, OKEMOS, MICHIGAN 48864, U.S.A.
TELEPHONE or FAX: 517-347-0944 or 24 hrs at 1-800-595-BEST

FAX COVER SHEET

DATE: 12-6-93

ATTENTION: Kevin Myron

FAX NUMBER: 617 787 5969

PAGES: 2

FROM: Paul Smith, Best Impressions International Inc

NOTES: **Want a holiday treat for your listeners? Try the "Shame Doctor." On-the-phone cures for holiday blues and feeling guilty.**

Invite Dr. Ruben, the "Shame Doctor," to show your listeners—

- how to stop being a people-pleaser
- how to rate their dates
- how to stop feeling guilty all the time

Celebrity psychologist Dr. Ruben, recently on DONAHUE, is author of *"No More Guilt: Ten Steps to a Shame-Free Life."* His ten-step advice is eye-opening; it hits the nail on the head. But best of all, he's entertaining. You won't find this mix of humor and compassion in most doctors today. But Dr. Ruben has it. And your listeners won't stop raving about it. Give us a call.

For information or booking telephone interviews, call 1-800-595-BEST

unusually generous air time to nonprofit organizations, especially for highly visible organizations such as the ACLU, United Way, and state offices.

Second, use your supervisory role on grants and research projects to negotiate a media budget. Allocate travel and publicity funds for radio, TV, and other promotions, drawing attention to consumer-benefiting programs. For example, under a grant to develop a transitional living center for multiply handicapped blind students, this author arranged a radio interview with *Radio Talking Book*. This is a local educational station serving the visually impaired statewide. State or federally funded grant regulations permit media exposure only after the granting period begins and according to certain stipulations such as getting prior approval of the press release or interview topics.

Voice-Overs

Your most precious commodity is your *voice*. Mental health professionals rely on language and voice command as persuasive tools in therapy. Words and intonation go into your vocal delivery, effectively defining your individual style. Now that style can reach radio audiences by promoting other products in a commercial by doing *voice-overs*. Voice-overs involve reading a prewritten script later mixed with a jingle, new music, and product descriptions. All radio commercials use voice-overs. Voice-overs may be soft-sell, hard-sell, narrative, and caricatures. Soft-sell is quieter, slower, smoother, and invites product curiosity without pressuring the listener. Funeral home ads use this format. Hard-sell is rapid speech pressuring limited-time offers on products going out of stock. Car dealerships and appliance stores lead the pack on this variety. Narrative is technical readings used in audio-visual, educational films. Videos on auto mechanics, flying, psychology, and other disciplines, all use one or two readers. Character voices, either as soft- or hard-sell, send a humorous message to listeners. Comedy, over force, entices potential buyers into product curiosity.

Doing voice-overs is for anybody, not just for actors or deep-voiced DJ-sounding individuals. First, find a printed advertisement in the newspaper or magazine. Read it aloud slowly until the words and your breathing flow naturally. Now record the reading a couple of times using the condensed microphone on a tape recorder. For instant effect, re-record the script against a background of quiet "elevator" music. Each spot is no more than 15 seconds long. Combine four to five spots on a single tape and contact your local talent agency for an interview. Talent agencies in smaller towns welcome new voice-overs to keep up with rising demands from local and state advertisement needs.

Once under contract, agents send out duplicates of your *demo* tape and wait for responses. Voice-over jobs involve (a) receiving and rehearsing the script, (b) punctually arriving at the recording studio for taping, and (c) compensation after 10 percent to 15 percent commission has been deducted. Beginners earn from $50 to $60 per hour, with one-year veterans earning up to $150 per hour. Fee requirements and job demands all depend on your locality and competition.

Interview Another Person

Another way to directly begin radio is by interviewing *somebody important.* Public officials, community leaders, shakers and movers–all of these people share the common denominator of being interesting. Get the scoop on their interpersonal lives or have them reveal secrets, and the doors of radio are wide open to you. Put the interview on cassette tape. Contact local radio stations by phone and ask to speak to the producer of certain shows (larger stations) or station manager (smaller stations). Pitch the interview as a segment and offer to send the tape for review. In return, expect no remuneration but be prepared if they use and like the tape that you might receive *future assignments from the station.* Compensation is appropriate for future assignments.

LOCAL RADIO SHOWS

The business of radio is simple. Disseminate information as quickly as possible, repeated over many segments of the day. Newscasts held every 15 minutes or every hour repeat headline stories, featuring one or two new pieces. Twenty-four-hour news repeats major stories every half-hour, but fills in the gaps with local weather, traffic reports, and talk shows. In all, find a local radio station meeting your product needs and reaching a loyal listening audience.

All News

All-news stations hold excellent opportunities for one- to three-minute segments. WWJ in Detroit, for example, invites newsmaking input from listeners, plus runs several spots for community events calendars. Send a press release about your product for mention in the calendar of events. Or, send a tape briefly describing the product and its benefits and availability to the community. For example, an author scheduled to sign books at B. Dalton in a local mall sent a promo tape one week ahead of the signing. The tape briefly pitched the book, who needs to buy it and why, the cost, and times and dates of the book signing. *Does that guarantee a large attendance at the book signing?* No. But it does announce *product availability.* Buyers may be busy that particular day but now know where to get the book another day.

All Talk (TALKNET)

Talk shows are the "in" thing. AM stations co-owned by FM stations make up for over 1,500 radio stations nationwide, the bulk of which feature guest talk shows. Morning editions, midday editions, nightly additions, and special editions all capture the morning, lunch, and after-work traffic tuned in for another ruckus exchange. Some hosts live for controversy. They deliberately interview high-profile guests and fuel debate for sensationalism and high ratings. But not all hosts do this. All talk stations are different. Other hosts, for example, on WGN-AM in Chicago, discuss city life and events happening in town. Those are the shows you want to appear on. Likewise, WJR-AM in Detroit offers a convention of public service informational shows focused on lifestyles, celebrities, and community events.

Interview and Call-In Shows

WLS-AM in Chicago has over 12 defined shows. What do the *Bill Garcia Show, Roe Conn Show,* and *Mike Murphy's FANTALK*

all have in common? They deal with business, finance, public affairs, entertainment, sports, and are heavy into guests. Interview and
call-in shows appear in every city, some even cover a statewide
radius. These are shows where the host introduces your product or
expertise and discusses it for the first segment. Segments thereafter
involve your improvisational replies to call-in questions. On
WCHB-AM in Inkster, Michigan, NAACP president and host
Joanne Watson, for example, is superb at "radio-acupuncture"; she
pinches the right listener nerve-endings causing a flurry of telephone calls. A show under her voice command is guaranteed to
knock the phone off the hook.

And then there are network shows. Network affiliated stations
and shows naturally are better known and gain faster recognition.
Bob Cudmore's show in Schenectady, New York (WGY-AM, a
CBS affiliate) broadcasts over 50,000 watts, one the largest in the
area. Networks other than CBS, ABC, and NBC include Associated
Press Radio (AP), American Public Radio (APR), Cable News Network (CNN), Mutual Broadcasting System, Moody Bible Network,
National Black Network, National Public Radio (NPR), Public
Broadcasting Service (PBS), United Press International (UPI), Sat-
ellite Music Network, USA Network (USA), and many more inde-
pendents.

Educational (Noncommercial) Stations

Public and educational stations are unusual. They are the last of a
dying breed who beg for your contribution during annual fund-raisers. "Marathon madness" describes the panic of long, unappreciated hours airing special shows and special music to attract new
patrons to keep the station alive and breathing. Last-minute donations have rescued more than one sinking budget from bankruptcy.
But when funding is secure, and programming occurs, talk shows
reach an unprecedented loyal audience, largely because listeners
feel as if they are *stock investors.* They paid for shows they plan on
listening to. Listeners tend to be more educated, middle to upper-
middle class, conservative, and *older.* Ages 35 and up may be
classical music lovers, and take great interest in creative and liberal
arts. Supporters not only are loyal patrons, but so are universities

and colleges. For that reason, most educational independents are located on a college campus.

Radio Personalities

Is there a local radio personality always in the news? Always the talk of gossip? Is he or she a household name? Dolly Parton was number one in the movie *Straight Talk*. But how about in your town? That's whose show you want to be on. Ask yourself, "Does my product or expertise respond to an immediate problem? Does it entice impulse purchases?" If so, one way to mobilize product sales is by media giants endorsing the product. Get the radio host to say "Yes, it works," or "What a good idea it is," and thousands of daily fans will agree exactly with the host. This is why popular hosts and esteemed sportscasters frequently are spokespeople for major commercial products. The recently retired and Hall of Famer Ernie Harwell, voice of the Detroit Tigers for over 30 years, is the hottest candidate for commercial promotion. Imagine if he got his own talk show. If your specialty is sports psychology, playing his show would be a *must.*

Timing Counts

Talk show hosts welcome guests on a regular basis and at different times of the day. Early morning shows are the most popular because *everybody* drives somewhere–to work, to daycare, school, and to the stores. AM shows are a premium and competitively harder to book over noon, PM (afternoon), or late night shows. While *any show* is better than none, AM and noon listeners (the lunch crowd) still have half the day to buy your product or apply your expertise. Listeners headed home after work want *nothing to do with more effort.* Likewise with late night listeners; they want brainless entertainment from slapstick comedy to police stories. Hearing about parenting or new advances in phobia control are too cerebral for these insomniac folks in the outer-limits. So, choose radio shows that strike the right hour for consumer interest and ultimately increase product purchases.

Live Appearance vs. Telephone Interview

Radio interviews have a distinct advantage over TV interviews. You don't have to be there in the studio. True, TV stations can satellite or microwave you across affiliate stations, but you still must appear in front of *some camera*. With radio, interviews frequently are by telephone. The station calls you or you contact the station five minutes before the interview begins. While on hold, rehearse your main pitch or answers to scripted questions provided ahead of time to the interviewer. Once introduced, your voice transmits from the telephone to the live interview and is heard directly over the radio. Muffled voices result from poor telephone equipment or from speaking improperly into the receiver. Regular hand-held telephones must be tilted "just right" over your mouth so that sound is static free. Hand-free telephones that act like intercoms for conference calls are equally as bad. Voice quality is choppy, tunnel-sounding, and incoherent. Even today's revolutionary headsets sound like amplifiers. So, choose one option and ask the host for feedback during commercial breaks. That way you can sit back and enjoy the interview.

Is there any advantage of doing studio over telephone? Yes. Studio is personable and builds instant rapport with the host which carries over to the listener's ear. Together you can laugh, exchange eye signals on bizarre telephone calls, strategize in between news or music breaks, and pass written notes that nobody but the two of you can see. If your product or expertise feeds on compassion, face-to-face dialogue will assuredly establish your honesty and credibility for a convincing pitch. In-studio interviews also show *you care*. But this is for radio studios within a 100-mile radius of your home. Any interview outside that perimeter involves a long and expensive drive, usually starting at the crack of dawn or returning when it's pitch dark. In either case, driving fatigue may defeat your excitement.

Alternatively, think like an agent thinks. When traveling out of town on business or pleasure, contact radio talk shows located in those vicinities and indicate "you are on tour and will be in their area on such-and-such dates." Schedule the shows back-to-back, leaving enough leeway for drive time. Announce in your fax or letter that after the show you will be available at a certain location for product sales. For example, national hypnotist Damon Reinbold told radio listeners to attend up for his weight loss and smoking cessation programs *that evening* at a certain hotel. Authors take the same approach. They let producers and hosts know ahead of time they'll be signing books at a bookstore and promote it again during the live interview (see Figure 4.3).

NATIONAL RADIO SHOWS

How do you stay awake during morning rush hour? With coffee? Maybe. Most early risers tune into *Morning Edition* on National Public Radio (NPR) for news updates and information. NPR is one among many nationally syndicated Radio Networks providing a full range of programs. Other network leaders include ABC radio, Associate Broadcast News Service (ABN), American Farm Bureau Federation, Associated Press (AP), American Public Radio (APR), Black Radio Network, Business Radio Network (BRN), CBS radio, CNN radio, Copley Radio Network, Financial News Network (FNN), Hispanic Radio Network, In Touch Networks, Longhorn Radio Network, Mutual Broadcasting System (MBS), Money Radio Network, National Black Network, North American Radio Alliance, Newstalk Radio Network (NTR), Satellite Radio Network, Sheridan Broadcasting System, Sun Radio Network, United Press International Radio Network (UPI), USA Radio Network, and *Wall Street Journal* Radio Network among others. Less popular radio syndicators include Arkansas Radio Network, Robert Braverman Productions, Broadcast Services of the American Association for Retired Persons, Christian Science Monitor Network, Consumers' Union, Family Radio, Minnesota Public Radio, and Moody Broadcasting Network, among others.

Each station broadcasts a variety of morning, afternoon, prime time, and late night shows, covering business, public affairs, entertainment, sports, and consumerism. Like TV, syndicated radio's prime objective is delivering messages with an angle. It's not subliminal, even though the humor, controversy, and blatant "say-it-as-it-is" approaches frequently imply deeper meanings. *Car Talk*, on NPR, for example, features two brothers who are expert auto mechanics turned cynics who answer call-in questions about car

FIGURE 4.3. Fax letter to radio show producer about upcoming book signing

Best Impressions International Incorporated

4211 OKEMOS ROAD, SUITE 22, OKEMOS, MICHIGAN 48864, U.S.A.
TELEPHONE or FAX: 517-347-0944 or 24 hrs at 1-800-595-BEST

FAX COVER SHEET

DATE: 8-31-93

ATTENTION: Denorris Myles, Producer, WJMO-AM

FAX NUMBER: 216 791 9035

PAGES: 3

FROM: President, Best Impressions International Inc

NOTES:

Want your listeners to know–

- why they might be people-pleasers?
- how to rate their dates?
- how to stop feeling guilty all the time?

Let the shame doctor join you live . .

Celebrity psychologist Dr. Ruben, recently on DONAHUE, will be at the Little Professor Bookstore (in Parma) on Tuesday, September 7, at 12:30. He'll be speaking about people-pleasers and shame, and will sign his new book, *"No More Guilt: Ten Steps to a Shame-Free Life."*

For booking telephone interviews on Wed thru Sun, call 1-800-595-BEST

problems. But they are more than Sears auto-repair troubleshooters. Each reply humorously attacks the "brain-dead" car industry from ignorant buyers to charlatan salesmen. Then, too, for a more serious edge on life, business reports or headlines on Capitol Hill heard on the CBS Radio Network is more your speed.

Expertise on News Story

Like TV, radio needs your input. Frequently you'll hear a 24-hour newscast advertise a 1-800 or cellular phone number to call if you have news and information. Call this number and describe how your product relates to local, state, or national events. For example, hearing about the tragic death of comedian Sam Kinison, you may call and offer a commentary on how his death affects fans and the entertainment world at large. Or, suppose you just released a book on recovering lives, from post-traumatic stressed celebrities to Indians in South Dakota. Use your book and expertise as strengths in pitching a segment or interview that ties together Kinison's life after leaving the Pentecostal ministry, hating women, reaching stardom, and finally, five days before the accident, getting married. The punch line is that "post-traumatic stress takes a toll on lives."

Treat syndicated shows the same way you treat local radio shows. First, send an inquiry letter to the executive or senior producer of the show that interests you. In the letter offer to send a demo cassette tape either of past interviews or on the topic proposed. Follow up with a phone call within two weeks. Even if producers reject the need for resident experts, don't despair. Try a new angle; offer a two- to three-minute interview segment *for free*. Your material may fit just perfectly in that time slot.

Send Tape of Local Interview

You probably don't have a library full of interview demos at your disposal. In fact, maybe you've never done a radio interview and have nothing to promise producers in your pitch letter. Well, never fret; there are always alternatives. Create your own interview following these simple steps. First, ask a colleague or good friend with a deep, natural-sounding radio voice to interview you on your expertise. Begin the mock interview with your friend saying, "Today we have Doctor so-and-so, author of so-and-so, who is going to answer the question, Why do people do so-and-so?" You fill in the blanks based on your product or expertise. Interview time lasts three minutes, followed by a closing line such as "Thank you, Doctor so-and-so, for joining us today." Record the tape using a double-condensed, microphone tape-cassette machine that allows for maximum stereo reception. In fact, most tape players with recording capacities have this standard feature. For copies, duplicate the tape at an audio studio or using your own rapid dubbing capacities that are also becoming standard on modern stereo equipment.

Make multiple copies of the original tape using standard high-speed dubbing recorders or through digital computer programs. Label the tapes neatly, for example, with Avery Laser or Ink-Jet printer labels especially designed for plastic cassette surfaces (Avery #5198). Besides enhancing quality, professionally printed labels look like the tapes were submitted by a publicity agency–a plus if you're facing stiff competition for an open slot.

Chapter 5

Your Own Spot and Syndication

Guest appearances are the first way to get into radio. But after paying your "dues" on-air, try the next daring step of proposing your own regular segment. Regular segments vary from two- to three-minute weekly spots on the same topic or theme pretaped for playback, to a live radio show. With demands still bursting for talk radio, live radio shows are strong possibilities even if you lack formal broadcast training. Remember, you're not interested in being a DJ. What you want is a chance to advertise your expertise and product in a fashion that helps people and stimulates listener ratings. That's what *Dr. Harvey Ruben* does on the Westwood One Radio Network. Figure 5.1 is such an example. Relate your experience to a current void in the radio world that you can fill with emotionally powered interviews exposing, explaining, and entertaining life's unusual problems.

PROPOSE A DAILY OR WEEKLY SEGMENT

Choice of Topics

Whether live or pretaped, what should you talk about? Your product, right? Maybe not at first. Self-promotion takes time. Do it gradually; do it methodically. Product promos during a daily or weekly segment are more effective if offered as one among many commercial solutions to a problem. Present facts, fiction, and problems on such consumer topics as child health and learning, elderly health, adult stressors, and general psychology. Several years ago the author did a segment called *Now You Know,* a three-minute

FIGURE 5.1. Letter to radio program director pitching a new show

BEST IMPRESSIONS INTERNATIONAL INCORPORATED

4211 OKEMOS ROAD, SUITE 22, OKEMOS, MICHIGAN 48864, U.S.A.
PHONE or FAX: 517-347-0944; PHONE: 1-800-595-BEST

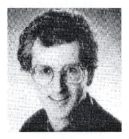

May 16, 1994

Mr. Bill Elliott
Program Director
WMMQ-FM Radio
913 W. Holmes Rd. #190
Lansing, MI 48910-0411

Dear Mr. Elliott:

I recently appeared on several AM radio stations promoting a workshop on "how to be a published author." But I'll tell you what I discovered and why I'm writing you. Most local AM talk stations did a great job pulling in current, political—even crime-beat headlines—but were light on personal and tabloid issues. Issues on lifestyles and hard-core family problems from addiction to marriages.

That's why I'd like to propose a 30 mn or 1 hr radio show during PM or late night that fills this local radio-talk void. Call it—*Secrets of Intimacy, hosted by Dr. Doug Ruben (or "Dr. Doug")*. No, not another "Ask the doc" show. *Secrets of Intimacy* opens the airwaves to hard-to-talk about and embarrassing subjects such as impotency, how to love again, infidelity, and choosing the right mate. *Secrets* is a call-in-show with interview guests who are real, off-the-street people sharing their secrets. And sure, we'll have a guest expert adding input. So, input isn't just from "Dr. Doug."

Not a bad idea? Okay, so how do you know I can pull it off? Here's why. I'm a family specialist turned national media consultant. I'm author of over 31 books including trades *Bratbusters, No More Guilt, Avoidance Syndrome, Family Recovery Companion,* and *60 Seconds to Success*. Recently on DONAHUE!, on local and regional TV and radio talk shows and even will be hosting a cable show soon. Plus, I've done a weekly taped segment for radio called "Now You Know." And the best part, I'd coordinate all the guests for each show. Your producers don't have to do it. That's what I do best.

As for what's in it for me? The chance to do it. We'll worry about pay when and if we get regular sponsors. But for now, how about spicing up your station with *Secrets of Intimacy?* Give me a call or fax. Perhaps we can meet and discuss a pilot show. And most of all, thanks for considering this idea.

Very sincerely,

Douglas H. Ruben, PhD

fact-filled update on emotional and substance abuse problems. One segment featured pros and cons on the "controlled-drinking" controversy. Another segment addressed what to look for in mismedicated and alcoholic elderly. Still a third segment revealed *Why support groups really work and why they don't work.* On the solution side, recommended consumer guides from books to tapes rounded out the segment. Featured among those guides were the author's own products.

In Minneapolis, for example, *Recovery Net* made its debut as a clearinghouse. Distressed callers reaching out for sober advice would hook into the 24-hour emergency line, later turned talk show, as listener support quadrupled and regular programming began. Self-help guides, tapes, videos, and spiritual retreats took to the airwaves, attracting a huge following. At last contact, *Recovery Net* said they were expanding the market on their product line and hoping to branch into TV. The same ripple effect is possible for your own show or segment.

Let your no-nonsense reporting follow the juicy excitement of TV's *Hard Copy* and *Now It Can Be Told.* Make the listener feel that only you hold the secrets to unleashed truths which each segment can expose in graphic detail. You're not just informing, you're also *performing.* So, make it entertaining. Interject humor, either by satirizing hard-core research on peculiar topics (e.g., "Did you know a study showed unsafe sex hits record numbers of older people? Why wait until you're older to be careless?"). Or, come up with off-the-wall "asides" as segues onto new topics. For example: "And speaking about research studies, did you know there's a study on how to trap a mosquito by its nose? Just tense your muscles as tightly as possible the next time a mosquito makes a plasma withdrawal on you. Pinch the skin around the skeeter and watch the bug bulge." They're weird comments, but they work.

Length of Segment

Pretaped segments for routine radio spots always are short–two to three minutes in length. Never longer. Even demos of your talk show capacities should remain short, five to eight minutes long.

Keep the topic flowing with a beginning, middle, and save the punch line for the end.

Format of Segment

Write out the script beforehand. Read it aloud several times, making sure you combine facts with humor. But keep to a general format. Standard formats begin with a "teaser," or opening line enticing the listener to stay tuned to the show. Follow that by introducing yourself and the topic covered. "Ever have your child rant and rave in the grocery store? You're not alone. It's the deadly curse of temper tantrums–This is Doctor so-and-so: Why tantrums occur and what to do about them in today's segment of *Raising Your Child* " (see Figure 5.2).

Pause for a moment, allowing for segment breaks to splice in network advertisements. Then begin your discussion. First explain the wrong things people do, then the right things, always injecting humor where possible, without going overboard. At the end, don't leave your audience hanging; give them resources to contact. For light and serious segments, be sure you sign off with a little humor.

Free, No Remuneration

Wouldn't it be nice to be paid for your talent? Of course it would. But promoting your public image begins as a voluntary undertaking at your own expense except for the perks now and again, such as attending studio parties and rubbing elbows with the big-wigs, or opportunities for longer and diversified radio segments. So, when is compensation possible? It is possible when your name and talents hit prime time, or you're featured in live talk shows and become part of the station's woodwork. Remunerative scales vary along union lines, depending on your contract; frequency of broadcast and number of stations you appear on make all the difference.

DISSEMINATE DEMO TAPE TO OTHER STATIONS

Why be content with one station? You have a quality demo and are enjoying regular air time, so why not contact other local or national stations to run your show? Here's how you do it.

FIGURE 5.2. Script for radio segment

SCRIPT:

Ever have your child rant and rave in the grocery store? You're not alone. It's the deadly curse of temper tantrums– This is Dr. Frederik: Why tantrums occur and what to do about them in today's segment of *Raising Your Child*. (Leave break for commercial).
Most choosy parents would choose Jif over a screaming child. You get embarrassed and can't stand those other shoppers acting like Olympic Judges while they expect you to stop your child's tantrum. So, you scream, spank, even threaten your child. Bribes ahead of time even fail. Now you feel like you've failed. But follow the three-step rule for beating tantrums. First, don't take them personally. Kids do what they do, but not because of you. Second, ignore the burst and let the burst fade like the wind. Third, a calmer child can be talked to. Ask your child after the tantrum is over to do something with you. Add to these three steps by reading *Bratbusters: Say Goodbye to Tantrums & Disobedience* or other self-helpers. But don't despair, because tantrums are not like Ever-Ready batteries. They don't keep going and going, until you drop. Only adolescents do that. We'll cover them next time. This is Dr. Frederik for *Raising Your Child*.

Cover Letter with Demo

After establishing yourself on one radio station, take a different approach in the inquiry stage. Duplicate ten to 15 copies of your original demo. Send a copy along with an inquiry (pitch) letter to a highly rated public or commercial radio station, or to a station in a geographically desirable location. Check the *Bacon's Radio/TV Directory* for state listings. In the letter, recommend the air time schedule you currently have with other stations. For instance, if your segment plays in AM, recommend that the station try the demo during AM. Also offer to tailor-make segments according to the producer's or station's needs. Some radio stations already may have mental health experts on board, or slated input on certain topics from certain people; should you find that out, propose a new angle consistent with the station's profile. For public radio, for instance, change your segment to "Secret Lives of the Masters of Classical Music"; here you reveal the untold or forgotten stories of emotionally distraught composers such as Mozart and Beethoven. Tidbits from the composer's psyche and emotional history add a new flair of appreciation to the classical pieces.

CONTACT NATIONAL RADIO SYNDICATION FIRMS

Doing your own legwork may not be financially rewarding but it accomplishes two goals. First, you learn firsthand the law of the land, the jargon, and feel in control of your public image campaign. You are the manager, marketing team, and sales force all in one. Second, strides made at any level reflect your own perseverance to be an entrepreneur. Still, there are drawbacks to being your own public relations manager. First and foremost is that it takes *time, energy, money, risk, and recuperation.* Time, energy, and money are obvious expenditures. But what are risk and recuperation? Risk is the daily and weekly salesmanship of pushing yourself, your product, and your expertise through unfamiliar and downright frightening doors. When the doors swing open, you feel your effort was worth the expenditures. When doors remain shut you feel defeated, angry, and decide to return to a monotonous life-style. You don't want to recuperate from failure. Bouncing back from rejection is plenty hard the first, second, and every time you knock on media doors, no matter what your track record is of success. This is why many mental health providers seek syndication firms to do the dirty work for them.

Terms of Agreement

Syndication firms are more than agents. Agents help to sculpt your talent for a price or hefty commission, and may find you radio spots in exactly the manner described above that you can do yourself. For example, Stephen Wright Agency (New York) accepts radio scripts and ideas from beginners for a reading criticism fee of $500 for 300 pages, with costs varying for shorter materials. This entitles agents to *tell you what's wrong with your radio script or idea and they may or may not do anything else for you.* By contrast, syndicates act as brokers for the material they handle. Radio demos are sold as a package; five to ten consecutive segments for one price. Syndicates promote and market the shows and keep careful records of sales. If picked up, there is reimbursement. You can earn 40 percent to 60 percent of gross receipts, receive a small salary, do work for hire, or a flat fee for one-shot items.

Syndicates aim for general or specific information. Editorial Consultant Service (West Hempstead, NY) solicits material with an automotive slant. General News Syndicate (New York, NY) is looking for entertainment-related material. Fotopress, Independent News Service International (Ontario, Canada) needs all subjects. It all depends on the focus and needs of the syndicators based on their distribution.

Resources

There are several places to begin. Syndicates who handle radio segments *also* handle column writing (political, humor, consumer, gardening, etc.). Best resources to contact for syndicate agencies are:

The Writer's Market
Cincinnati, OH: Writer's Digest Books
F & W Publications
1507 Dana Avenue
Cincinnati, OH 45207

How to Write and Sell a Column
Cincinnati, OH: Writer's Digest Books
F & W Publications
1507 Dana Avenue
Cincinnati, OH 45207

The Editor & Publisher Syndicate Directory
11 W. 19th Street
New York, NY 10011

Single vs. Multiple Syndicators

Is it unethical to send your demo and inquiry letter to multiple syndicators simultaneously? No. The number of recipients is limited only by your marketing budget and sales ability, not by a protocol in the field. Some syndicators promptly reply within a week to two weeks, while others never reply. Failure to reply means many things, from not interested in your material, to not reading the over-the-transom mail. Whatever the reason, let hurt feelings go away as you pursue hot new leads.

Chapter 6

Prerequisites and Roadblocks for Radio

Does your voice sound hoarse all the time? Does it sound choppy with noticeable gulps of air to breathe? Or, do you have that nasal-sounding *Laverne* snort from *Laverne and Shirley?* Well, you probably have all of the above. But so does everybody else. Nobody is a natural radio announcer. Even Paul Harvey groans and moans, has funny pauses and awkward pitched tones. And he's as much a national pastime in journalism as baseball is to sports. So what separates the men from the boys? Are there super skills necessary for effective delivery in the radio medium or that increase your segment's salability? For starters, there are some basic pointers to remember. This section covers the bare essentials, although fine-tuning even these characteristics does not guarantee perfection or an instant radio winner.

CLARITY OF VOICE

Talk Slowly, Casually, and in Simple Words

Radio conveys only one of your features across the airwaves: Your voice. Deep, loud voices suggest anger and rigid authority. Light, soft voices are passive and lack integrity and credibility. Forced "DJ" voices create a facade, picked up instantly by all listeners. But voices that sound casual, relaxed, humble, and gentle draw listener support and an earful of interest. Voice inflexion further adds youth and energy to words, casting an image of the speaker as knowledgeable, fun, and exciting.

Word choice equally affects impact. Be sure your vocabulary is middle school to high school level; words are one to two syllables, in simple sentences, and used with many idioms or "expressions of speech." For instance, rather than say, "kids do appropriate behavior," say instead "when the kids are angels." Rather than say "parents have low frustration tolerance," say instead "parents lose their cool (or composure)." Turn technical or complex phrases into simple one- to two-word descriptions using speech colloquialisms or patterns found within the listening audience.

Learn the Audience

When preparing tapes or doing out-of-state or national radio shows, take a moment to consider the listeners. Shows aired in Manhattan are very different from shows aired in Birmingham, Alabama. In Sioux Falls, South Dakota, AM and FM stations are more conservative, entertainment-oriented, without slapstick and crude comedy. Using idioms and slang on, say, KELO-Radio, probably would backfire and turn the audience against you. Get a feel for the people–the *demography*–first before launching into a set radio routine. Rehearsed routines that played well in Minneapolis, Cleveland, Chicago, even Dallas, may fare poorly for nonmetropolitan cities. The best way of sampling listeners is to ask the producer who comprises their top-rated audience groups–kids, younger adults, older adults, employed, unemployed people? Where, generally, do they listen to the shows–in the car, at work, at home, or on the farm?

MAKE INTERVIEWER LOOK GOOD

The general rule in radio is the same as in TV: You are a privileged guest in another person's home. When interviewed, be polite, receptive, and diplomatic. Casual replies under pressure sustain your credibility, dignity, and maintain rapport with the host. In talk shows by telephone, you neither can see the host, nor his cue cards, nor any other feedback that typically guides your performance on TV (e.g., stage manager's directions, TelePrompter, television screens). Robbed of all cues, you must improvise your lines following the interviewer's lead, no matter what direction he or she goes in.

Interviewers look at your material ahead of time, may even read your interview questions as back-up, but expect impromptu. Expect unscripted questions literally pulled from thin air or from a call-in question. Suppose you're talking about when "your lover hates your children." An interviewer says, "That reminds me of my old girlfriend's hang-up with aggressive men. What do you think about women who hate men?" *Oh my God! That has nothing to do with my product or expertise; I haven't the foggiest idea how to answer that.* Wrong. You'll have an answer. Even if it takes you a second longer to reply, come up with an answer that ties the topic back together.

Agree and Keep It Flowing

Never debate or stop the discussion because of feeling criticized, insulted, or confused. Just keep the words rolling, and repeat key phrases or ideas you believe are generic and safe. Shift back to relevant issues by saying, "That may be true in that case, but. . . . " There is no shame in admitting the interviewer or other guests are partially correct, even if you believe they are dead wrong. *Agree only as a transition to return to your own product promotion.*

Never Take It Personally

Forensic psychologists learn never to take personally the prosecutor's cross examination. The same is true for media experts. You must never take personally the interviewer's criticism, conflicts, or insulting comments perceived to undermine your integrity. Hosts may raise the roof during interviews for entertainment effect, to build up listener participation with call-ins, or to augment their own celebrity image. *People are not interviewing you, personalities are.* Be especially ready for the unknown during a ratings week. During off-weeks, hosts still have a stake in maintaining their "personality" and will use you as bait, if necessary, to reinforce their audience image. Bite the bait but never feel exploited; you still can communicate your message in a calm, civil manner and enhance your product image at the same time.

For instance, one interviewer talking about bribes and rewards said, "Hey I bribe my dog to do things like that–do you mean people are really pets?" *Now, stop for a moment; forget feeling trapped, misunderstood, and defensive.* Say this instead: "It seems like that, doesn't it? But that's because people and pets learn the same way. Rewards get pets to do things, and people learn faster with incentives."

You see, you just turned the tables around, regained your composure, and came out smelling like a rose.

Use Person's Name and Express Gratitude

Show respect to the host by frequently saying his or her name before answering a question. "Well, Bob, you're absolutely right." On TV game shows you'll notice contestants chatting with the host as if they are best friends. They speak to each other on a first-name basis, shake hands, even kid around about personal topics. This is deliberate. The producer made a very strong effort to assure contestants talk this way and create the impression for home viewers that the host is personable, and the show is perfect for family entertainment. Make your show perfect for family entertainment by treating the host as your best buddy and making listeners feel you're right at home with them. This makes listeners like you, trust you, and *believe in your product.*

PART III.
BECOMING A BEST-SELLING AUTHOR:
THE PRINT MEDIA

You've heard of "writing phobias." For mental health workers there's a worse writing fear; it's called *I hate paperwork.* Years of ulcer-producing term papers, masters' theses, and doctoral dissertations were bad enough. You burned the late-night oil churning out paper after paper, recycling old ideas into new words, hoping the teachers never caught on. Then graduation came and you were free of the paper mill. Thank God. But a cruel joke happened; the writing panic returned. Endless clinical notes, state and federal forms, release forms, medical forms, social histories, and reports, reports, and more reports consumed your life. You were buried in paperwork hell. No escape this time; now you were doomed for eternity.

So, why in the world would you want to do *more writing?* It's simple. You're trained to write. Part of graduate school slavery was the merciless task to write *on command.* You wrote *when* you didn't want to write and *what* you didn't want to write. You just *had to write it.* And for what? For one reason: to make writing easier. Words flow easily because you know how to construct sentences, paragraphs, and many, many pages of text. It's not a big deal. Nobody says you love it; it's just not a big deal. So, imagine making a big deal out of a skill that will always stay with you such as riding a bicycle. Imagine doing something with your *writing skills.*

The benefits of writing and using print media for product exposure are numerous. Printed pages can be read, and reread. They can be saved, consulted later, and picked up by other writers who cite your terrific ideas. Print media reaches far more people than television and radio and is a cheaper and simpler process to get started.

Self-promotion depends on using every medium within your grasp, and overusing any medium you're comfortable with. For most providers, that means the print media.

Chapters 7 through 10 walk through different ways print media can accelerate your expertise and produce sales in clinical and media circles. Books, newsletters, newspaper articles, and computer media all are for the lay reader, not the academic reader. Many of you already are avid editors and authors of articles, professional handbooks, and treatment casebooks. Much talent goes into compiling these works, from recruiting and coordinating contributors and writing and rewriting the chapters, to perfecting indexes according to a publisher's specs. It's a very time-consuming process and usually pays a poor dividend. It's even harder if you're solo author. But that's not the type of writing you need to promote your product and expertise. So, if you haven't written articles and books, you may be better prepared for this chapter.

Chapter 7

Writing Your Ideas for Local Circulation: Newspapers, Newsletters, and Handouts

Writing is never as difficult as knowing what to write about. Ideas can be original or in response to newspaper articles. Routes to boost your product and expertise are infinite and all depend on your preferred range of exposure. Larger exposure comes from circulated metropolitan newspapers, some only citywide and others covering the entire state, even sold in other states (e.g., *The New York Times, Chicago Tribune,* etc.) Less circulated papers are shopping guides that serve local interest. Shopping guides or "shoppers" are great for product promotion because 90 percent of the paper is merchandise ads (furniture, books, farm equipment, used cars, etc.) and 10 percent is regular columns on local events. Shoppers also reach a larger readership since they are free; homeowners usually receive one or multiple complimentary copies every week.

Shopper and newspapers are for mass appeal. But that may not be your market. Perhaps you have a product or expertise benefitting only a limited or specialized group of people, such as your former, current, or prospective clients. In-house newsletters and handouts are your best bet. Three- to six-page newsletters can describe self-help insights and your new office resources (e.g., 1-800 number, computer testing, information clearinghouse, support group meetings, etc.) Handouts are also for tailor-made readers. These are shorter versions of methods, techniques, and services provided not only to readers in your lobby but also for the lobbies of allied health professionals (physicians, dentists, nutritionists, hospitals) willing to display your materials.

NEWSPAPER SUBMISSIONS

Writing copy for a newspaper is a tricky business. If at first you don't succeed, *don't try, try again.* Find out why you don't succeed by contacting the department head or regular columnists who may offer pointers on rewriting the article. Articles must be brief, have a catchy theme, and swiftly flow across the page like water. Ellyce Field, columnist on weekly family events for the *Detroit News,* writes the way she talks–a conversational flow of small words, short sentences, and expressions making you feel like you're saying and doing the activities with her. You see what she sees, hear what she hears, and smell what she smells. You're there *with her.* That's a perfect impact. Draw the readers into your opinions by vicariously tapping their sensitive experiences and desperate needs. Style-wise, this is very different from objective, journalistic news reporting that spits out facts. Stick with a personable style that every reader can relate to. Let readers *identify.* Seeing it through your senses is merchandising at its best. Remember, like TV and radio, your primary goal is to sell the product by selling yourself.

Contact Section Editor and Propose a Topic

Begin by sending an inquiry to the section editor. Your pitch should propose a single piece or series of consumer pieces locking in on newsworthy events, controversies, and celebrities. Stay current. News on Chappaquiddick is old, for example, even if Senator Kennedy again hits the front page. Whereas, Bosnia is today. From the pitch explain your expertise and product, and why *you can help the public.* Always describe how your proposal is compatible to other regular features. Choose topics that follow the same principle of popular appeal: greed, vanity, success, and power. Enclose along with the inquiry two additional items. First, a picture of yourself. Second, a sample double-spaced page article (two pages). Proposals alone are too hollow unless you offer solid proof. Your picture should be a professional portrait, an 8" x 10" glossy or smaller. Editors want to know *who this person is and what you look like.* Pictures later can be shrunk down and placed alongside your signed column. The sample article is your greatest pitch (see Figure 7.1). Editors *will read it.* After two weeks, follow up with a telephone

FIGURE 7.1. Sample article for submission to newspaper

Self-Help Groups: Do They Really Work?

An interesting phenomenon of the past few decades is the increase in peer self-help groups–that is, groups of people who share a special problem and meet to discuss that problem with or without mental health professionals. Take Alcoholics Anonymous (AA). When AA was founded in the 1930s, people were skeptical about whether they could obtain from one another as much help as they could obtain from experts.

Today AA is much more widely accepted and there are now self-help groups for hundreds of different kinds of problems: groups for dieters, stutterers, drug addicts, dialysis patients, cancer patients, families of cancer patients, single parents, parents of the closed-head injured, and so forth.

More than anything else these are "social-support groups." In some groups like Weight Watchers, that social support combines with other techniques to help members overcome a specific behavioral problem. In others, social support is itself the primary goal, giving members the opportunity to air their problems. A group of mastectomy patients, for example, may discuss everything from problems of buying clothes to postoperative sexual inhibitions to fear of death. The group may not actually "solve" these problems for any individual member, but it can offer encouragement, a sympathetic ear, and the knowledge that she is not alone.

For most anyone with a serious problem, such support may be very helpful. But for those without other sources of social support, it can be absolutely crucial.

In both kinds of groups, the goal-directed type and the pure emotional support type, the assumption is that no one can help you or understand you better than someone who has been through what you have been through. This assumption may be correct to some degree, but not in all cases. Male gynecologists and pediatricians advising on post-partum depression, for example, of course never experience labor and delivery. But they are certainly skillful in this matter.

Another assumption is success rate. Do self-help groups bring about therapeutic gains as great as those of mental health services? I admit, it is hard to tell, since the anonymous membership prevents clear and valid evaluation. Nevertheless, self-help groups are undoubtedly the best alternative to the therapy marketplace, and they probably reach many people who would not otherwise seek professional help.

call and request an opportunity to meet personally with the editor, columnist, or person in charge.

Local vs. Metropolitan Newspapers and Magazines

What is the paper you read every morning with coffee? Maybe you only get it on Sundays. Or, how about that glossy local magazine–the one you never get to read in your lobby? Believe me, your office is a receptacle tank for each type of print media. In every city, town, and province there are daily or weekly local papers featuring two to three sections on national news, local and community news, business, and sports. Community-supported magazines cover the same topics on a monthly or quarterly basis, plus highlight prominent figures or businesses in town. Somewhere in those sections lies your treasure chest for widespread product exposure.

In smaller papers (one section), condensed sections abbreviate the national news and leave more space for community events. Smaller papers have smaller staff–less reporters, editors, and columnists. Circulation is smaller and so is frequency of publication; most papers publish once weekly. This type of paper is the best place to start. Figure 7.2, for instance, was a regular column appearing in *City Scene,* a Battle Creek (Michigan) freebie available in most offices, restaurants, and stores. *City Scene* is a typical, moderately urban city paper covering civic and community events, culture and the arts and entertainment, business, personal profiles, and hot shopping spots. Reader interest is stronger and develops into a faithful following on current trends or shake-ups affecting local life.

By contrast, regular columns in monthly periodicals take longer to pique reader attention and delays between publication lose precious dateline information. That's why magazine columns should be generic with nondated materials that editors can use or shelve until space is available (see Figure 7.3). On the positive side, invited or regular columns are longer, printed pages are glamorously more attractive than newspaper, and copies have a longer shelf life; you'll find one to two months of back copies in every doctor's lobby.

Larger circulated papers with several editorial departments and reporters equally share interest in new material but there are miserable obstacles encountered before you talk to the right people. Editors are under deadlines, reporters and regular columnists are out

FIGURE 7.2. Weekly column in local newspaper. *(City Scene*, 1985, Vol. 3, No. 4, p. 12. Reprinted with permission.)

Self Help

Self-Esteem

by Douglas H. Ruben, Director of Substance Abuse Services Mental Health Professional Associates

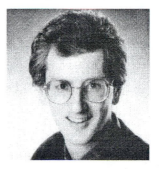

Some say that no psychological need is more fundamental than the need for self-esteem. People who exist in the state of self-distrust and guilt are badly crippled in facing the challenges of life. A healthy self-trust, self-reliance, and self-respect is the necessary foundation for a well-actualized and fulfilling life. Authentic self-esteem has nothing to do with boasting or bragging, or being pushy or arrogant; in fact, such behaviors generally reflect some lack of self-esteem.

What is the important message here? Is it that self-esteem is essential for survival? No. How about, self-esteem is essential for something. But what is that something? A better commitment to life? To have a good feeling about ourselves? No, none of these will do. These reasons are too general to mean anything. The virtues of self-esteem are also like the virtues of happiness–unless they refer to specific things, nobody can really achieve them in any realistic way.

Being specific about self-esteem gets to the heart of what people say or do when interacting with others every day. "Esteem" is the pride we feel after fulfilling personal social needs. But when needs are unfulfilled it doesn't mean we lack "esteem." It simply means our abilities to communicate the needs and change people's behavior are weak. Correcting these abilities is a matter of learning better assertive social skills, which is different from thinking we need a new personality.

To put us in contact with our highest possibilities, we must first recognize what we can and cannot do. Through strengthening weak behaviors, that sense of pride or esteem becomes highly visable in our behavior.

and about, and those minding the office *can't make the decision for you.* It sounds defeating. But there are ways around red tape roadblocks. First, contact a columnist doing a series on your expertise or close-to expertise, offering research and writing assistance. You will instantly become the godfather of his or her next child.

FIGURE 7.3. Invited column in monthly community magazine. (*Active* magazine, 1985, Vol. 2, No. 3, p. 15. Reprinted with permission.)

HEALTH by Douglas H. Ruben, Program Director, Substance Abuse Services, Mental Health Professional Associates

Mother, Mistress, or Manager? Roles of Women in Business

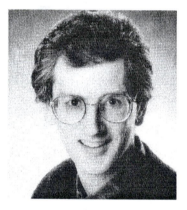

Mother, mistress or manager? Which one is she? Hired by the organization as manager, she regards herself as a manager. She sees herself as a manager, *first*, and a woman *second*. Her role as manager is defined by the managerial positions she holds. Or so she thinks.

Unfortunately, her employees fail to perceive her as she sees herself! They view her–not as a manager–but as a *woman*. Their feelings about her as a woman affect their willingness, or lack of it, to cooperate with her as

their manager. She might wonder why this is so. And this is where her problem begins.

Her ability to manage is threatened by the employees' perception of her as a woman first–stereotyped identities create this bias. Women in management-levels face this grueling reality that people see and think of her either as a mother, mistress or manager.

Take the mother-image. Employees respond to her as they would to their own mothers. Age differences are irrelevant. Whether they are older or younger than she is, she is still their mother. They seek advice from her about their personal lives and confide in her about their hopes and dreams for the future. When they are upset, they turn to her for comfort. When she gives advice they dislike, they rebel against her childishly.

Of course, as their manager, she is puzzled by this reaction. She doesn't understand their wounded pride or hurt feelings. She thinks they take her advice "too seriously" or "personalize" it. She believes that as their manager, she can dispense advice and they will grasp the logic of it.

She is also seen as the "mistress." Many men in the organization identify with her in this role. Not a real mistress, of course, but a mistress in their minds or "mental mistress."

Their interactions with her hint toward sexuality. While it is easier for her to ignore the "come-ons," she runs a terrible risk in doing so. Men may continue making innuendoes to her and chuckle over their cleverness to expose her "real nature." But she ignores it because she is a manager—she thinks it will pass in time. But it never does. This is because innuendoes draw tremendous social attention and are reinforcing to all who hear them. What's worse, a woman manager may accidentally encourage this behavior through her smiles, and "play-along-with-it" attitude.

Some women managers discover it is easier to relate to men in a sexual way. This is not to say they have romantic relationships. Rather, they simply couch their requests in a "cute" or "seductive" way. Of course, such women will deny their intentions are provocative and that nothing they say or do is openly sexual.

Denial by women managers can take the opposite extreme, too. Here they are regarded as being "cold." They may not realize it, but employees start remarking about this disposition. They explain her coldness or austerity in terms of sexual deprivation, not once attributing her business actions to a managerial role.

Realizing that others view her in the roles of mother or mistress enables her to face this issue. She must realize that her efforts to manage, to gain respect and control are all affected by how others perceive and react to her. One solution, some women feel, is by holding weekly staff meetings for better and more open communication. But rarely, if ever, will biased perceptions be the topic of discussion.

And so, where does she turn? How can the woman manager recognize when this problem exists and how to solve it? Strategies that stimulate behavior-change in people are the most direct route, but only after she learns how to catch the situation when it happens. Consider the context of the employees' behavior. Getting the facts straight in the early stages can save time and trouble. Here's how to do it.

Strategy 1: Observe who says or does something. Observe to whom they say or do something. Cues for this observation are in statements and gestures. What do the facial expressions or gestures indicate? What happened moments before these statements and gestures?

Strategy 2: What action or behavior is occurring when this problem occurs?

Strategy 3: What follows this behavior? In other words, is there some pattern to things that happen immediately after the woman manager's behavior?

Take Carolyn, manager of a new retail store who was invited repeatedly by the company's vice president to meet after hours to discuss "business." Her refusals launched a series of embarrassing insults and ruined her career at the store. In looking back at which events took place, she realized that her own actions played as much a role in sustaining her appearance as "mistress" as the vice president's. Rather than taking blame for her "poor management skills," she discovered that managing was not the issue. The real concrete issue was to identify and change how this vice president and other employees perceived her and her actions. (Excerpts from a book in preparation, *Mother, Mistress, or Manager: Overcoming Mistaken Identities of Women in Business,* by M. J. Ruben & D. H. Ruben.)

Second, run an ad regarding your product or expertise for a limited time. As a paying client, you now have the unusual privilege of reciprocity.

Many newspapers and magazines acknowledge your patronage by running an article about you, your business, product, and expertise. Of course, you may have to remind them of this "good faith" gesture. Use this publicity route to launch your own column ideas. "Paying for a break" is not always the best inroad to guest writing, especially if your budget is tight and past advertising efforts proved futile. Prioritize your costs by asking if paid advertising will earn you a signed byline, generate lucrative product sales, and stimulate client referrals that will recover the initial investment. On the belief it will, go for it.

Shopping Guides

Never underestimate the shopping guide. This advertising tradition is a mecca for expansive publicity. Shoppers deliver from 100,000 to 500,000 homes in your residential area and always stimulate bargain hunters. Why do you think grocery stores pay large bucks to run full-page ads in shoppers over regular newspapers? *It's the impact on impulsive buyers.* Shopper readers flip through household items, recreational vehicles, building and home improvement, real estate, and cars searching for fabulous coupon-cheap discounts. That means they usually *skim* the paper rather than make a serious study of it. Scattered above and between paid ads are self-help columns written by specialists, doctors, and politicians. *You can be one of those specialists* (see Figure 7.4).

Writing for "shopper mentality" does not mean that you should undercut the integrity. It means keep the article easy to read and the advice easy to follow. Use eye-catching phrases, cliches, and capitalize words to add emphasis. Follow the stylistic guideline of telling the reader *who, what, when, and where* about the product. For example, "Dr. Smith has a parenting book immediately available at your local bookstores." Drive the impulsive buyer into temptation by using "contrasts," "testimonials," and discounts. Contrasts first describe awful problems, followed by how the product cures them. Testimonials, you recall, are case examples validating your product. Say, for instance, that "Ms. Jones of Charlotte,

FIGURE 7.4. Bi-weekly column in a community shopper. (*Shopper*, Thursday, February 7, 1985, p. 43. Reprinted with permission.)

Health Services in Town
By Douglas H. Ruben
Mental Health Professional Associates

Health Services in Town is a new bi-weekly column offered in the Shopper News. It is being submitted by Douglas H. Ruben, a psychologist with Mental Health Professional Associates.

"Seniors and Medication"
by Douglas H. Ruben

"My mother is over 60 and forgetting to take her daily medications. Will this be a problem?"

Indeed, it will. Persons 60 years and over who have trouble managing their prescribed medications are prone to overuse, underuse, and "erratic" use of pills. Taken incorrectly, medicines can cause sudden physical symptoms and possibly reverse the positive effects of the drug's proper use. Such medication errors do not mean the person is "sick," or has a "drug problem,"

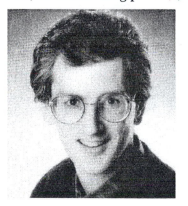

but rather that adherence to the doctor's prescription is poor.

Many agencies in town specializing in substance abuse or gerontology now provide training for seniors to manage their medicines better. Services to Seniors (Volunteer Center) is an information and referral source for helping programs, plus it provides case managers for transportation and in-home care. Call Someone Concerned in Adrian sponsors a senior citizen substance abuse program for groups and is educational. Treatment specialists for elderly and medication problems include the ELDERMED program at Mental Health Professional Associates, and services at Nine-Hundred Myrtle Recovery House in Sturgis. ELDER-MED provides individual and group therapy, consulting, and inservice training for hospital and direct care staff. Myrtle House, largely alcoholism treatment, is participating in the State's medicare-medicaid pilot project for low-cost, inpatient service. Have a question? Call D. H. Ruben, 968-9280.

NC breathes easier every night because 'I know my child behaves better.' " Of course, be sure this is exactly what Ms. Jones of Charlotte, NC said. Testimonials must be unpaid, authentic accounts of product effectiveness. Let the rapid reader also see this product is on sale for a limited time offer until–"noon this Friday." Capitalize on the rush-to-get-it concept that mobilizes buyers to act as if there is no tomorrow. Other tempting bites include 1-800 numbers and purchase incentives, such as "You receive a free 30-minute session with every book purchased."

Deadlines

The trouble with shoppers or newspapers is that copy must be received several days ahead of publication. Deadlines are unchangeable with very few exceptions: *Stop the presses! Hold the front page!* Deadlines for most papers run 24 to 48 hours before press runs for regular weekly columns, but not if the article is for a special series. Editorial review may take longer, or keylining it in different sections of the paper may require more time in the graphics department. With computer desk-top publishing replacing older graphic procedures, preparation time is shorter and under less pressure. Still, once you are a regular contributor, plan on sending your copy by mail, fax, or modem a day in advance of the deadline. Adherence to editorial schedules is professional, and it also builds trust in your ability to *deliver the goods*. This allows printers to reserve a weekly spot on the page knowing you will always come through.

Expect Editing on the Copy

If you thought the reviewer's comments from refereed journals were harsh, beware of the news editor. Mr. Grant in *The Mary Tyler Moore Show* was a bit stereotyped but not entirely off center. Editors have a duty to keep the copy clear, precise, ethical, and informational at the expense of chopping your best quotation or punch line. Brevity demands simple phrases, easily grasped concepts, and consumer opinion or advice that compatibly fits as many readers as possible. Your submitted copy may undergo one or several modifications, including being rejected, before it appears in print. But this is normal and should be regarded as routine.

No Remuneration

Regular self-help columns featuring your latest advice are voluntary contributions in exchange for free publicity. *People now know who you are.* Compensation for this luxury is nearly impossible for three reasons. First, shoppers and smaller papers lack the budget to reimburse freelancers. Second, even papers with freelance budgets reserve funds for established or degreed journalists, hired to report *needed* stories. Third, the paper is *doing you a favor, you're not doing the paper a favor.* Valuable, highly competitive space is earmarked for your weekly input after you solicited it. Papers that instead seek you out for articles or input may, on occasion, offer meager compensation. But even then, I wouldn't count on it.

Exceptions include the larger metropolitan and nationally circulated papers (*USA Today*) that agree to run or reprint your articles at a flat fee. As with radio shows, syndicated agencies exist that package and market your columns and pay royalties on the number of packages sold or number of times weekly the column(s) appear.

NEWSLETTERS

Identify Audience, Length, and Frequency of Circulation

Pros and cons clutter the field with reasons for starting your own newsletter. Advantages are numerous: publicize your clinic and product; draw new business; gain social recognition; and generate paid subscriptions. Marketing books replete with this advice (e.g., Brown & Morley, 1986; Sachs, 1986; Winston, 1985) boast about giant leaps into community awareness and that it polishes your professional image. However, keep in mind the hard-to-swallow disadvantages: high costs; upstaging competitors; outdated mailing lists; limited time for writing; limited circulation; and accountancy system.

The biggest hang-up is time and cost. Creating copy for, say, a four-page newsletter produced monthly or even quarterly involves tiring research and editing efforts. What does the public really want? Why do they want it? Do you have the time to dig up juicy consumer-conscience tidbits, transcribe them for simple reading, and edit them before press time? Is your cash-flow expendable in the neighborhood of $500 to $1,500 start-up and printing costs? The answer is: Yes, if you use the newsletter efficiently as a sales device for product promotion or selling your expertise.

Use Newsletters to Generate Sales Only

Using newsletters to generate clientele really is a waste of time. Office referrals largely rise or fall through word-of-mouth and from established network agreements such as with EAPs (Employee Assistance Programs), HMOs (Health Maintenance Organizations), PPOs (Preferred Providers Organizations), among others. Newsletters instead have a better purpose; they are your door to a mass of consumers needing your expertise or product but who are either unaware of or afraid to obtain more information on it. So, turn your newsletter into a big ad. Design the newsletter as an enlarged advertisement, featuring articles, testimonials, or graphics affirming the benefits and simple utilization of your ideas

For example, Damon's user-friendly newsletter for "mental powers" is a commercial powerhouse (Figures 7.5 to 7.7). His suave picture mesmerizes you underneath the thunderous headlines "Your Mind Is More Powerful Than You Think!" The first two pages highlight symptoms that anybody can experience. He inserts short sales pitches from local experts or excerpted from national experts (citing the reference) on the epidemic proportions of panic. The next two pages combine product description with order information. The last page repeats testimonies of his product, with the ironclad guarantee of a full refund if buyers are unhappy.

In addition, offer a toll-free number to purchase products by credit card, or an order blank to be cut out and sent in. Order blanks vary in size and contents but all contain what the consumer will receive, plus address, phone number, and credit card information if desired. Going the "Damon-way," or fancier depends on your pocketbook. Examples of high-gloss newsletter advertisers currently in public circulation include *The Wall Street Jungle* ($5.00/issue, from Phillips Publishing), *Tax Avoidance Digest* ($4.75/issue, from

FIGURE 7.5. Damon's cover for product-sale newsletter

Your mind is more powerful than you think!

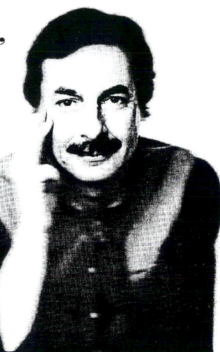

DAMON REINBOLD, renowned expert in "Perception Therapy," will expand your mental powers so that you can reach your greatest potential!!

For fast paced people who know what they want and want it instantly! Perception Therapy is one gigantic step beyond hypnosis.

FIGURE 7.6. Inside description of Damon's newsletter

Approximately 10 percent of the human mind is used consciously and the remaining 90 percent constitutes what we call the subconscious. . .

The subconscious is the most sublime and sophisticated computer in existence and it efficiently carries out whatever it is "programmed" to do! Damon will show you how to take advantage of your own subconscious to turn positive thought into positive action in four dynamic presentations:

Knowledge Is Power–Memory Is the Key
You are What You Think–The Subconscious Computer
The Key to Success–Get What You Want from Others
Miracle of the Mind–Real Magic!

These fascinating presentations are outstanding individually or combined for their motivating and entertaining qualities. When incorporated with sales meetings, trade shows, conventions, staff enrichment seminars, or luncheon meetings, you and your organization will benefit personally and professionally from learning Damon's unique mental tools. Each presentation is independent from the others. To gain the full benefit from any workshop, it is not necessary to take all of them.

Throughout each presentation Damon will prove his command over the subconscious with many astounding and highly entertaining demonstrations:

☐ Damon memorizes a current issue of a popular magazine and dares anyone to call a page number he can't describe!

☐ Damon asks someone to pick an imaginary playing card from an imaginary deck and place it in a real envelope. When the person calls the name of the (freely?) imagined card, Damon draws a real card from the envelope and it is the correct card!

☐ Doodles or drawings made by various persons out of Damon's sight are returned by him to their rightful owners without so much as a question asked by him!

☐ Damon shows 4 envelopes and allows 3 audience members to freely(?) select one for themselves, leaving one for Damon. When they tear open their envelopes, each of the 3 have received a 50¢ off coupon, while Damon's envelope contains a $20 bill!

☐ Damon races a calculator in mentally adding a series of large numbers accurately! All this and much more!

KNOWLEDGE IS POWER–MEMORY IS THE KEY!

Most successful CEOs agree that memory makes money. The more information you command with your memory, the more successful you can be! Damon will show you how to easily enhance your own memory and recall abilities by using simple tricks of "mental shorthand." By the end of this thought-provoking and laughter-filled series of demonstrations, you will be able to instantly recall a long list of items or appointments after quickly reviewing a list one time. You will know how to successfully apply this mental shorthand in other areas of your life.

Can you imagine using just your mind as a daily planner? Would you enjoy making speeches or presentations without referring to notes? Not to mention remembering colleagues' names and companies; recalling quotations, prices, and facts from reports; and easily recalling data from important meetings! Imagine how these skills will benefit you and your organization!

Damon has used his memory-enhancing techniques with witnesses in aiding police department investigations of major crimes and is a qualified expert court witness on the subject of memory and recall.

Everyone has a good memory and Damon proves it. Never again will you say "I forgot" when you don't want to!

FIGURE 7.7. Testimonials from Damon's newsletter

Who IS Damon?

Damon Reinbold's expertise lies in understanding and maximizing the use of the subconscious mind. He is considered one of the world's foremost authorities in neuro-linguistics, hypnosis, memory, subliminals, and motivation. Over the past two decades Damon has spoken to and entertained literally millions of people.

Damon's unusual demonstrations have been featured on these television programs:

ABC's 20/20	The Tonight Show
A.M. Los Angeles	Merv Griffin Show
Mike Douglas Show	Live with Regis and Kathie Lee
Larry King Show	Sally Jessy Raphael Show
Oprah Winfrey Show	Cable News Network
Dr. Sonya Friedman	Entertainment Tonight

. . . and numerous local and regional shows

> *"Damon is one of the finest hypnotists in the country today."*
> **Regis Philben**, WABC-TV, New York

Damon's skills have been recounted in these publications:

USA Today	Time Magazine
Woman Magazine	US Magazine
Cosmopolitan	Playgirl
National Enquirer	New York Times
New York Newsday	Chicago Tribune
Detroit Free Press	AP News Service
UPI News Service	Gannett
Knight Ridder	Philadelphia Inquirer

. . . and many others

> *"Damon is amazing...interesting!"*
> **Richard Sher**, WOR-TV, New York

For bookings contact:

These movie and television celebrities have sought out and benefited from Damon's unique brand of mind-bending techniques:

Don Johnson	Melanie Griffith
Kathie Lee Gifford	Sally Jessy Raphael
Heidi Bohay	Patti D'Arbanville
Anne Marie Johnson	Jayne Mansfield
Thelma Houston	Debra Shelton

. . . and the list goes on

> *"I liked Damon from the first moment I met him. Most people do. He's one of the most genuine people I know—utterly sincere, completely open, and possessor of a gentle, warm, and spontaneous humor that makes him extremely comfortable to be with."*
> **Jim Cash**, screenwriter of *DickTracy*, *Top Gun*, etc.

Among the many corporations that have utilized Damon's services are:

General Dynamics	Rockwell International
IBM	Northwest Airlines
General Motors	Southland Corporation
Chevron Chemical	Gulf Oil Company
Continental Airlines	Owens Corning Fiberglass
Scott Paper Company	

> *"Thank you for making our Human Resources meeting a great success!"*
> **Jim Notarnicola**, Human Resources Manager
> 7-Eleven Food Stores, The Southland Corporation

Damon belongs to numerous societies involved with neuro-linguistics, hypnosis, memory, subliminals, and motivation. He is past president and a founding member of the Michigan Society for Investigative and Forensic Hypnosis and a member of the elite International Platform Association which was founded by Thomas Jefferson. Damon was educated at Marquette University and before that he had studied for the priesthood at St. Francis Seminary in Milwaukee, WI.

Baltimore, MD), and *The Doctor's Office* ($96/yr., from Wentworth Publishing Company). But don't despair. Glitz doesn't sell the product. *You do.* Shiny or plain paper–it doesn't ultimately matter as long as the written copy propels your product or expertise with compelling force.

Desk-Top Publishing

Style dimensions vary considerably and the best route for creatively choosing your dimension is with desk-top publishing software. True, not all mental health providers have computers and so the luxury of self-producing newsletters may be limited or depend on using a cheap printing house. However, users of print media are finding that inexpensive computers networked with laser printers produce quality outputs that save printing costs and preserve originality. Tandy, Omega, IBM-compatibles, and Apple–all are aggressively lowering costs on new machines for faster availability. Apple Macintosh computers lately announced reduced prices for new portables and large-size multi-megabite hard drive units that used to cost in the upper thousands; now prices are hitting below the thousand mark. Affordable computers means more access to desk-top software that allows you to manipulate graphics and text without hours of manual pasting, drafting, and editing.

Among the most powerful desk-top-publishing software for newsletters are *PageMaker, Ventura, ReadySetGo!,* and *X-Press.* Newsletters formatted on these software programs are identical to work done at a printer, from the types of letters (fonts) and color used, to placement of art and graphs. So, if you haven't joined the computer revolution yet, spend your next lunch hour at a local Apple or IBM retail store and see why many people stay in during their lunch hour to work on computers. I promise, you won't become a cyberpunk!

Specifics of Layout

Layout design follows some protocols. For advertising products, follow the structure described above when generating sales only. Newsletters intended only to inform the public have greater latitude. The *Health Letter* (Public Citizen Health Research Center) and *MHPA DIGEST* are good examples (see Figure 7.8). On the first page under the Mass Head is the headline followed by the lead story. Lead stories must get readers to "bite the bait" by impulsively drawing their attention. An hysterically funny or unrealistically inflated heading–"Man discovers body inside of him through therapy!"–is overdoing a good thing and is best left for tabloid shoppers. Still, catchy titles, clever word uses, and hard-hitting facts about daily problems are eye-catchers and may prevent readers from tossing your newsletter into file 13. "How to deal with mean neighbors," for example, pinches the sensitive nerves of most frustrated urbanites. Just as "How to talk to your teenager" pitches to "tough love" parents bewildered by their hormone-bouncing adolescent. Snappy titles generate first impressions long enough to have the first paragraph read. After that, readers may lose interest.

Captivating writing is one way of sustaining interest. But newsletter experts rely more heavily on graphic integration than on pros. Next to the opening article place a humorous picture or artwork. Comical enhancers entertain readers and give depth and variation to format. Line art used throughout the newsletter underscores key points and enlivens your ideas for faster reading and comprehension. Original artwork is especially tasteful but greatly time-consuming and requires advanced preparation. A better choice is "clip art" that covers many themes and is sold separately on diskettes and CDs. Clip art is available for medical, psychological, and business themes, for adults, children and elderly, and for specialty needs such as arrows and other symbols. A third resource is pictures from either books in the public domain (over 75 years old) or printed clip art designed for public consumption. Books published in mid- to late-1900's featured beautiful color plates that are duplicable using today's modern scanners. Likewise, Dover publishing house, among others, sells books entirely of clip art on different topics. To scan pictures, first find out who has a rentable or usable scanner. Convert the scanned file into a "TIFF," "PICT," or equivalent file name. This allows it to be imported or transferred into your desk-top publishing program.

FIGURE 7.8. Informational newsletter

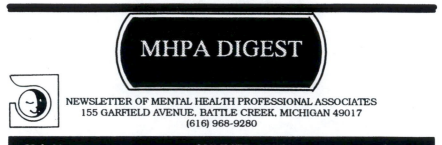

MHPA DIGEST

NEWSLETTER OF MENTAL HEALTH PROFESSIONAL ASSOCIATES
155 GARFIELD AVENUE, BATTLE CREEK, MICHIGAN 49017
(616) 968-9280

Vol. No. 2   **SUMMER 1985**

ELDERLY ALCOHOLICS: A SPECIAL PROBLEM

–Douglas H. Ruben

OLD alcoholics never reform: they just fade away. . . .there is no such thing as an old alcoholic; alcohol takes care of that. . . .old people don't develop an interest in alcohol, if anything they lose it along with their ability to metabolize it.

These are a few of the damaging misconceptions about alcoholism among older people that have prevented professionals from dealing with it, even when identified. Elderly alcoholics may be somebody's grandmother or grandfather. They are often ignored by the outside world and free to drink to excess and take too many pain pills. They are able to often conceal their alcoholic condition behind an array of other ailments of old age. But the facts are clear–some 90,000 alcoholics in Michigan are elderly.

But the facts are clear–some 90,000 alcoholics in Michigan are elderly.

Some of them have newly come to the condition–through a process of personal loss and grief; loss of job, loss of social status, loss of financial security, loss of spouse and friends, and, that final indignity, loss of physical powers. According to a recent national survey, at least 15% of elderly alcoholics develop their condition after retirement.

Common signs attributed to aging can actually be indicative of problem drinking.

For example, brain damage, heart disease, and gastrointestinal disorders that frequently result from problem drinking are also characteristics of old age. Such changes as depression, memory loss, mood changes, dramatic changes in employment, and economic or marital status are also included. Therefore, problem drinking in the elderly is not always a clear diagnosis.

Another problem for the elderly is their decreased tolerance for alcohol. This results from the natural slowing down of the metabolic process.

Another problem for the elderly is their decreased tolerance for alcohol. This results from the natural slowing down of the metabolic process. Even though senior citizens drink less than younger individuals, they often experience increased effects of alcohol. These include:

(1)   Drinks to the point of psychological and psychomotor impairment at least once a week;

(2)   Stays intoxicated for several days at a time, at least once a year; stays intoxicated for over 24 hours at least twice a year;

(3)   Exhibits symptoms of psychological withdrawal when alcohol is removed or is unable to consistently control time and extent of drinking.

COMMUNITY CORNER
Building Ties: Something New

SINCE 1979, the Office of Services to Aging (OSA) and Department of Mental Health (DMH) have worked cooperatively to address the mental health needs of older adults. Now this endeavor is possible with the assistance of an Administration on Aging Demonstration Grant in FY '79. Under this grant, the "Building Ties" Project developed and evaluated materials and techniques to promote effective local level interagency cooperation between mental health and aging in Calhoun County. In addition to Mental Health Board staff, committee members also include Volunteer Bureau, Calhoun County Medical Care Facility, County Commissioners, Community Action Agency, Visiting Nurses Services, Department of Social Services, Mental Health Professionals Associates (substance abuse), Leila Hospital, First Christian Church, Battle Creek Housing Commission, and consumers.

The committee task force already has identified the major need as establishing or enhancing outpatient/outreach diagnosis and treatment in the following areas: the bad image of "seeking help," medication misuse and abuse, and service delivery programming. At present the task force will consider a new outreach-elderly program under Community Mental Health. Further recommendations look toward expansion of existing services. Suggestions and consumer input are welcomed and should be directed to Sandra Withers, Chairperson of Building Ties (962-7523)

Circulation

Just exactly who will receive your newsletter? There are several points to consider. First, who needs your product or expertise? Second, what mailing lists are cheaply or immediately available? Third, how many newsletters do you send out? First, decide on the consumer groups: Parents, grandparents, students, teenagers, youngsters, or professionals–educators, physicians, lawyers, or mental health providers? Who can either directly purchase your product or expertise or rapidly generate referral leads for you? Second, think what's available in-house. Your immediate mailing list is your previous and current client caseload. Relatively reliable addresses are at your disposal and generally will produce a fair market return since clients *know you or trust your correspondence.*

Third, mailers to other consumer groups can be a headache or a simple process depending on your budget and creativity. It involves first tracking down the addresses; you can rent or buy them. Many direct marketers rent and sell bulk mailing labels sorted by demography, profession, or other choice characteristics. Mailing labels are also obtainable from your local county and township office. For a moderate fee, clerks can generate lists of apartment tenants or single-family dwelling homes on adhesive labels, on diskette, or on hard copy. Still another inexpensive system of list collection is lifting the newly announced businesses and their addresses published regularly during the week in your local newspaper under the headings of "NEW DBA's and CORPORATIONS."

Be creative on tracking down viable mailing lists but always check if the lists are *confidential.* Unauthorized lists protect personal, financial, or other security information for which there are no releases, and consequently sending mail to people on that list constitutes a federal violation. Examples of confidential lists better left alone include a physician's or psychologist's caseload. But where names are in the public domain, for example, on ballots or in directories, permission for use is implicit.

Buying Mailing Lists

Buying mailing addresses gets very expensive and unreliable. Hundreds of brokers nationwide will compile and sell consumer group addresses for fees ranging from $40 to $500 per 1,000 names. For instance, suppose your target audience was working mothers between ages of 25 and 45. Groups such as Meredith List Marketing will sell you up to 3,500,000 active subscriber addresses of *Ladies' Home Journal* at $60 per thousand. All names are for one-time mail usage and may require minimum orders of 2,000 to 3,000 names; additional usage may be priced separately. Specialty groups may be cheaper, such as Christian parents (e.g., Doug Ross Communications, Inc., SMS Publications, Inc., etc.) and students (e.g., American Student List Company). For assortments, consult the industry giants such as *Dun and Bradstreet's Catalog of Business Mailing Lists and Direct Marketing Services.* Another fabulous resource for starters is the *DM News.* This is the official newspaper of direct marketing that provides priceless, updated stories on postal regulations, new marketing campaigns, agency assignments, new creative approaches to direct marketing, alternative media, and information on mailing lists–where to get them, how to select them and how to use them effectively. Best of all, *DM News* is free if you fill out their small subscriber application form, available by writing to 19 West 21st Street, New York, NY 10010/(212) 741-2095.

Limit Circulation

The last concern is "How many newsletters do you send out?" Not many. Save costs of initial press run by test marketing only 50 to 100 copies in high sales areas within your state. Hitting the national trail early in marketing is wasteful and immeasurable. If inquiries or purchase orders are minimal, you'll be happy the first mailing was a small one. Low returns also signify three things. First, there are defects in the newsletter (writing style, layout, content, order blank). Second, the mailing list is unreliable or outdated. Or, third, the product is a problem: it's too costly, too intangible, or everybody already has one or doesn't need one. For example, diet books are a dime a dozen. Unless your book is unique, cheaper, or beats the competition in some other way, all the glossy hype in the world won't sell it.

HANDOUTS

What about in-house reading material? Plenty of doctor's lobbies supply brochures, pamphlets, or fliers describing the services provided or background on relevant pathology. Many professional organizations (e.g., American Ophthalmological Association, American Dental Association, etc.) print consumer handouts. But independent publishers also get into the act. They discount large quantities of products for lobby reading. Leaders in mental health materials such as scriptographic booklets (Channing L. Bete Co., Inc.), The Economic Press ("Bits & Pieces"), Positive Promotions, Ohio Psychology Publications, among others, sell coffee table readers individualized with your name on them. But don't forget the free resources. National clearinghouses (National Council on Alcoholism, Consumer, etc.) provide materials either free or at rock-bottom prices by writing or telephoning a request. Free quantities are limited to first-time or annual orders but in a small practice that amount may be plenty.

So, why do it yourself when others can do it for you? The reason is simple: you like to write. Nothing beats original material. Desktop published materials tailor-made for your office add marketing savvy to running a business. The same feeling of esteem doubles when colleagues or clients request copies of your handouts for their own office distribution.

What Do Most Clients Need?

This is a good question. Naturally clients want to know *what you do and how you do it.* So, a professionally based brochure briefly describing the tricks of the trade is a good beginning. Little if any research is necessary since you intuitively know this information and can crank it out rapidly. Now turn to your product or expertise. What is your clinical specialty? Do you work with children or adults? Is your expertise in addictive disorders, parent-child problems, anxiety or compulsive disorders? Maybe all of these things? Handouts prepared on these topics will be picked automatically because *that's why clients came to see you in the first place.* You may also give out these items as part of therapy.

Lobby Handouts

Lobby handouts are more narrative, descriptive, and inform consumers on exactly how things work. They may be clinically specific or product specific. Clinically specific handouts tell how to spot and what to do about behavior problems such as tantrums, lying, poor reading, obsessive compulsions, among others (Figure 7.9). Keep the reading level at about the eighth grade, very easy, in simple words, and entertaining. Product specific handouts are advertisements for tapes, books, videos, and related bibliotherapeutic paraphernalia (Figure 7.10).

Therapy Handouts

Course of treatment varies for each professional and his or her orientation. Directed therapy (reality therapy, behavior therapy, etc.), for instance, teaches skill exercises and involves homework

FIGURE 7.9. Lobby handout on reading

LYING !

What to do when children lie . . . .

"Telling the truth is always better than lying." A simple rule to understand. But a hard rule to follow for many children. How come?

Lying delays getting into trouble. It's that simple. He steals a cookie; she hides her mother's keys. Both lie about where the objects disappeared. This is because mom and dad *automatically* get angry when the objects are lost. And then get angry if the kids tell what happened.

What gets "punished" is not the stealing or hiding. Punished is what kids tell you; so they learn to tell you nothing or will make up stories. They're afraid.

FOLLOW THESE STEPS:

1. Never take it personally. Kids lie to avoid, not to get you mad.

2. Praise kids when they answer your questions. First let them learn it is *safe* to talk.

3. Encourage them to talk about something you just did with them. This teaches them to describe things accurately and you can verify it.

For more information or appointment call Dr. Ruben, 517-482-1102

© 1987 Best Impressions

FIGURE 7.10. Lobby handout on ordering reading materials

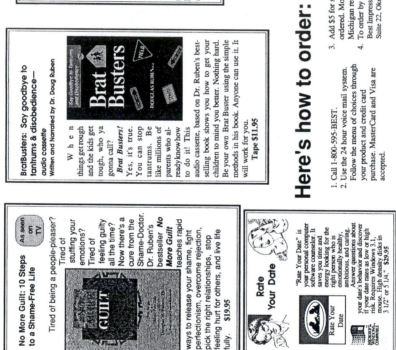

No More Guilt: 10 Steps to a Shame-Free Life   *As seen on TV*

Tired of being a people-pleaser? Tired of stuffing your emotions? Tired of feeling guilty all the time? Now there's a cure from the Shame-Doctor. Dr. Ruben's bestseller *No More Guilt* teaches rapid ways to release your shame, fight perfectionism, overcome rejection, stop feeling hurt for others, and live life fully.   **$19.95**

Rate Your Date

"Rate Your Date" is your personal computer software counselor. It saves you time and energy looking for the right person who is emotionally healthy, ambitious, and caring. Answer questions about your date's behavior and discover if your date rates as low or high risk. Requires Windows 3.1, mouse. High density disks in 3 1/2" or 5 1/4."   **$29.95**

BratBusters: Say goodbye to tantrums & disobedience—
audio cassette
Written and Narrated by Dr. Doug Ruben

When things get rough and the kids get tough, who ya gonna call? *Brat Busters!* Yes, it's true. You can stop tantrums. Be like millions of parents who already know how to do it! This audio cassette, based on Dr. Ruben's best-selling book shows you how to get your children to mind you better. Nothing hard. Be your own Brat Buster using the simple methods in his book. Anyone can use it. It will work for you.   **Tape $11.95**

Get rid of fear
Now and forever!

Douglas H. Ruben, PhD.
AVOIDANCE SYNDROME
Doing things out of fear

Are you afraid of doing things? Is it hard to breathe in crowds or elevators? Do you worry what people think of you? Do you hate conflict? Do you doubt your own abilities? If so, then Avoidance Syndrome is your answer. Dr. Ruben's bestseller tells you what avoidance is and how to conquer it.   **$29.95**

Here's how to order:

1. Call 1-800-595-BEST.
2. Use the 24 hour voice mail system. Follow the menu of choices through your product and credit card purchase. MasterCard and Visa are accepted.
3. Add $5 for shipping and handling for each item ordered. Money back guarantee within 30 days. Michigan residents add sales tax.
4. To order by mail, send check or money order to: Best Impressions International 4211 Okemos Road, Suite 22, Okemos, MI 48864

Call 1-800-595-BEST
Use our 24 hour voice mail system
7 days a week for rapid ordering.

MasterCard

VISA

assignments. Reading books, filling out forms, checklists, and using other self-monitoring devices play a crucial helping role. Lessons of therapy are structured, pragmatic, and immediately targeted for healthy recovery. The materials you hand out can equally impact on healthy recovery.

Handouts are of two types. The first type is interactive. That's when clients use it like a crossword puzzle; questions are answered until the "ah-hah" or gestalt hits them between the eyes. Marital, sexual, and work-related questionnaires accomplish this result (e.g., Figure 7.11). The second type of therapy handout elaborates on skill learning. For example, treating adult children of alcoholics begins with a crystal-clear picture of their patterns of behavior, and why patterns develop. A handout describing these facts is a great reference tool (Figure 7.12). Borrow the same computer template or layout to rapidly format a new tear-sheet on, say, employee job stress (Figure 7.13).

Professional Handouts

The most polished, graphically appealing handouts are those prepared for or distributed to hopeful referral sources. Your cheapest commercial outlet is marketing a product or expertise to buyers who already like you and can put in a good word about your services. If your name in town is popular, use that status for merchandising. First ask, "Who needs help out here *besides regular clients?* Who can benefit from my product or expertise?" How about consumer organizations and businesses? Send fliers or handouts to presidents, executive directors, and human resource offices eager for assistance.

When panic hit corporate America in downsizing trends, outplacement firms popped up overnight offering employment testing, relocation, and job training skills. That's what prompted the author's *Employee Selection Practice* (Figure 7.14). This combined screening and risk management service and was described in a flier and cover letter mailed to over 300 outplacement firms, and companies facing cutbacks and stringent rehiring criteria or showing high turnover. Using a similar template, response was quick to the deluge of elders placed in Adult Foster Care (AFC) homes. Home managers tired of transporting residents hither and thither could now receive on-site services via *Geriatric Services Plus* (Figure 7.15).

FIGURE 7.11. Page 1 of therapy handout questionnaire on dating the right person

Questions To Ask Yourself About a New Woman
(Adapted by DH Ruben, PhD)

Questions

General Rule Not to Repeat Bad Relationships:

If you meet somebody and instantly feel "you've known her all your life or you can't believe how comfortable you are around her" that's a warning sign. It means you're doing things that are too familiar, because you did them before in a bad relationship. Instead, if you feel nervous, intimidated, or even inferior around somebody, thinking she's so much better than you–you probably are on to a good relationship. She's not any better than you are. But her actions are making you do new things you are not familiar with and should learn for a healthy relationship.

1. Can you state particular characteristics of her that you love? (good)
2. Can you give examples of them? (good)
3. How many essential characteristics of your "ideal" woman does she have?
4. Does she accept your right to discuss if you'll use contraceptives? (good)
5. Does she think it's a wife and mother's right to decide whether to work at a paid job? (good)
6. Is she willing to have you spend time alone, even if she'd like to be with you? (good)
7. Is she glad you have other friends? (good)
8. Is she pleased with your accomplishments and ambitions? (good)
9. Does she think women and men have equal potential to be wise, worldly, confident, strong, decisive, and independent? (good)
10. Does she sometimes ask your opinion? (good)
11. Does she both talk and listen? (good)
12. Does she tell you when her feelings are hurt? (very good)
13. Does she think it's okay for women to show they're weak or vulnerable and to cry sometimes–aside from right after she's abused or hurt you? (very good)

FIGURE 7.12. Therapy handout on patterns of adult children of alcoholics

Do These Things Describe You?

1 Trouble Expressing Feelings

5 Fear of Losing Control

2 Can't Seem to Relax

6 Difficulty with Relationships

3 Are Loyal Beyond Reason

7 Fear Being Abandoned

4 Are Overly Responsible

8 Are Overly Self-Critical

Are you afraid you might:

1. Make an error
2. Cause somebody grief
3. Embarrass somebody
4. Look stupid
5. Lose control

Does this fit your parents?

1. Very critical and angry at you
2. Insisted you'd never be anything
3. They fought all the time
4. Real strong parent/real weak parent
5. Blamed you for their mistakes
6. They drank or had bad tempers
7. Ignored your good qualities
8. Refused to hear your reasons
9. Told you not to think you're better than anybody else
10. Told you must please everybody
11. Punished you for being independent
12. Told never to relax–keep busy

When your parents got angry, was that anger-

1. Random-aimed at anybody
2. Arbitrary-never could predict it
3. Continuous-always happened
4. Accompanied by criticism
5. Signalling the worst was yet to come

For more information, contact Dr. Ruben, 1-515-347-0944 or write 4211 Okemos Road, Suite 22, Okemos MI 48864

FIGURE 7.13. Therapy handout on job stress

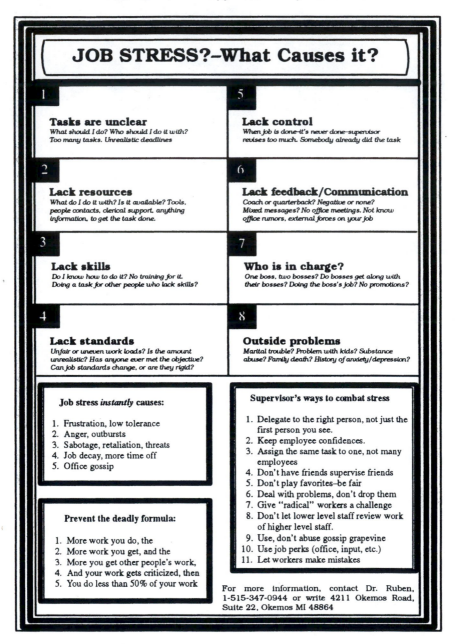

JOB STRESS?–What Causes it?

1

Tasks are unclear
What should I do? Who should I do it with?
Too many tasks. Unrealistic deadlines

5

Lack control
When job is done–it's never done–supervisor
revises too much. Somebody already did the task

2

Lack resources
What do I do it with? Is it available? Tools,
people contacts, clerical support, anything
information, to get the task done.

6

Lack feedback/Communication
Coach or quarterback? Negative or none?
Mixed messages? No office meetings. Not know
office rumors, external forces on your job

3

Lack skills
Do I know how to do it? No training for it.
Doing a task for other people who lack skills?

7

Who is in charge?
One boss, two bosses? Do bosses get along with
their bosses? Doing the boss's job? No promotions?

4

Lack standards
Unfair or uneven work loads? Is the amount
unrealistic? Has anyone ever met the objective?
Can job standards change, or are they rigid?

8

Outside problems
Marital trouble? Problem with kids? Substance
abuse? Family death? History of anxiety/depression?

Job stress *instantly* causes:

1. Frustration, low tolerance
2. Anger, outbursts
3. Sabotage, retaliation, threats
4. Job decay, more time off
5. Office gossip

Supervisor's ways to combat stress

1. Delegate to the right person, not just the first person you see.
2. Keep employee confidences.
3. Assign the same task to one, not many employees
4. Don't have friends supervise friends
5. Don't play favorites–be fair
6. Deal with problems, don't drop them
7. Give "radical" workers a challenge
8. Don't let lower level staff review work of higher level staff.
9. Use, don't abuse gossip grapevine
10. Use job perks (office, input, etc.)
11. Let workers make mistakes

Prevent the deadly formula:

1. More work you do, the
2. More work you get, and the
3. More you get other people's work,
4. And your work gets criticized, then
5. You do less than 50% of your work

For more information, contact Dr. Ruben,
1-515-347-0944 or write 4211 Okemos Road,
Suite 22, Okemos MI 48864

FIGURE 7.14. Flyer on "Employee Selection Practice" sent out to companies

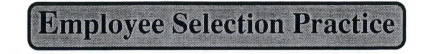

What is Employee Selection Practice-ESP?

Admit it. Hiring new people is a pain. You need them yesterday, not today or tomorrow. They say they can do anything. Okay, you believe them. You have to, you're on a tight schedule. Sure, they have references. You even check them out. Fine, they're hired. But it never fails. Problems pop up every day. They don't show up. They're hung over. Their quality stinks. On top of that, they got an attitude problem. And their temper is wild.

Wouldn't it have been nice to know what they were like ahead of time? Before hiring them?

Employee Selection Practice (ESP) tells you this information within 24 hours. And it's not expensive. Screening the worker for emotional or chemical problems can be an important step in your selection process.

"ESP tells you if the applicant is high, medium or low risk in drug use, temper, following instructions, reliability, and in other things you need to know."

Call today to plan ahead for tomorrow 347-1811

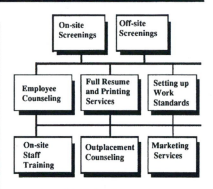

Services of Employee Selection Practice

Call today to plan ahead for tomorrow 347-1811

TWO TYPES of SCREENING	
on-site $50	off-site $25
per applicant	

Service rates set by customary fees but are negotiable.

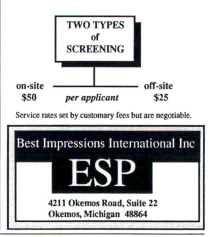

FIGURE 7.15. Flyer on "Geriatric Screening Plus" sent out to AFC homes

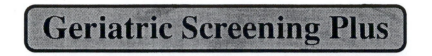

Geriatric Screening Plus

What is Geriatric Screening Plus-GSP?

Geriatric Screening Plus (GSP) is an emergency relief service for mental health problems. Residents showing gradual or rapid shifts in mood, memory, behavior, thought, and personality need quick attention. Something may be wrong with them.

GSP provides **eight (8)** on-site services. They evaluate the resident and tell you the next step you or the family need to take. They help find and contact physicians, arrange for psychiatric hospitals, provide personal therapy, and follow-up with treatment plans.

GSP can also train your staff to handle tougher patients.

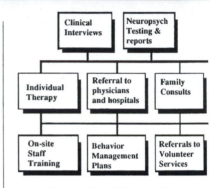

Services of Geriatric Screening Plus

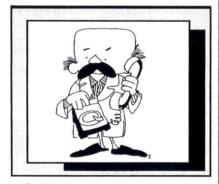

Call today to plan ahead for tomorrow 347-0944

Call today to plan ahead for tomorrow 347-0944

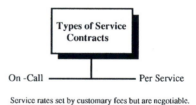

Service rates set by customary fees but are negotiable.

Dr. Douglas Ruben is a family and geriatric specialist.

He is neuropsychologist for the Geriatric Unit at Lansing General Hospital, and consultant to nursing homes and Adult Foster Care. Author of two books on aging.

Chapter 8

Writing Your Ideas for Magazines: From Start to Finish

Are you tired of being your own freelancer for lobby handouts? Yes? Well, it's time to be a bit more daring. Now you're ready to step outside the four corners of your office and see if people beside your clients and close colleagues like your stuff. It's worth doing and here's how to do it. Begin with newspapers. Then go to magazines. Magazines are usually local and national self-help periodicals ranging from health and fitness to good parenting. They are not academic or trade journals and so writing style and submission requirements vary greatly. The only stable requirement is that you *know what you're talking about.* Professional credentials open the editor's door, but your inquiry (pitch) letter and orginal article really close the deal. Many consumer magazines such as *Self, McCall's, Glamour, Cosmopolitan,* and *Psychology Today* assign articles in-house to salaried writers, or accept freelance written articles. Magazines working with first-time or seasoned freelancers may have sliding payment scales depending on manuscript length or column inch. Lengths of 1,000 to 2,000 words may pay as low as $50 and as high as $3,000. Some larger magazines even pay the expense of writers on assignment. So, opportunities for sharpening your public image are endless.

LETTER OF INQUIRY TO MAGAZINE EDITOR

Begin by sending a letter of inquiry that pitches your idea for a short article. Resist the academic temptation to first write the article and circulate it around the city or department for feedback. *If you do this, that step comes later.* Hold off on writing anything until you get the green light from the buyer. Indicate in the pitch what you propose and why you know your subject matter, similar to writing pitches for TV and radio. Address the letter to either the editor in chief or department editor (see Figure 8.1). If you're pushing your product, let the editor know how a product-oriented article directly feeds the subscriber's hunger for solid insight.

REQUEST AND FOLLOW WRITING GUIDELINES

There is no shame in asking for the obvious: writing guidelines. No two consumer periodicals are alike even if they are published by the same company. Standards for writing style, length, choice of topic, and submission vary so widely that the blurb on the editorial page about submissions either is incomplete or outdated. Never trust that guideline alone. Call the publisher ahead of time and request their style sheet. Once received, treat it as you would your first grade teacher. You listen to nearly 90 percent of what it says without praying to it. It's not the Bible, just a guideline. Deviate only marginally, and where you believe your creativity is still compatible with the magazine's theme and yearly direction. However, when it comes to submission, do take the guidelines seriously. If guidelines call for SASE (self-addressed, stamped envelope) to assure return of the manuscript, do it. It looks professional and can be processed through regular channels without exception. It's not as though manuscripts without SASE are refused; they're just confusing. Volumes of over-the-transom (not invited) mail forces company clerks and editors to follow some standard procedures. If your submission out of 200 submissions is wrong, they push it aside until later–much, much later. By age 80 you'll receive your rejection notice.

WHERE TO GET MATERIAL

Okay, you're ready to go for the gusto. So, what should you write about? Look inward to your product and expertise. You sleep, eat,

FIGURE 8.1. Letter to magazine editor pitching an article

BEST IMPRESSIONS INTERNATIONAL INCORPORATED

4211 OKEMOS ROAD, SUITE 22, OKEMOS, MICHIGAN 48864, U.S.A.
PHONE or FAX: 517-347-0944; PHONE 1-800-595-BEST

January 28, 1994

Ms. Lynn Varacalli, Editor
AMERICAN WOMAN
GCR Publishing
34th Floor
1700 Broadway
New York, NY 10019-5905

Dear Ms. Varacalli:

I have enjoyed reading your upbeat and highly informative articles, and frequently will recommend them to my patients. In fact, topics are right up the alley of what I usually write about in my books and articles. Or, when I do talk shows, these are topics I speak on or arrange panels of guests to talk about.

So, I hope you will kindly consider the enclosed article, *How Can You "Rate Your Date?"* for publication in your department of MEN/ SEX & RELATIONSHIPS or in other areas.

I would be happy to speak with you should you have questions on format, length, or regarding other editorial changes.

Please also feel free to fax me for a faster reply.
Looking forward to your thoughts.

Very sincerely,

Douglas H. Ruben, PhD

and talk about that knowlege and thus can represent it the best. But market your material by linking it to important topics in a heavily circulated magazine. In *Expecting,* for instance, much of the articles are health-related–written by nurses, doctors, and infant specialists. A prenatal care product or expertise is right up their alley. In *Christian Parenting Today,* focus is on evangelical Christian family practices, looking for solutions to childrearing issues with a clear biblical basis for advice. A pastoral expertise, even using secular parenting methods, is bound to hook the editor. Another way to get material is by directly asking the magazine editors what they want. This is not an opportunity for you to pitch your ideas, but rather to narrow down your options.

SINGLE VS. MULTIPLE SUBMISSIONS

Trade and academic journals discourage multiple submissions. They feel it undermines the carefully crafted referee process. "Be patient," they say, "the process may take several months," in spite of optimistic claims by editors to accelerate review steps and seek rapid publication of research data. Well, in the pop-magazine industry, you can't wait for a reviewer to rub his beard and say, "No, rewrite the paper and let me see it again." Incentives for writing are financial, not scholastic. You deliberately set out to sell your product and expertise for profit and image expansion. That is why multiple subsmissions are *a must for magazine writing.*

Plan on simultaneously shipping your inquiry letter or manuscript (if already written) to ten or more editors. Initial replies range from one to three weeks, but never exceed one month. Busy as they are, editors know the fierce business side of freelancing, and generally treat cooperative writers with punctual correspondence. When two editors reply favorably for an idea or article, maximize on mileage. Offer one editor your original idea and the other editor a variation of it. Never ignore the other editor. After authoring two or more articles for a magazine, ask the million-dollar question to the editor you worked with: "How about freelance assignments?" You can join their ranks of team players who work on assignment or receive a part-time salary.

Chapter 9

Writing Your Ideas for Self-Help Books: From Start to Finish

Scholarly writing is no more an art than writing self-help books. It starts with a germ, an idea, fermented in the prospectus, and ultimately given birth by interested publishers. Ideas that make it from draft to the finished book, sealed and delivered, go through eons of editorial changes and wind up looking different from the original proposal. Academic publishers are selective, they push brevity, and still expect a comprehensive scope. So, when editing or authoring a technical book on addictive disorders or any psychiatric disorder, remember that persnickety publishers are par for the course. After a while, seasoned authors get into the habit of proposing to publishers what they want and then delivering a solid product as promised.

But when you switch gears and write for self-help markets, suddenly the laws of gravity disappear. Rules of writing no longer apply. Academic precision goes out the window. Third-person, active voice, using "may" instead of "is," and nearly the entire *APA Writing Manual* (whatever edition) is obsolete. That's because there is a trade secret in self-writing implicitly carved into stone: *Anything goes.* There are no hard and fast rules for self-help writing. First person ("I") is okay, but so is third-person ("we"). Metaphors are okay, personal stories are okay, humor is okay. Subjective opinions–the "no-no" of scientific composition–also are okay. *Most everything is okay as long as it moves the text and meaning along to main points.* Self-help readers seek direct, practical, "nuts and bolts" solutions to problems of everyday life. Providing that in clear prose is a challenge and can be the best marketing vehicle for your product or expertise.

GREAT, SO HOW DO I WRITE
FOR THE SELF-HELP MARKET?

Writing for the self-help market naturally is an exciting challenge filled with eagerly awaited rewards. You see your book in paperback, and can find it alongside bestsellers in a national chain bookstore. It adds credibility to your clients, and makes a great coffee table conversation piece. You wrote it–*and it has the potential of being in everybody's household.* Well, sort of. Before your newborn book can really grow to maturity and become a household word, it must pass its own right-of-passage test. Think of it as a book barmitzvah. The test is simple: Your audience has to know what you're talking about.

Easy as that sounds, writing for self-help markets after years of serious scholarly scribing is no cinch. Books with tabloid titles may hook readers into flipping open the cover but once they scan the pages and can't understand one word or stumble over technical language, it's all over. The book is put back on the shelf and *killed.* And in a bookseller's business, dying books do not get a hero's funeral. They are buried fast by returning them to the publisher with a "Dear John" letter attached. Booksellers are not alone in canning self-helpers. Therapist writers also pick and choose the best of the lot among their colleagues' products in trying to sort out recommended books for "bibliotherapy." Dr. Gerald Rosen, for example (1976; Glasgow and Rosen, 1978, 1979) made no bones about rejecting popular titles because they were profoundly boring, confusing, and lacked scientific integrity. By "scientific integrity" he meant the anatomy of the book, no matter how well presented, didn't have a scientific basis.

Rosen's advice sounds like a megaphone–it's loud and clear but many writers just don't listen to it. Preferring their own styles, authors frequently jumble up well-intentioned self-help prose in three ways (e.g., Ruben, 1989). First, they make assumptions about the readers. Second, technical points mistakenly get translated, not explained. Third, design of the self-help book is still too academic for lay readers who want a beach-reading book that takes little effort to get through.

Assumptions About Readers

New converts to self-help writing make the assumption that writers already are familiar with their topics or theoretical orientation and will naturally understand the advice given. Wrong! Start with a *tableau rasa* way of thinking: readers don't know what you're saying or where you're coming from unless you spoon-feed it to them intravenously. That does not mean your audience is ignorant, uneducated, or nonprofessional. Trade book buyers span the knowledge spectrum and writing style.

Technical Points Get Translated, Not Explained

Rewriting technical terminology into conversational speech is like converting Russian word by word into English. It doesn't work. Meanings get lost in the translation since each word does not have a counterpart in another language. Similar confusion arises when academic words scramble for vernacular cousins. For example, advising parents to "reinforce your children for good behavior" seems pedantic; so, authors frequently flip to everyday familiar expressions, such as "reward your children for good behavior." But "reward" is a weak substitute for "reinforcer" and loses precious information about motivating behavior. For example, the statement, "Say or do something your child likes right after he cleans his room and watch how fast he'll listen to you the next time you tell him his room is messy." Now you've described exactly what *reinforcer means in its technical sense without losing your reader's interest.*

Design the Book for Your Audience

Writing style is a matter of taste and habit. Some authors write in the "active voice," flowing their words from phrase to phrase exactly as they speak. Other authors, preferring archaic prose, combine active with passive voice, using many commas (breath marks) and dangling modifiers to stretch the sentence ad infinitum. Scholars who break away from textbook writing are particularly guilty of thinking what was good for one audience will work, with some modification, for another audience. And that's how design problems occur.

For instance, in academia, students get an accelerated learning through programmed instructional texts, now on interactive computer software. They can answer questions and score their answers immediately. This feedback advances their performance, their retention of concepts takes a quantum leap and largely replaces the traditional instructor, proctor or lecturer. Self-instruction books also were tried on a commercial basis, thinking the technology would carry over to mass media. It didn't. They were too dry, too boring, and left on bookseller shelves to rot. Programmed texts bombed, in part, because consumer readers expect stories or anecdotes, look for a personal introspective views of the author, and regard self-help reading as taking an adventurous journey into the unknown, holding the author's hand for security.

If that sounds odd, you haven't heard anything yet. Design of self-help books should follow a theme or metaphor personifying a life-problem into a tangible, visual object able for the reader to hold, look at, and fully appreciate in relation to his or her own life. *Coping with Difficult People,* for example, classically used this gimmick in labeling stubborn or aggressive people with military names and vehicles such as Sherman Tank and Bulldozer. Another example is a Hollywood celebrity actress revealing hidden truths about her disastrous relationships and pointers for healthy romance-building encounters. Readers readily identify with her message, her cyclical emotional plight, or the terms she uses to describe destructive men (e.g., "down-dating losers"). As in Stephen King horrors, readers can vividly picture the people being described by the author within their own workplace or home life. Your book should create a similar virtual reality.

SELECT A POWERFUL TITLE

Even before you write words on paper, come up with a title. *Titles sell, words don't.* But so does the author's popularity. If you are not today's toast of Manhattan, titles *must* sell your book. Ideas set the title in motion. For example, suppose you want a book on shame and feeling bad. Over the years you notice clients complaining of guilt, anxiety, and humiliation they cannot shake no matter how perfect they make their world. So, you think: "That would make a great book!" Fine, now what do you call it? Multimillion copies of shame-type books already exist. *The Shame Within, Healing the Shame that Binds You, Understanding Shame, Guilt-Letting Go*–and the list goes on. How does your title capture the right angle of attack, beating out the competition? It must be simple, eye-catching, and must say a mouthful in one expression. Any ideas? How about *No More Guilt!* It sounds boring at first. Does it need more "punch" to it? Titles such as *The 60-Minute Manager, Sixty Seconds to Success, Women Married to Alcoholics, Women Who Love Too Much, Recovery from Rescuing,* and *Little Miss Perfect,* implicitly say exactly what the book promises to deliver. Titles do this.

Brainstorm a title by asking the following questions:

1. What sounds funny? (*Bratbusters, I Can't Be Fat*)
2. What are common phrases or expressions? (*Too Good for Her Own Good, Little Miss Breadwinner*)
3. Can something be turned into a "syndrome?" (*Avoidance Syndrome; Good Girl Syndrome; Chronic Fatigue Syndrome*)
4. What do you want the reader to do? (*Overcoming Eating; Panic Attack Recovery Book; How to Avoid Your Parents' Mistakes; Survival Skills Against Violence*)
5. What strikes a chord for special populations? (*Adult Children of Alcoholics Syndrome; Family Addiction; After War*).

Try the topic out on your clients. Don't think they will humor you with unconditional agreement; bad or overly technical and formal titles stick out like a sore thumb and clients will let you know it immediately. Think *not in terms of what your doctoral chairman or supervisor would like, but what the next-door neighbor would like.* My wife once said, "Picture the type of books people read lying on the beach–now, does your book fit in their hands?" It will if you lighten up the title. Take your working title over to a bookstore chain (e.g., Walden, B. Dalton, Barnes & Noble) and compare it with existing books on the market. Is your title more clever? Does it have a humorous or sensitive ring the other books lack? Then you're on the track to begin locating a publisher.

Here's a hurdle most authors trip over in their rush for exciting titles. They've come upon a great idea, introducing a brand new phenomenon or new twist on an old theme for the popular press.

That recently happened with my co-editors on *Little Miss Bread-winner.* Two insightful authors approached me with the idea that today's ambitious, upwardly mobile women are going backwards by selecting intimate partners below their standards–educationally, financially, socially–you name it: Mr. "A" is Mr. "Wrong" because he lacks integrity, anatomy, and a career appetite. They called this phenomenon "Down-dating." And, consequently, their running book title was *Down-Dating: And Those of Us Who Do It.*

Now, on the surface, you might feel this title explicitly spells out their self-help purpose and simultaneously has that eye-catching "bite" for five-second title-browsers. For two solid years these authors struggled to pitch their proposal to New York and Los Angeles agents, many of whom enthusiastically gobbled up the concept but rejected the book nevertheless. Why? Here's one reason: Who knew what the authors were talking about? Suppose you're that five-second title-browser. Do you automatically know what "down-dating" means? Probably not. *Never introduce your new phenomenon in your book title. Only you will know what you mean. And you're not the one buying your book.* On analyzing where these authors were headed and how I might spice up title and book for them–here's what I suggested: *Little Miss Breadwinner and the Crumbs She Dates.*

Now apply the same principle to shame and guilt. *No More Guilt* is on the right track but a little heavy on cliche. Add a subtitle feature to it, qualifying exactly what the book will do: *No More Guilt: Ten-Step Guide to a Shame-Free Life.* And there you have it. Readers now know what the book is about, how they can reach this goal, and what they'll feel like after taking your medicine.

LOCATE PUBLISHERS

One of the first rules of writing self-help books is: *Never write a page until you find a publisher.* Publisher specifications and expectations vary widely and what one publisher adores, another finds repulsive. Extremes are very normal in perception. *Gone with the Wind* was rejected by a number of first-run publishing houses before it got picked up by a small firm. The same happens with many first-time authors ignored by the Cadillacs of the book industry.

Publishers first want an inquiry letter and proposal, both introducing the book concept, table of contents, and author credentials. Wait for the publisher to request more information such as your vita or sample chapter. Then, and only then, does drafting original material begin.

Small Publishers

First-time authors incorrectly believe that safe gambles in publishing mean finding a large, well-known publisher. They choose the Rolls Royces such as Macmillan, Random House, McGraw-Hill, Warner Books, William Morrow & Co., among others. Chances of newcomers breaking into these edifices without twisting a leg or good-old-fashioned nepotism using a reputable agent are next to impossible. You won't do it. Even academic-turned lay publishers whom you would think are sympathetic to the heartaches of beginners may close their doors. *Research Press, Impact Press, New Harbinger Publications,* to name only a few, face stiff competition from cutthroat publishing giants who muscle in on market areas. The best bet, then, is to try a small publisher.

Small publishing houses are not all shoestring operations. Many companies publish from three to 50 books a year, gladly read over-the-transom submissions, and eagerly work with new authors. Some are less enthusiastic about first-timers but still publish 80 percent from unpublished or nonagented authors. Skidmore-Roth Publishers, for instance, averages ten trade paperback originals per year on consumer health. Ten Speed Press prints under the different names (imprints) of *Celestial Arts* and *Double Elephant Books,* and averages 100 books a year. Small presses spend more time and energy working with authors and asking author input on every stage of production, from editorial to distribution. In fact, small presses represent 70 percent of the book industry, independently gaining ground on rough terrain. The number of books they publish annually is only one statistic reported. There is more you need to know about. Before signing on the dotted line, find out answers to the following questions:

1. *What advances on royalty do they offer?* Six-digit advances are only for celebrities, not first-time authors. Most small publishers

do not offer advances against royalty sales. Those that do offer from $100 to $1,000 contingent upon different stages of manuscript production. For instance, $300 is paid upon returning the signed contract. Another $300 is payable after submission and acceptance of the manuscript. The remainder follows the book release. Advances are meager because small presses rarely budget for author expenses, figuring there are other contract incentives to loyally stick with the schedule. However, *everything is negotiable.* Experienced self-help authors can bargain for advances even when the fine print says "no advances." Feeling your manuscript is a winner, publishers may agree to pay middle to high hundreds, even $1,000 offset by other concessions such as reducing the marketing budget.

2. *What royalty agreement do they offer?* Standard royalty agreements specify that authors receive 5 percent to 8 percent of the net price, after returns, of the units sold. Some publishers offer gross earnings as well. In other words, on every book sold for $10, you may receive between 50 to 80 cents. That's not very much on one or two books, but should the entire press run (3,000) sell, royalty earnings jump to $1,500 to $2,400. Royalties are usually also incremental with subsequent press runs. Runs of another 3,000 books may raise the royalty from 5 percent to 8 percent, averaging 3 percent jumps on all press runs up to 15 percent. Of course, by the time your book sells some 15,000 copies it may come to the attention of reprint publishers (e.g., Bantam), who buy out the copyright and establish an entirely new author contract. Buy outs are split 50-50 between author and publisher. Earnings also come from subsidiary rights. These are other mediums requesting the publisher's permission to reprint or convert your book for their own use. Books converted into audiotape, videotape, or excerpted for magazine serialization all earn dividends because the copyright belongs to the publisher.

3. *What distribution network do they use?* Small presses use a wide variety of distribution systems. Some presses directly sell books through brokers or wholesalers who distribute books to the large bookstore chains. Such wholesalers as Baker & Taylor Partners, Ingrams, and West Publishing "carry the book" and market it to retail stores who order it on commission. Retailers deduct a

percentage of sales after the wholesaler deducts another percentage of sales per unit. By the time publishers make money on the book, actual dollars and cents are subtracted from costs of wholesaler and bookseller. Other companies have their own in-house distribution system. Still, many companies, discouraged by the financial distrust and ineffectiveness of distributors, sell directly to bookstores or other outlet centers. Mail-order options exist for all publishers, although it is usually a secondary market approach.

4. *What type of marketing budget do they have?* Know what the publisher is willing to spend on promoting the book and your publicity. Small firms are reluctant to dish out funds for first-time authors unseasoned in the media. Even experienced media authors may run up against resistance. Budgets for travel and lodging to go *on tour* are unavailable since most small firms rarely get authors who feel comfortable with this exposure. Even travel reimbursement for book signings may be scarce or unavailable. Specifically, then, find out if the publisher or its publicist plan on scheduling and paying you for TV appearances, radio appearances, and book signings.

5. *What type of editorial support do they offer?* Publishers accept your book on *spec,* that is, on the speculation that your finished product will turn out as good as promised. (Some publishers, incidentally, require the full manuscript before making a decision; this author discourages pursuing business with that company.) Proposals that turn into 200- to 300-page double-spaced manuscripts may go through a series of cooperative publisher-author steps. Editors may wish updates on writing progress by seeing a chapter or having chapters sent out for impartial review. Be willing to work with editors and agree on most changes they request, rather than bullying their suggestions. *You may be the author expert, but you're not yet the expert in book marketing.*

Let the editors' insights guide style, format, and audience-enticing elements in early stages of book preparation. However, not every editorial staff is so supportive. You may be the Lone Ranger, expected to wallow through writer's block, unmet deadlines, and the writing style guidelines without assistance. Don't despair; if asked, most editors are glad to offer direction.

6. *What computer capacities do they use?* This is a new question for small publishers. Most large publishing houses already use computers for typesetting and layout functions. Authors can send their manuscript on diskette (3 1/2," 5 1/4") rather than as a printed hard copy. Publishers copy the disk documents onto their own hard drive and, if need be, convert the program into compatible operating programs. Most IBM programs, for example, are transformable into Macintosh programs using a super-drive and certain software. Likewise, Macintosh programs can be converted into IBM and IBM-compatible files. Computer facilities expedite editing and typesetting stages and rapidly get the book ready for release. But small publishers may be behind the times. If so, follow whatever manuscript policies they employ. This is not a major reason to dismiss the publisher for your book.

7. *What timeline do they offer to complete the book?* Polished manuscripts take time. But realistically, time is part of the deal. Standard deadlines for completing the manuscript are one year following a signed contract. Earlier deadlines depend on shortcuts in production, such as camera-ready and camera-ready preparations. In all, three factors dictate timeline. First is the advance against royalty sales. If publishers give you money, deadlines are shorter to ensure against your default. Second, timeliness of material may require fast turn-around time. Writing the psychohistory of President Clinton or of Hollywood celebrities, especially if any are embroiled in controversy, speeds up the production schedule. The faster it's in, the faster it's out. Third, publishers are stricter with new authors. Six months to one year for first-time authors, again, is an insurance policy. Publishers liked your pitch, bought your spec, but don't know you from Adam. So, they spice up the financial end of royalties with the bittersweet news of rushing the manuscript to press.

8. *What is the initial press run?* This may seem unimportant but it really is. Most first-time authors, even veterans, take homage knowing their book is in print and available in bookstores. But how many bookstores carry it depends on how many books are in the press run. The press run is the first inventory produced at the publisher's expense, representing the initial financial risk. Runs for self-help books range from 1,000 to 10,000 copies, unless the book or author (first-time or veteran) has celebrity status. For example, Football great Joe

Namath appeared in several TV commercials and even in feature-length movies. But once his name appeared on a book spine, consumer excitement soared. He's not an experienced author, but his name alone generated powerful sales.

A first run of 2,000 copies is average for small presses, trying to limit their overhead expenses and break even. Once 2,000 copies sell, minus returns or complimentary copies, publishers cover their expenses plus enjoy a small profit. The decision to run another 2,000 (or more) copies is both an economic and psychological one. How book-hungry is the public for this manuscript at such and such a price? If test marketing shows brilliant sales over three months, projections are that lucrative sales should continue over the next three months; thus another press run is worth it. But good fortune never lasts forever. Just as a shelf life is five months maximum, so it is that hot streaks lose their vitality in five to six months.

9. *What things are negotiable?* Interested publishers project dollar signs in your proposal and offer you a contract based on sales. But they are not misers. Contracts that look "standard" are always negotiable. *Everything is negotiable.* First-time authors usually feel overjoyed by contract offers and will sign anything to get their name in print. Others take extreme caution, distrusting any contract and thinking every publisher is a dishonest slime-bucket turning the screws on them at every corner. Neither extreme is healthy. First, never sign on the dotted line until you understand or feel satisfied that the contract terms are fair and represent the best interests of both parties. No harm comes from having an entertainment attorney review the contract for loopholes. Attorneys may suggest higher royalty percentages, guarantees of publication, or first author rights of the returned manuscript should publisher refuse it or go bankrupt before production is completed.

But if you rewrite the contract, think in *bargain-mentality.* Negotiating *more or less* of the standard clauses must have reciprocity. What can you do *in return for the publisher?*

There are many things you can do. First, if you are a computer whiz and love desk-top publishing, propose typesetting and graphic layout of your manuscript; send the document in camera-ready form. Computer publishers may buy it and save nearly $5,000 in typesetting and keylining costs. That's a lot of money saved. Another bargaining chip is publicity. Publishers that lack big budgets for public relations may welcome your willingness to contact and appear on TV and radio. They may agree to send complimentary copies to your media contacts plus boost your royalty percentage. This is because you're doing the expensive footwork. You're saving the publisher the expense of a salaried or commissioned employee by self-promoting your book and probably doing a more efficient job of it. News releases, contacts with producers, booking schedules, and appearances not only is a deal *the publisher can't refuse,* you'll double your chances of going into a second press run and quadruple your chance of asking that publisher to contract your next book.

Large Publishers

Okay, so you don't want a small press. You've heard nasty rumors about their shady character and you've decided it's either Disney World or nothing. You figure, "Look, if illiterate athletes can publish their biographies (courtesy of their ghost writers), I most certainly can break into the market." You're buzzing with energy and ready for the kill. You feel it in your bones. That habit-control book of yours is a guaranteed blockbuster. You write to Bantam books. They say, "No, thank you." You write to NAL Penguin books. They also say, "No, thank you." You write to Harcourt Brace Jovanovich. They never respond. So, you get sneaky. You directly call the editor of Houghton Mifflin. They ask what your agent's name is; you freeze and hang up. But that's nothing. You become more clever by the hour, this time disguising your voice as an agent. Macmillan falls for it. They ask about your "clients" and other book prospects. One lie was fine, but this is getting out of hand. So you abandon ship at the first port and say you'll call them back.

You're running out of ideas; except for one—it's your best poker hand yet. You tell an editor at William Morrow that you're a best-selling author putting your next book up for open auction. Highest bidder publishes it. They say, "Okay, send us the prospectus and two chapters." You feel victory in your bones. You spend the next two weeks pumping out chapters and send the whole package over-night express to William Morrow. They never reply.

Sounds like a wild goose chase, doesn't it? How about a true story retold by nearly every first-time writer, including this author. The time, energy, and lies invested in drilling for oil in large book publishers is not worth it. They are "good-old-boy" clubs surrounded by a network of loyal agents and reputable, reliable authors who keep their wheels in motion. Breaking into this deeply entrenched establishment is not impossible, but greatly improbable and can discourage a writer's ambition. Rather than fight City Hall, try trusting a small press. They are efficient, personable, and can produce royalty earning rewards equal to the big boys if marketing and distribution channels hit the mark.

Packagers

Packagers are a new breed in the United States. Actually they first emerged in England in the 1940s. They're not exactly publishers, not exactly agents, and not exactly writers. Book packagers develop a book proposal, assemble the writers, illustrators, and editors to prepare it, and submit it to a publisher. Once the product is accepted, packagers act as coordinators of the entire project and liaison to publishers. In-house staff comprise 80 percent of writing assignments but contracts with freelancers are also needed. First, identify packagers whose line of book projects are compatible to your writing interests. Send an inquiry letter describing your abilities, previous writing record, and how you can help out on their forthcoming projects. While none of their slated projects may fit exactly with your idea for a book, topics such as health, exercise, and self-control do strike a familiar bell. Pursue those leads based on writing on *their topics*. This is the time to toot your horn. Writing for a packager gets you into the business, gets you a book credit, and earns you money. Royalties, perhaps; but more frequently packagers make outright purchases or work-for-hire agreements.

Subsidy Presses

Never get tired of trying. Persistence is the name of the game. Disillusioned authors usually give up when they feel their work really is unsaleable or they cannot stand another rejection letter. That is *not the time to seek a subsidy publisher.* Never pursue a subsidy publishing arrangement when you feel defeated. Subsidy publishers produce more than 50 percent of their books on a financially shared or *cooperative* basis. You pay either half, 75 percent, or all editorial and production costs and they deliver the book in a shiny book jacket ready for distribution. Subsidy arrangements cover many services, from editing to marketing, and can cost several thousand dollars ($10,000 to $15,000) before the final bill is paid. Companies also offer to store the inventory and ship book orders, under contract. However, no matter how generous their provisions, it still boils down to *you and your pocketbook.*

Legitimate subsidy companies can be a viable alternative to traditional publishers under three circumstances. First, your employer (university, hospital, clinic, etc.) plans to foot the bill in return for free publicity and control over distribution. Working with subsidy publishers secures this control and assures your employee the product will be tailor-made according to individual specifications. In fact, many cooperative publishers (e.g., Ginn Publishing Company) will not charge you money, per se, if given guaranteed purchase orders of 200 to 500 copies. Instructors who teach large lecture hall classes year long seize this gold-mine opportunity to gain book credit because the "student bookstores" agree to make this financial commitment; instructors walk away with a book and royalty stipend.

Second, you are actively on tour; you give lay or professional workshops nationwide and use a text as part of the purchased materials. Subsidy groups are perfect because you can mastermind the book design and press runs based on projected workshop attendance. Third, joint publishing agreements are arranged between yourself and some large industry capable of mass distribution and a 90 percent guarantee of recouping your expenses. For instance, a book on "Driving safely with children" (from seat belt use to when they have tantrums) may be picked up by GM, Ford, and Chrysler, who sell the book or give it away as a premium for every car purchased. Automatic distribution routes include the thousands of car dealerships nationwide.

Resources

Where do you find publishers? Naturally you can spend hours at the local bookstore, hunting down your favorite topics and flipping inside the book cover for a publisher name. But there are easier and more efficient resources at your disposal. The list below directs you to mainstream magazines and nationally available books:

Canadian Writer's Journal
Gordon M. Smart Publications
PO Box 6618
Depot 1, Victoria, British Columbia
V8P 5N7 Canada

New Writer's Magazine
Sarasota Bay Publishing
PO Box 5976
Sarasota, FL

Publishers Weekly
R. R. Bowker Company
205 E. 42nd Street
New York, NY 10017

Small Press, the magazine of independent publishing
Small Press Inc.
Colonial Hill, RFD #1
Mt. Kisco, NY 10549

The Writer
120 Boylston Street
Boston, MA 02116

Writer's Digest
F & W Publications, Inc.
1507 Dana Avenue
Cincinnati, OH 45207

The Writer's Market
Writer's Digest Books
F & W Publications, Inc.
1507 Dana Avenue
Cincinnati, OH 45207

INQUIRY LETTER AND PROPOSAL

Now that you know which publishers to send proposals to, it's time to put together a persuasive proposal package. Sending a chapter is too premature. Assemble your proposal with brevity in mind. Simple, to-the-point proposals take the publisher by surprise, since most first-time or seasoned authors never are that organized.

Key Factors in the Proposal

Writing the proposal is more crucial than any book chapter you later compose. This is what busy, "I-don't-want-to-be-bothered" editors first see. First impressions count. If it doesn't stimulate their interests immediately, the proposal dies. No second chances. So, here's a template for producing this document that can answer nearly every question editors may ask upon receiving your inquiry. First, let's look at the cover letter. Second, let's look at the proposal.

Cover Letter

Cover letters must grab the editor like a sales pitch (Figure 9.1). The first paragraph asks a rhetorical question or strikes a tender chord:

> Frustrations in adult children of alcoholics and codependents sabotage healthy relationships and smother personal growth. Unless, or until the enemy within–Guilt–is attacked head on without fear.

Follow this emotional statement by introducing the title of the book. The next paragraph briefly overviews the book and why it is important. The third paragraph is a biographical note. Keep it short and relevant; who you are, what your expertise is, and why the publisher can trust that you'll deliver. End the letter by saying you're looking forward to a reply.

Proposal

Plan on three to five pages of a carefully worded and organized report, headed by a cover or contents page (Figure 9.2). On the next

FIGURE 9.1. Book proposal letter to publisher

BEST IMPRESSIONS INTERNATIONAL INCORPORATED

4211 OKEMOS ROAD, SUITE 22, OKEMOS, MICHIGAN 48864, U.S.A.
TELEPHONE: 517-347-0944

February 20, 1992

Ms. Georgia Mills, Publisher
Mills & Sanderson Publishers
41 North Road, Suite 201
Bedford, MA 01730-1021

Dear Ms. Mills:

Frustrations in adult children of alcoholics and codependents sabotage healthy relationships and smother personal growth. Unless, or until the enemy within–Guilt–is attacked head on without fear. How to do this is as simple as **No More Guilt: Ten Steps to a Shame-Free Life**.

I invite your company to consider **No More Guilt** for publication. **No More Guilt** consists of systematic steps to cope with agonizing anger, self-hate beliefs, toxic shame, fear of rejection, and avoidance/escape actions. Steps are in direct, simple-to-read form, ready for immediate use. Adults attending my many seminars and behavioral practice over the last ten years are ecstatic over how easy it is to follow these guidelines. Now I wish to make these steps available in more detail in a book designed for your product line.

An author, researcher, and clinician, I have published over 100 professional articles and 28 books in adult/pediatric topics including for the popular press. Currently I am touring for my parenting book, *Bratbusters: Say Goodbye to Tantrums and Disobedience*.

Enclosed is a prospectus of **No More Guilt**. I will be happy to forward a vita and sample chapter upon your request.

I look forward to hearing from you.

Sincerely,

Douglas H. Ruben, PhD

page, begin the first section. Headings should be in bold print and in 14-point size (or larger) if composed on a computer word processor. Otherwise, underline or bold the headings. Text underneath headings is in 10- to 12-point size. Here is how the sections appear:

1. General Description and Specification

Give an abstract of the book describing its content, relevancy, and general intended audience. For example:

> Life traumas are tragic enough. But enduring the grief of shame every day is worse because the solution to it seems elusive. *No More Guilt* offers a stepwise approach directly suited for individuals faced with disabling fears of rejection, self-anger, and worry, and whose suffering is beyond simple anxiety. These are people perfectly able to function in jobs, at home, but who secretly disguise being overly sensitive to their faults, their impositions upon others, and resistance to risks.
>
> Adult children of alcoholics or of dysfunctional families are prime targets for shame and it permeates all avenues of their lives. Following the ten-step approach, readers can identify and immediately apply methods proven in clinical practice to defuse fears and build a productive repertoire. Such skills promote risk taking above safe boundaries at home or in personal relationships. Readers of all adult ages and walks of life will be excited over the rapid improvements in their behaviors in just a short time.

2. Length of Manuscript, Estimated Completion Date, Computer Capacity, and CD-ROM

Identify how long you project the manuscript will be in double-spaced pages. Estimate, as well, a reasonable date in the future the completed manuscript can be delivered to the publisher. Start your first round of negotiations here. Describe any advanced capabilities you have to save publisher production costs, including your camera-ready facilities or programming literacy in designing a book on software (CD-ROM):

FIGURE 9.2. Cover page of contents for prospectus

PROSPECTUS

No More Guilt
Ten Steps to a Shame-Free Life

Douglas H. Ruben PhD
Best Impressions International Inc.
Okemos, Michigan

Contents

1. General Description and Specification.

2. Length of Manuscript, Estimated Completion Date, Computer Capacity, and CD-ROM

3. Table of Contents

4. Competitive Market

5. About the Author

Manuscript length estimates at 300 to 500 double-spaced pages (excluding frontmatter, backmatter). Estimated completion date is six months to one year following contractual agreement. Considering computer capacities on the Macintosh/IBM and laser printer, photo-ready preparation is available based on higher advances against royalty sales and higher royalty percentage on net sales. On computer, manuscript can be completed on Microsoft word (5.0) or Pagemaker. ALSO, disk submissions can include programming instructions for multimedia on CD-ROM combining audio, video, or animation, depending on your conversion software and multimedia distribution needs.

3. Table of Contents

Give a cursory outline of heading and subheadings, without elaborating on each section:

Step 1. What Is Guilt?

Step 2. How to Spot Guilt

Step 3. No More Taking It Personally
    a. How you read into things
    b. Basic steps to prevent assumptions
    c. Basic risks to prevent assumptions
    d. Roadblocks to look out for
    e. Reversal of guilt

Step 4. No More Avoidance and Escape
    a. What is avoidance and escape?
    b. Different types of avoidance and escape
       (excuses, defenses, blaming, apologies,
       compensating, aggression, withdrawal, sex)
    c. Setting up opportunities for conflict
    d. DESC assertiveness for offensive behavior
    e. Basic relaxation for staying in situation

Step 5. No More Fear of Rejection
    a. Facing the need for hurt
    b. Risks for disapproval
    c. Letting it go–the delay process
    d. Why rejection doesn't equal abandonment

Step 6. No More Fear of Failure
    a. Why perfectionism doesn't work
    b. Exposing vulnerability in risk situations
    c. Acceptance and soliciting of compliments
    d. Reversing imposter situation

Step 7. No More Toxic Shame
    a. When it is okay to be *wrong*
    b. When it is okay to be *bad*
    c. When it is okay to be *defiant*
    d. When it is okay to be *independent*

Step 8. No More Need for Control
    a. Why controlling is really protecting
    b. Sharing control
    c. Abandon control

Step 9. No More Feeling Hurt for other People
    a. Why feeling sorry is really out of fear
    b. What is a caretaker?
    c. Resisting the caretaker role
    d. Urge control

Step 10. No More Repeating Bad Relationships
    a. Stop sign on "comfortable" relationships
    b. Criteria for selecting significant others
    c. Testing the criteria
    d. Why sex restarts the guilt cycle

4. Competitive Market

This is your strongest pitch for a spec purchase. Tell the publisher in no uncertain terms why your book is better than competitive books on the market. Explain mistakes other books make by comparing how your book solves those mistakes. Make your product the doctor to the competitor's illness. And save the best for last. Book sales depend on a *marketing angle*. How can you merchandise your book faster, reaching cash-paying consumers in your target group? If you can, don't be shy. Offer a full-scale marketing blitz on why contracting with you as author is a risk-free guarantee through use of your mailing lists, contacts in radio, TV, and print media. Clearly state that your reader network is a diamond for widespread publicity and can save the publisher the cost of hiring a PR team.

Consider *Little Miss Breadwinner.* Here we have a unique combination of authors from different walks of life talking the same language and hitting readers from all sides as experts, celebrities, and victims. Surely there must be a marketing angle somewhere. There was, and here's how it sounded:

> *Little Miss Breadwinner* is a winner on all fronts. First, hard-hitting books on dating are popular but lack the author prestige and scientific principles found in this book. Readers either get one or the other: bestselling authors who give general or nebulous advice or unknowns who hit the nail on the head. *Little Miss Breadwinner* gives you both elements for the price of one book.
>
> It goes beyond *Women Who Love Too Much* by showing women precisely how they trip into unhealthy, abusive relationships and why they couldn't spot the warning signs beforehand. It's not like *Smart Women, Foolish Choices* for two reasons. First, that book blames women for arrogantly looking for the perfect Prince Charming and advises, "Hey, get a life; they're not out there." Second, that book is too superficial on revising dating choices. If it were that simple, who'd need therapy? It's also not like *Codependent No More, Beyond Codependency* AND *Sexual Strategies: How Females Choose Their Mates.* Here's why: All three books personify the slang "co-dependency" into a "Gotcha, men-bashing" roast using the Alcoholics Anonymous philosophy for dressing. Mary Batten's *Sexual Strategies* lightens up on men, saying, "Give them a break, they're only trying–so what if they're age 40, never been married and know nothing about relationships– they'll do just fine." Well, sorry, no they won't. And *Little Miss Breadwinner* will tell you why and what to do about it.
>
> The second angle of *Little Miss Breadwinner* is its phenomenal potential for exposure. Hollywood TV star Martha Smith, former *Playboy* centerfold, and today's in-demand guest on hundreds of talk shows, is a powerful plus to marketing. Reruns of her *Scarecrow and Mrs. King,* frequent appearances on *Lifestyles of the Rich & Famous*, her roles in the daysoap *Days*

of Our Lives and opposite John Belushi in *Animal House* keep her in the public eye. Martha also had horrible down-dating experiences during Universal Studios days; sizzling stories that would play well on *Oprah, Sally, Phil, Jenny Jones,* and others. Adding to the ménage à trois is a feature film and commercial actress Carole Field, who is now a love-addictions therapist. Carole is on the lecture circuit able to sell copies of *Little Miss Breadwinner* by the droves. And that's not all.

When publicity speaks, it hears the name of Dr. Doug Ruben. After some 32 books, self-helpers from marriage and relationships to addiction, Ruben spends every year touring on at least two books and is frequently on TV and radio. Bookstore sales following his appearance on national tabloid talk shows will generate second and third printings and easily stimulate audiotape and possibly videotape adoptions. But best of all, Dr. Ruben assembles and markets his own media package and makes the media contacts through his Best Impressions International Inc. So, if your publicity division is small or on a tight budget, Dr. Ruben can help you reach the top market for this book.

5. About the Author

Finally, it's ego time. Describe your credentials and past publications relevant to your expertise on the proposed book. Be proud but humble. State attributes that are publicly or universally recognized such as inclusion in *Who's Who* books, previous books authored, appearances on TV, radio shows, on editorial boards of consumer magazines, and your major community leadership roles. Editors want more than she's a "PhD with lots of clinical experience." They look for the marketing angle on why this PhD with lots of clinical experience can be the goose that lays the golden egg.

THE WAITING GAME

How many days must it take before writer's depression sets in? Waiting the terrible weeks, months, even years for a publisher's reply or a "yes" reply can be tiresome and discouraging. Rejections pile up like unread newspapers; you'd stop the subscription, so why not stop sending inquiry letters? Are you a glutton for punishment? Of course not. Most of us are not into pain and suffering. Writing for remote rewards is bad enough, but how remote does the reward have to be before there is a light at the end of the tunnel? In most cases, publishers failing to reply by three weeks will not reply at all. While backlogs of over-the-transom mail do account for delays, the two-month-late reply only has one message in it: "Sorry, try another publisher."

When Is It Time to Call the Publisher?

Thus far your modus operandi has been through inquiry letter and proposal. Lack of correspondence for over one month means the publisher disliked the proposal and is too busy or lazy to send a rejection letter. But if that publisher is an especially desirable one, or you have contacts mediating a review in your favor, telephone follow-ups are perfectly acceptable. Contact the publisher or editor to whom you sent the inquiry package. Ask about the *status* of your proposal, in terms of its editorial approval, disapproval, or needing additional material from the author. Frequently, a talking relationship is just the right medicine to get the proposal over the proverbial waiting list and into editorial processing.

Use this brief opportunity to further plug your book, reiterating cost-saving options described in your proposal. However, use the time fairly and succinctly. Don't overplay a good thing. And tricks never work. Threatening the editor to make a decision *because there is another publisher ready to sign a contract with you* is a waste of time. Should another publisher *really* offer you a contract, softly present the idea to your first choice publisher and allow a reasonable deadline (two weeks) for their deliberations.

When Is It Time to Give Up and Start Over?

Is there ever really a time to give up the search for publishers? Yes. Persistence can go so far until you've exhausted publishers and different routes of entering the industry. That does not mean you should give up on the project forever. Take a break from it and begin another project. Use your expertise in another capacity, fine-tuning it along other marketable dimensions. Unpublished books occur for many reasons, but five reasons stand out prominently. First, the book is too esoteric for the self-help market. Second, the topic is overdone and has saturated the consumer. Third, the book poses ethical or moral controversies too risky for the publisher's pristine image. Fourth, the writing style is too scholarly, archival, or technical and does not fit the lay market. And fifth, author credentials are too weak to satisfy the publisher's celebrity taste.

GETTING AN AGENT

So what, then? Get an agent? The law about agents, much like syndicators, is this: If you really did your homework marketing your manuscript, and not a single publisher bit the bait, agents probably will be ineffective. Even shoe-in contacts they have in publishing can't repair an irreparable manuscript. Author representatives or "reps" who do welcome you on board charge a tariff; unpublished authors pay a reader's fee plus additional telephone, mailing, and other clerical expenses. Full service reps may also serve as interim editor, offer ghost-writing services, even collaborative authorship. Your bill reaches into the hundreds without knowing how far ahead the agent's work really promoted your book. But for every drawback there are positive gains in using agents. Let's consider both pros and cons.

Pros and Cons

Advantages are numerous. Agent representation is a rapid transition into the heavyweight of publishing. Manhattan reps know the scuttlebutt; who is looking for what, when, and how much they'll pay. Insider information that is essential to sell your manuscript may save you months and years of scrounging for the "right publisher." Agents also can *negotiate*. A vote of higher royalties for you means a higher commission for them. Agents charge percentages of 10 percent to 15 percent against your royalty earnings, which means for every $10.00 you earn, they yield $1.50. Sounds like peanuts for the work they do, but percentages pay off on larger royalty payments. Suppose you earn $50,000 on a relatively strong-selling book; your agent profits $7,500. And that's only from one author. Most agents represent 20 to 30 authors on a continuous basis. And what's good for the agents ultimately works out the best for you.

That's the good news. The bad news is: *who really needs agents?* Author reps are valuable commodities for writers who dislike beating the bushes for self-promotion. They stick only to writing and let *another person handle the business side of writing.* Entrusting agents or attorneys to manage your affairs is perfectly fine if you travel a lot, are too busy in clinical practice and running workshops, or touring TV and radio shows. They act as your spokesperson and forge new opportunities in your absence. But no matter how busy you are, effective agents will *increase* your load of responsibility. It's a pipedream to expect agents to relieve your hectic lifestyle of annoying publisher negotiations. Every deal mediated by agents must receive your approval or disapproval before consummated, just as a real estate agent negotiates and confirms with you on a bid to the seller of a house you're buying.

Agents expect that you will accept all reasonable contract offers and career stepping-stones researched. They build a reputation on promising and then delivering the goods at the best price. Refusal to take their deals may constitute an agent-author violation resulting in arbitration, compensation, or litigation. Either way, agents win because they performed a service according to an agreement and they did not anticipate your indecision. While this may not ever happen to you, be prepared for some unpredictable scenarios during the agent-author relationship.

Where to Find One

Who is the best agent around? Intuitively you might ask a friend who he used for his published works. Or, call a local author support group. They provide an amazing clearinghouse of places and contacts and problems never found in any text. On record there are thousands of agents located nationwide. Research them in terms of services provided, service fees, percentage against book royalties, and how long the contract is binding (six months to two years). Resources below represent the best places to look first:

Guide to Literary Agents and Art/Photo Reps
F & W Publications, Inc.
1507 Dana Avenue
Cincinnati, OH 45207

Literary Market Place
R. R. Bowker Company
1180 Avenue of the Americas
New York, NY 10036

International Literary Market Place
R. R. Bowker Company
1180 Avenue of the Americas
New York, NY 10036

Chapter 10

Writing for Multimedia, On-line Computer Databases, and Related Electronic Media

Writing newsletters, handouts, magazine articles and books all champion the print media. Your ideas in print highlight the product and expertise, and add versatility to your clinical image. But print media is not enough to keep up with burgeoning technology. Ten years ago the fad for "talking books" (audiotapes) caught on like wildfire. Five years ago video markets sprung up from nowhere, claiming 15 percent entertainment purchases and closing in on the book industry. Now people can watch Jazzercise, aerobics, and self-help videotapes easier than reading a book. Mediums are turning electronic, from audios and videos to computers. Already personal computers can replace shopping. Imagine it–buying your groceries, clothing, airplane tickets, and financial investments all at the touch of a button. That's what computer databases such as *Prodigy, CompuServe, and America-on-Line* can offer. These interactive software programs link into vendors who sell merchandise and services directly over the computer. You just charge what you want to your credit card. Credit information stored in the memory is activated the moment you make and affirm a purchase order.

Talking, reading, and buying via computer is an electronic paradise for the jet-setting public who has no time for domestic chores. Odd hours of the day are the only stress-free times for shopping, learning, and entertainment. Late night and early morning computer uses are heavy, and frequently lines are tied up for two hours before subscribers can sign on. But when they do, unlimited franchises vie for a piece of the action. This is where you come in.

Welcome to the electronic intergalactic highway. Information travels at lightening speed through computer hyperspace using today's advanced adult toys from CD-ROMs to E-Mail bulletin boards. Seconds pass as your brainchild product is sent from your homebase computer outward among literally millions of subscribing cybernuts nationally and internationally, all with fax-modum capabilities either to buy, reject, or improve upon your product just as quickly as they received it. And why? Because electronic publishing in all forms, from on-line databases to multimedia, is no longer a sacred idol. The product is not immutable. It can be changed, improved upon, and returned to you entirely unrecognizable from readers after they surgically reconstruct it using combinations of text, sound, graphics, animation, and video. What you put on diskette or send through the hyperspace pipeline, in other words, may be very different by the time it's a finished product. That's due to your audience. Computer users, by and large, are not just consuming new material; they're not like tabloid-reading junkies who have a large appetite for how-to words. By contrast, computer junkies are a breed of their own; they absorb your words so they can *revise, revamp, and reproduce your ideas with greater glitter and sophistication.*

That means your intended audience is not passive. They are active, do-it-now shakers and movers who are on the prowl for good material that can showcase their own multimedia insights. It's not that your copyright is lost forever; they don't steal it. Like patents, once your product is copywritten, you own the rights to it–but you don't own the rights to any and all variations of your product ingeniously manufactured through electronic techno-surgery. And that's what electronic readers will eagerly do to your precious materials. So, don't fight city hall on a common practice; get into the spirit by cashing in on the publicity and commercial market of this New Age communication.

BOOKS IN HYPERSPACE

By now the hoopla is over concerning the merge of giants Apple and IBM Computers to form a larger electronic nation–and why? To corner the market on advancing technologies that are giving traditional publishers a run for their money. It's called the *CD-ROM.* This

1980s brainchild of discontented disk-users springboarded the potential for audio CDs into computerland. The result was a viable business tool for storing extensive information beyond the 800-K or 1500-K limits of double-sided diskettes'–now storage capacity was astronomical: try storage of up to 680 megabytes of data. That's equivalent to 136 *million* typed pages.

Still, in spite of CD-ROM madness, some unenthusiastic critics want to nail the coffin on CD-ROMs, calling them a faddish "eight-track player" and blame their demise on the National Information Infrastructure (NII). NII promises a 500-channel interactive television to the Internet for a whopping boost to the information superhighway. But news of CD-ROM's death are greatly exaggerated. Why? Because most skeptical scenarios overlook that CD-ROMs are the *only practical way of publishing digitally.* CD-ROM is an incredibly cheap medium for mass production of large digital titles such as archives, databases, manuals, brochures, and *books.* That's right: CD-ROM books.

The CD-ROM is an electronic publishing gold mine headed to revolutionize the print media industry (cf. Newmark, 1994). Consider the facts. The Optical Publishing Association (OPA) recently released figures highlighting significant growth in CD-ROM manufacturing. According to the OPA, approximately 100 million CD-ROM disks were manufactured worldwide in 1993. Representing a large share of the manufacturing were traditional publishers turned cyberspecialists. HarperCollins, for example, one of New York's most respectable adult trade publishers, launched a new imprint called *HarperReference Interactive,* which will produce software and CD-ROMs for the consumer market. Running parallel to this initiative are Putnam, Random House, Penguin, Paramount Communications, and Reader's Digest Books. Take Putnam, for instance; they plan to create a complete framework for the development, distribution, and marketing of new media "family" titles. Reader's Digest Books is onto something better; they won't just dump the book on disk, but plan to produce original series of books containing videos, illustrations, footage, and reference materials in the Do-it-Yourself genre.

Because many trade publishers are taking risks to aggressively enter the upward computer market, authors will have to re-think their proposals when scribbling for big bucks. Dictated by market demand, your product or expertise can go beyond the printed page to include sound, video, animation, and virtual reality. Proposals can creatively describe how your book would integrate multimedia elements without sounding too program analytical. You do not need to specify computer language or write out logarithms for the pitch. Just focus on content and imaginative ways that computer users can be educated, entertained, and economically sold on your product.

Submitting for CD-ROMs can go the traditional publisher route or, on better advice, can be a self-publishing venture. In-house hardware for converting your own material into CD-ROM is becoming price-friendly at an alarming speed. One year ago conversion technology was at $15,000. Now it's around $5,000. And by the time this book reaches your eyes, CD recording devices will be affordable at under $1,000. Data storage, archival, and data distribution requires a management software that both digitally records and allows for retrieval. Imagine producing CD-ROMs at home on your DOS or WINDOWS PC and selling your creation to anybody with a CD-ROM. That's what programs such as *Alchemy* (Information Management Research, Inc.) and companies such as *MicroRetrieval Corporation* and *M3 Dimensions* do. They either show you how (for a fee) or enable you on your own to operate a complete CD-production system including a computer management database, premastering and mastering software, a CD-recorder, a SCSI interface (sound board), and some recordable media.

Showcase your multimedia products on CD-ROMs. This technology is a stock paying high dividends for traditional publishers or for outlet stores and distributors who may carry your in-home products. To get started, find out which publishers and software companies are shifting over to CD-ROM divisions and in the market for new ideas. The best resources are trade magazines on CD-ROMs, for example:

CD-ROM News
Pemberton Press Inc
462 Danbury Road
Wilton, CT 06897-2126

CD-ROM Professional
Pemberton Press Inc
462 Danbury Road
Wilton, CT 06897-2126

CD-ROM Pocket Guide
Pemberton Press Inc
462 Danbury Road
Wilton, CT 06897-2126

CD-ROM Multimedia
Universal Multimedia Inc.
100 Ballantyne S.
Montreal West
Quebec, Canada H4X 2B3

CD-ROM Today
GP Publications Inc.
300- A South Westgate Drive
Greensboro, NC 27407

Multimedia World
Subscription Department
PO Box 58690
Boulder, CO 80323-8690

Electronic Entertainment
PO Box 7969
Riverton, NJ 08077-8669

PRODIGY, COMPUSERVE, AMERICA-ON-LINE, AND STILL OTHER INTERACTIVE SERVICES

There are several ways of breaking into on-line services for a high-profile product promotion. Let's consider some initial steps that parallel the traditional publishing routes.

Propose a Weekly Column

Consumer on-line services share a common denominator. They are for young, upwardly mobile professionals looking for rapid solutions on everyday issues from daycare and parenting to converting computers into mini-orchestras. Travel, arts and entertainment, and sports also fill the encyclopedic volume of weekly columns written by specialists who answer subscriber questions. Ann Landers-style columns are easy to do if you feel your area of expertise is missing from the on-line directory. Take a column called *You & Behavior.* Suppose it provided inexpensive, valid, and sensible tips on all sorts of adult problems, from habits and stress to addiction and marriage: "Computer-shrink" at your service. Staying ethical, probing answers are kept simple, frequently on how-to subjects such as "How do I stop biting my nails?" Deeper answers or needs for catharsis are referred elsewhere: "You should contact your local mental health expert for that answer."

"You and Behavior" is an example of what you might propose to the program manager of editorial and business affairs. To do this, send an inquiry in one of two ways. First, send it on-line using the system mailbox or E-Mail; this saves you postage. Second, send the inquiry in more detail through the regular mail. On-line replies are relatively fast, considering the millisecond input and output transmissions. The reply may refer you to the correct person or office able to consider your proposal. In Prodigy, for instance, the mail message requested that you direct a letter of interest with a resume to another address; transmission took less than one day. But computer operators are more efficient than bureaucrats. The administrator replied one month later. If the reply is favorable, submit an outline of weekly topics and types of write-in questions projected. Then, once the weekly column is a regular on-line feature, use this medium to announce your new products or expanding expertise.

Communicate on "Bulletin Boards"

Heavy user traffic also appears on the bulletin boards. These are communication exchanges between subscribers. Topics, again, are widely diverse and frequently the same people tend to reply to the inquiries. You can become one of those regulars who offer advice and solve a subscriber's dilemma. Know something about parenting? Explain to a frustrated mother of twins why her one child yells constantly while the other one is a silent mouse. Place your credentials after your name (e.g., MD, PhD, MA, etc.) to support content validity and help repeated users to identify who you are. On occasion, your advice may stimulate adversaries. Don't get defensive; opposing views can draw closer attention to your ideas and ironically fortify your dignity.

Product Sales

Use the on-line service for its *interactive* quality as well. *Computers talk to you, and you talk to them.* Interactive technology is the mainstay behind merchandising; products and services are advertised in between and during each program to maximize buyer exposure. For example, while selecting an airline, ads for a travel agency and car rental discounts appear in the left- and right-hand corners. Promos sneak in everywhere and anywhere they can be seen. And you can do the same. Why not have your product exposed to buyers? Books, tapes, videos, or even equipment for clinical practice (timers, charts, billing and diagnostic software) all can be sold through a vendor agreement with the on-line company. Contact the buyer or acquisition department handling your product and work together to develop a marketing plan or contract entitling you to a larger percentage of sales.

In all, take advantage of the vastly increasing print media sources from hard copy to electronic services. There are endless ways to advertise your products and elevate your professional clinical status by writing original material designed for any number of special groups. Your clients or consumers at large can read and reread how-to's, treating you as the newest authority on self-help facts. Undertakings that broadly cover in-house writings and authoring paperback books really are not difficult to do; they're just new and take a toll on frustration. That is why a guiding principle to follow is this: *expect more rejections than acceptances. Even when you finally win a publisher's contract, expect the next publisher you contact not to know who you are and what you do.* That's unfortunate. Starting over each time you seek publishers seems painfully redundant. But there is good news. *Publishers do not have to know one another, nor the word be out that you're a hot writer, for your books to sell big and for you to prosper professionally.*

PART III.
REFERENCES AND SUGGESTED READINGS

Brown, S. W. & Morley, A. P. (1986). *Marketing Strategies for Physicians: A Guide to Practice Growth.* Oradell, NJ: Medical Economics Books.

Glasgow, R. E. & Rosen, G. M. (1978). Behavioral bibliotherapy: A review of self-help behavior therapy manuals. *Psychological Bulletin, 85,* 1-23.

Glasgow, R. E. & Rosen, G. M. (1979). Self-help behavior therapy manuals: Recent developments and clinical usage. *Clinical Behavior Therapy Review, 1,* 1-20.

Newmark, E. (1994). The New York Trade Publishers and CD-ROM: Where are they heading? *CD-ROM Professional, 7,* 55-63.

Rosen, G. M. (1976). The development and use of nonprescription behavior therapies. *American Psychologist, 31,* 139-141.

Ruben, D. H. (1989). Bibliotherapy: Practical considerations when writing for substance abuse readers. *Journal of Alcohol and Drug Education, 34,* 70-78.

Sachs, L. (1986). *Do-It-Yourself Marketing for the Professional Practice.* Englewood Cliffs, NJ: Prentice-Hall, Inc.

Winston, W. J. (Ed.). (1985). *Marketing Strategies for Human and Social Agencies.* Binghamton, NY: The Haworth Press.

PART IV.
SCRIPTING YOUR TALENTS IN MOVIES

You've just returned from seeing a movie and can't get this wacky idea out of your head: "Gosh, that was awful. I bet I could do better." Days later you see a horrible made-for-TV movie and it's dejà-vu. The story stinks, the plot is lousy, and characters were totally fake. Just a worthless one million dollars down the drain. And so you wonder–really wonder–could I do any better? Probably you could. And that's not 100 percent blind optimism. Most of today's aspiring screenwriters started off in other careers and turned to television or feature-length writing realizing they had displaced talents. Talents are not only for the grade-school thespian or English major who landed a mental or medical health job instead. Talents appear in *knowing what commercially works and communicating it in a compelling story.*

Bob Newhart was an accountant. Then a comedy writer–and finally he hit big-time as comedian and television star. Kurt Luedtke started as a Detroit journalist. His unprecedented Hollywood success included writing credits on *Absence of Malice* and *Out of Africa.* Bob Cochran was a Stanford-educated lawyer, writing in his spare time. He rose to executive story editor of *LA Law* and *Falcon Crest.* Same with attorney Melinda Snodgrass. Her meteoric career led to executive script consultant on *Star Trek: The Next Generation.* Todd Langen was a systems engineer hired at Hughes. But he, too, dabbled in screenwriting and later wrote the summer hits *Teenage Mutant Ninja Turtles (I & II).* And there is speech teacher Bruce Joel Rubin. Years of doing industrial films lead to such movie magnets as *Ghost* and *Jacob's Ladder.*

So, it's not always the bright pupil of UCLA film school who achieves the lifetime dream of scriptwriting success. Out of Hollywood, would-be writers number in the thousands but never undertake the risk of drafting and submitting a script because they expect instant rejection. But many touted writers started as nonmovie writers outside of tinsel town, and continue their new careers away from Hollywood. John Hughes, writer, producer, and director of *Sixteen Candles, Uncle Buck,* and *Home Alone,* resides in Illinois. Jim Cash, too, believes in the homestead. He's a Michigan resident who wrote *Top Gun, Secret of My Success, Legal Eagles,* and *Dick Tracy.* In other words, you don't have to quit your job, pack your bags and relocate for the ultimate experience of studio assignments. There are fax machines, E-Mail, modems, and overnight express that keep your finger on the pulse of the movie industry.

Chapters 11 and 12 provide the first steps in really deciding whether your expertise has potential for industrial, television, and feature-length screenwriting. There's no question that it does. It's just a matter of following basic steps, trusting your instincts, and stepping outside that safe boundary of routine clinical practice. Your insights into human behavior already are exceptional. Intuitively you know about human motivation and predictable patterns of behavior; that's what *character development* and *storyline* are all about. But you need to know how to package and sell these ideas. For starters, then, consider the many different writing avenues available to you in film entertainment.

Chapter 11

How to Write a Technical Script

Technical scriptwriting begins with an idea. Whether writing for industrial or full-length movies, first figure out *what sells.* Saleable educational scripts cover the basics–Math, English, Science, History and Social Sciences. Topics vary considerably, from first alphabet letters and animated adventures of historical heroes, to documentaries on AIDS prevention. Nonprofit or for-profit organizations with production budgets independently contract with freelance writers experienced or competent in these areas. Established educational publishers such as Macmillan, McGraw-Hill, Prentice-Hall, and Random House frequently recruit scriptwriters. *The Writer's Market* contains a small but informative section on educational film companies for starters.

Scripting needs especially arise in business and industry. Videos on human resource (HR) issues are selling like hotcakes. In the last ten years, corporate personnel policies took a beating for undersensitivity and lack of formal planning. Lawsuits tragically exposed the slack, disorganization, and inequities mounting in private and public sectors. Now HR management is in its reformation. State and federal mandates for policy development of fair and equal practices affect a gamut of long-time office problems from unethical conduct and employee burnout to health benefits. And that's where industrial movies get their origins.

The Anita Hill-Judge Thomas controversy electrically stimulated market needs for videos on sexual harassment. And with recessionary blues, videos sprung up all over on the messy task of laying off the workforce. Other labor blunders calling for video solutions included discrimination against disabled workers (i.e., the new American Disabilities Act), drug testing and employee selection, employment safety liabilities, and securing jobs for returning Persian Gulf veterans.

HR (Human Resources) executives now take a bottom-line approach: A class-act training is *demonstrating* new techniques to workers. That is why Five and Dime companies on up to Fortune 500 giants allocate big video-buying budgets, and are the central force behind industrial scriptwriting opportunities. Let us first consider how to pursue this avenue of writing before looking at the Hollywood connection.

FIND OUT WHAT'S NEEDED

Never guess what's hot in the market. Read up on business trends by skimming through several trade magazines and video catalogs. But don't be afraid to send inquiry letters, feeling out the market direction, tempo, and hunger for new scriptwriters. Landing an opportunity is far greater in industrial films because production turnover is faster and market demands can't keep up with supply.

Contact National and Local Video Production Studios

Take two approaches for national firms. First, figuring your expertise is saleable, send a general letter soliciting freelance writing assignments. Briefly describe who you are, why you contacted them, and previous scripts completed or expertise for scriptwriting (see Figure 11.1). Support your credentials with a tailor-made resume highlighting your scriptwriting, film, theater, or drama-related expertise (Figure 11.2).

But shooting into the wind may not be your style. Replies may vary, from "Sure, we'll keep you on file," to "No, thank you." So, alter the inquiry with a purpose in mind. Propose writing an educational video on your product or expertise, pitching its strong market potential and compatibility with the company's line of merchandise. For example, suppose a company specializes in safety and maintenance of foster care homes for developmentally disabled. Realizing the deinstitutionalization movement is still big news, pitch a videotape for fire safety instruction sold to home managers and community mental health centers (Figure 11.3).

FIGURE 11.1. Inquiry letter to industrial video producer

BEST IMPRESSIONS INTERNATIONAL INCORPORATED

4211 OKEMOS ROAD, SUITE 22, OKEMOS, MICHIGAN 48864, U.S.A.
FAX or PHONE: 517-347-0944; PHONE 1-800-595-BEST; local 347-1811

November 20, 1989

Mr. Kurt Anderson
Executive Vice President
Westwind Productions
1746 1/2 Westwood Blvd.
Los Angeles, CA 90024

Dear Mr. Anderson:

Looking for writers to work on assignment? I can offer you the best of two worlds.

Experienced writer (books, articles) and screenwriter plus research and professional degrees. Specialty in comedy, romance fantasy, and documentary/educational. From feature length to cable specials.

Ever try writers outside the California area? There's a special freshness to them. It's that Midwestern energy.

Synopses or treatments available upon request. You name the genre. In the meantime, please see the resume enclosed for your perusal.

Hope to hear from you soon.

Very sincerely,

Douglas Ruben, PhD

FIGURE 11.2. Resume for industrial video producers

Douglas H. Ruben, PhD

4211 Okemos Road, Suite 22
Okemos, MI 48864
517-347-1811/1-800-595-BEST

EDUCATION

PhD Clinical Psychology
MA Clinical Psychology
BA Psychology
Specialty Degrees

EXPERIENCE

Psychologist

Private practice
Instructor at colleges
Consultant for hospitals
Workshop/seminar trainer
Consultant for Businesses
Consultant for Government
Consultant for Education

Writer/Literary Agent

Consultant for Theater
President/Best Impressions,
   Intl./Speakers Bureau
Radio/TV Show Host
Self-help columnist
Greeting Cards/gags
Screenplays

PUBLICATIONS

Author, co-author, and editor of over 80 professional
articles and 16 books on adult and child psychology,
management systems, and rehabilitation. Citations
provided upon request.

REFERENCES

References provided upon request.

Never underestimate your talents for local firms. Around the corner are small video production studios doing local advertisements, campaign promotions, and contract jobs with TV news programs. Letter or telephone inquiries, there, are less effective than a face-to-face interview. Walk in and ask to speak to the president of the organization or talent director. Frequently they are on the premises or may return that day or within the week, available for a scheduled appointment. Introduce yourself as a local provider ("Just down the street from you . . . ") and media consultant branching out into technical scriptwriting. Check out their needs for freelancers.

Talent recruiters usually find actors and voice-overs from theatrical agents, local or statewide; writers do not have a broker to negotiate deals. They fend for themselves or gain visibility through industry word-of-mouth. Writers also are in-house staff who double as producer-editors and scriptwriters, done primarily to save money. But most producers prefer to be producers; most editors prefer their editorial duties only. That is why you may be surprised how interested a video shop may be in your pitch.

Resources on Educational/Training Video Trends and Companies

What should you read to get leads on what's hot and what's not? There are many avenues to take. First, pick up authoritative information on trends in personnel and human resource management, training, and development. Second, contact primary and secondary school librarians for the latest wave of educational videos. They know firsthand what grabs the attention of teachers and principals and what school districts consider prudent and moral purchases. Librarians can provide you with publisher and company names, addresses, and contacts guiding your initial groundwork. Third, in video stores, keep your eyes peeled to videoplayers running one-to two-minute trailers of upcoming CD-ROM and video releases using the showcase method used for theatrical motion pictures. Electronic press kits (EPKs) are catching on quickly as product displays. Fourth, make an inquiry at hospitals, agencies, or facilities you consult with regarding their choice for training videos and video companies.

FIGURE 11.3. Inquiry letter to educational video producer on fire safety

BEST IMPRESSIONS INTERNATIONAL INCORPORATED

4211 OKEMOS ROAD, SUITE 22, OKEMOS, MICHIGAN 48864, U.S.A.
FAX or PHONE: 517-347-0944; PHONE 1-800-595-BEST; local 347-1811

November 20, 1989

Mr. Julian Olansky, Manager
Fire Prevention Through Films, Inc.
Box 11
Newton Highlands, MA 02161

Dear Mr. Olansky:

Looking for a different slant on fire safety prevention? One with strong interest and guaranteed commercial success? I may have the answer.

How about fire prevention for the mentally retarded? Sure, training programs exist—but few if any exist in film and video. Imagine it. A training program sold to states, counties, schools, hospitals, group homes, foster homes—the list is unlimited. It presents basic method on teaching the retarded steps in (a) residential evacuation, and (b) safe use of appliances.

And here is the best part. You would have an experienced writer (books, articles) and screenwriter plus research plus human service degrees. Specialty in documentary/educational films. Full range from 10 mn to full-length.

Synopses or treatments available upon request. Work on assignment preferred. In the meantime, please see the resume enclosed for your perusal.

Hope to hear from you soon.

Very sincerely,

Douglas H. Ruben, PhD

In human resource videos, the best directions come from the following resources:

Human Resource Executive
An Axon Magazine Group Company
Circulation Department
747 Dresher Road
PO Box 980
Horsham, PA 19044-9787

Training & Development
American Society for Training and Development
1640 King Street, Box 1443
Alexandria, VA 22313-2043

The Writer's Market
Writer's Digest Books
F & W Publications, Inc.
1507 Dana Avenue
Cincinnati, OH 45207

Producers of educational, occupational, and technical videos are widely diverse and may change their specialties overnight in response to the buyers' market trends. Rating high in the human resource market are such topics as organizational engineering, accepting change, empowering employees, eliminating internal conflict, customer service, managing cultural diversity, developing caring leadership, and avoiding workplace violence. Here is a list of frequently consulted video firms either producing, distributing, or selling high-profile training videos to private and public industries:

American Media Inc.
1454 30th Street
West Des Moines, IA 50265-1390

Barr Films
12801 Schabarum Avenue
PO Box 7878
Irwindale, CA 91706-7878

Blanchard Training & Development, Inc.
125 State Place
Escondido, CA 92025

BNA Communications
9439 Key West Avenue
Rockville, MD 20850

Cally Curtis Company
1111 North Las Palmas Avenue
Hollywood, CA 90038

Charthouse International Learning Corporation
221 River Ridge Circle
Burnsville, MN 55337

Copeland Grigs Productions
302 23rd Avenue
San Francisco, CA 94121

Corporate Health Policies Group Inc.
7201 Wisconsin Avenue Suite 620
Bethesda, MD 20814

Dartnell
4600 Ravenswood Avenue
Chicago, IL 60640-9981

Development Dimensions International
1225 Washington Pike
Bridgeville, PA 15017

Ethics Resource Center, Inc.
600 New Hampshire Avenue NW
Washington, DC 20037

Films Inc.
5547 N. Ravenswood
Chicago, IL 60640-1199

Hospitality Television
609 W. Main Street
Louisville, KY 40202

Human Resource Development
Coronet/MTI
Film & Video
108 Wilmot Road
Deerfield, IL 60015-9925

Nathan/Taylor
535 Boylston St.
Boston, MA 02116

Personnel Decisions Inc.
2000 Plaza VII Tower
45 S. Seventh Street
Minneapolis, MN 55402

Salenger Films, Inc.
1635 Twelfth Street
Santa Monica, CA 90404

United Training Media
6633 W. Howard Street
Niles, IL 60648

Video Arts, Inc.
Northbrook Tech Center
4088 Commercial Avenue
Northbrook, IL 60062

Video Learning Resource Group
1000 Thomas Jefferson Street, NW
Washington, DC 20007

Just a word about *Hospitality Television (HTV)*. This uniquely innovative cable channel has capitalized on reaching overlooked job sites where staff training is next to impossible: in restaurants and hotels. Imagine it: a closed-circuit television network transmits training programs to restaurants and hotels by satellite. It delivers training to nearly nine million viewers who work irregular hours or whose shifts change seasonally. The network delivers five hours of programming a day, five days a week. Satellite receivers installed by HTV at the subscriber's sites pick up the signal, and devices similar to cable TV boxes unscramble the broadcast. Programs cover food and alcohol safety, customer-service issues, management skills, basic literacy, and other matters (sexual harassment, time management, etc.).

So, if this represents the *Jetsons* of tomorrow's high-tech training networks, stay tuned in for how you can become a part of it.

TECHNIQUE

Writing *certain things* can be very easy. Take a research paper. Manuscripts for publication follow clear and defined standards. You need a cover page, abstract (so many words), running head, title (so many words), introduction section, methods section, results section, and discussion section. Even figures and tables have specific instructions. Logistics are crystal clear and laid out in the authoritative bible called the *APA Style Manual.* How simple can you get? And, where professional journals slightly deviate from *APA* guidelines, editors kindly detail the different formats in the *author guidelines.* Everything is neat and tidy. So, enjoy it while it lasts.

Because it doesn't exist in this field, scriptwriting has no definite guidelines. No matter who defines the three-act structure, the 15- to 30-page turning point, 120-page limit, or dynamics of character development, some other writing guru will tell you these things are completely wrong. Video, TV, and movie writing is not a science. Writing follows some format standards, some principles of storyline, and manuscript presentation is uniformly in a three-hole bindery. But that's it. The writing masters who lecture or publish on scriptwriting all agree on this disagreement (e.g., Helitzer, 1986; Sautter, 1988; Seger, 1987; Wolff & Cox, 1988). They settle on one obvious fact: Technique lies in the individual's imagination and finesse at creating believable dialogue and storyline. Lecture maven Richard Walter (1988), for example, pushes the *art* or creative processes underlying script development before serious writers should really focus on the *craft.* But Walter is not an exception to the rule. Most Hollywood and industrial scriptwriters subscribe to this general belief that idea formation is the foundation of great success.

This approach may have its aesthetic benefits, but not for most scientifically trained mental and medical health providers. For them, it is a nightmare. Not having a cookbook on writing rules is like doing therapy without techniques. It simply isn't done. At least, not until you learn how to do it. So, where does one begin? Scriptwriting books offer an excellent starting point in spite of their conflicting advice. Books by Field (1979, 1984) particularly contain logistics on page set-up, organization of headings, paragraphs, actor/camera directions, and storyline strategies. Second, get insight on formatting, plot developments that sell, and pitching strengths and weaknesses directly from the horse's mouth: Take a weekend seminar on scriptwriting.

Workshops

Workshops are *experiences you've never had before.* No workshop at professional conventions will ever compare to the entertaining lecture and unbelievable wealth of do's and don'ts that make or break a million dollar deal. Even no-money-down real estate seminars will seem boring after finishing an electrically charged "here's-how-to-do-it" scriptwriting session. Think seriously about attending one when it comes to your town. Below are the headliners in the industry who run monthly, bimonthly, or frequent classes depending on their own schedule and preenrollment figures. Contact them directly to receive a list of class dates and locations, and preliminary materials explaining why their training course is better than the competitors'.

African-American Screenwriters
Bill and Camille Cosby have established the Guy Alexander Hanks and Marvin Miller Screenwriting Program at the USC School of Cinema-Television. This 15-week workshop is to help experienced African-American sceenwriters to complete a film or television script. First workshop begins in March, 1995. Instructor: varies. Contact: 213-740-8194 for application (participation is free of charge to those selected).

The Craft of Comedy Writing
Eight weekly classes, three hours each (or three-day weekend class) covers (a) overview of comedy television writing, (b) methods of selling comedy, and (c) learning comedy that works. Instructor: Danny Simon. Contact: Danny Simon, 15233 Magnolia Blvd., #302, Sherman Oaks, CA 91403 ($300).

Creative Workshop
David Freeman's two-day workshop demonstrating over 200 powerful techniques and hands-on exercises to (a) develop saleable ideas and plots, (b) write luminous dialogue, (c) create unforgettable characters, and (d) improve your pitching ability. Instructor:

David Freeman. Contact: David Freeman, 310-478-6552 (price not listed).

Heidi Wall's Fast Forward
An eight-week seminar for the entertainment industry that teaches structure for theatrical writing, selling, pitching, and career-hunting in Hollywood according to its implicit rules of the game. Also offered as intensive two-day workshop. Instructor: Heidi Wall. Contact: Fast Forward, 235 N. Valley Street, Suite #230, Burbank, CA 91505 (eight-week = $295; two-day= $195).

Making a Good Script Great
One-day workshop teaches (a) troubleshooting script problems, (b) basics of scriptwriting following a creative process, (c) guidelines on reaching the studios. Instructor: Linda Seger. Dr. Linda Seger, 2038 Louella Avenue, Venice, CA 90291 ($75 to $95).

Screenwriting: The Whole Picture
Two-day workshop covers (a) plot development and basics for screenwriting, (b) using creative process, and (c) the pitch and selling the screenplay. Instructor will read all screenplays by participants. Instructor: Richard Walter. Contact: UCLA Department of Film and TV, Los Angeles, CA 90024-1622 ($250).

Screenwriting: Writing from the Heart
Two-day workshop covers (a) three-act structure and character development, and (b) pitching the screenplay to producers. Instructor: Jurgen Wolff. Contact: Jurgen Wolff Seminars, c/o *The Hollywood Scriptwriter,* 1626 N. Wilcox #385, Hollywood, CA 90028 ($150).

Scriptwriting for the 90s:
Selling Your Script to Hollywood
Two-day lecture covers (a) steps to begin career as screenwriter, (b) essential components of saleable, quality script, and (c) selling

script in commercial market. Instructor: Michael Hauge. Contact: Hilltop Productions, 5250 Lemona Avenue, Suite 1000, Van Nuys, CA 91411 ($145-$185).

Story Structure
Three-day workshop covers (a) essential writing concepts, (b) editing and plot development to final manuscript, and (c) stage direction and analytical screening of classic movie. Instructor: Robert McKee. Contact: Two Arts, Inc., 12021 Wilshire Boulevard, Suite 868, Los Angeles, CA 90025 ($375).

Writing for Hollywood
Three-day workshop covers (a) how to structure your screenplay, (b) how to market your screenplay and yourself, and (c) mini-workshops and networking. Instructors: Rachael Ballon; Carole Bennett; Scott Frank, and Don Halperin. Contact: G/R Advertising, 1030 N. State, Suite 46A, Chicago, IL 60610 ($199).

UCLA Extension
Classes offered every term are taught by producers, writers, and agents who share their knowledge and Hollywood insights with aspiring students. Information on enrollment, tuition, and residency may be obtained by contacting The Writer's Program, UCLA Extension, 10995 Le Conte Avenue, #313-W, Los Angeles, CA 90024-2883. Send it ATT: Terry, to receive a free copy of the *Writer's Program Quarterly,* with information about upcoming classes, the Certificate Program in Writing for Film and Television, and the Writing Consultation and Manuscript Evaluation Programs.

How to Write the Feature-Length Movie Script

A screenplay for a typical two-hour television or feature-length movie is about 120 pages long. That's one minute per page. The majority of scripts range from 110 to 115 pages in length. Timing of a script is an art in itself. Over the years, taking into account variations in camera work and production techniques, it has become customary to think of pages of a screenplay as the visual rehearsal of actors and directors. Words dictate physical movement, scene changes, camera angles, stage direction, and dialogue. Scenes are numbered. This usually occurs during the final stage of preproduction rather than in initial draft of the screenplay. But standards vary according to studio preference.

You can describe camera angles at the left corner, in capitals, such as INSERT, REVERSE ANGLE, and DISSOLVE, although scenes commonly open with inside or outside shots (INT. or EXT.), the location, and whether it is daytime or nighttime (DAY or NIGHT). Other fancy angle shots such as CLOSEUPS and POV (point of view) get too mind-boggling for first-time writers and are unnecessary for drafts. Unless you have a very definite vision of what a particular shot has to be and know the jargon for it, leave all the fancy camera angles to the technical staff. Directors, editors, and cinematographers devise imaginative cuts that you may never think of. Figure 11.4 gives you an idea of how the page appears.

Plot development goes in all different directions. Probably the best advice on learning story line twists and turns, from Hitchcock horror to Neil Simon comedy is to directly consult books that elaborate on style. Formula plots really do not exist, although daytime soap operas come close to making us believers. How "girl-meets boy" and "boy gets caught in espionage" takes more than a devious bit of mental gymnastics. Careful reasoning and subplot twists go into the total chemistry of characters who rise and fall through scores of predictable and ironic events. *True Lies,* the Schwarzenegger-Curtis romance spy-thriller, for example, detours along several subpaths, building up suspense in the happy couple's lives.

Some writers use notecards to organize plots and subplots, entirely formulating the events before typing away. Other scriptwriters regard notecards as mental impediments. They instead improvise along from one line to the next. You can choose which is the best way for yourself.

The value you bring to rendering a clever story and character is your insight on human behavior and motivation. For example, suppose you're scripting a story about an abused wife of an alcoholic who threatens to leave her husband if physically assaulted again.

FIGURE 11.4. Page from film screenplay

EXT FRONT DOOR OF SAM'S APARTMENT BLDG.
MORNING

SAM waiting nervously outside. Car arrives. JENNY is
32 yrs. old, pretty. Dashes into JENNY'S car and scene
opens with two riding together.

                    SAM
        (Sarcastic)
        Glad you made it.

                    JENNY
        Get off it, Sam. You knew I'd
        be here, didn't you?

                    SAM
        Getting here and getting here
        on time are worlds apart.

                    JENNY
        Oh, take it easy. We're still on
        time.

                    SAM
        You could have told me you were
        running late. Or were you still
        sleeping?

                    JENNY
        No, I didn't sleep this morning.
        Remember? I was listening to
        Cinderella talk about her royal
        ball.

                    SAM
        Fine, I'll never call you again.

                    JENNY
        Promises, promises.

                    SAM
        Lay off it, Jenny.

You write an assault scene, and in the next scene you have her *still refusing to leave her husband.* Now, lay readers might say your character is unrealistic, that *all people would leave after repeated brutality.* But you know better. You know that caretakers or "enablers" suffer through intolerable odds hoping to rescue the alcoholic spouse and are afraid to leave out of guilt. That's statistically the valid motivation for this behavior. And your insight assures an accurate character portrayal.

How to Write the Industrial Script

Educational and industrial scriptwriting is less formal and much shorter. Character development, story line, and many other variables forming the 120-minute script are dropped. Technical scripts vary from 15 minutes (15 to 30 pages) to 30 minutes (30 to 60 pages). One page, including camera instructions, equals about two minutes. Scripts use several animation and graphic overlay features. Animation softens the brute facts about some idea, while graphics illustrate the idea numerically for easier learning. Dialogue is used sparingly, usually in "vignettes" or "demo" scenes that act out solutions to a problem. Industrial scripts instead describe different SHIFTS in camera angles and when the spokesperson is talking while action takes place or as a Voice-Over (V.O.). Note in Figure 11.5 the scene opens up and is followed by camera instructions about one person's actions, while another person is heard as a voice-over.

Computer Scriptwriting Programs

Scripting by images and with ambiguous guidelines is cumbersome. You must have a vivid imagination and good retentive memory to keep first level and second level plots distinct and the story line in order. Imagination is just as taxing in educational and industrial films. Here you teach new concepts, present new facts, demonstrate those facts, and must keep the material simple and logical for comprehension. So, the last problems in the world you need are mechanical hassles. A bad typewriter or old word processor will drive you crazy, with all the indentations, capitalizations, up

FIGURE 11.5. Page from educational script

INT. KITCHEN–DAY

PARENT 7 WALKS INTO KITCHEN, THEN
SITS DOWN. SHE TIGHTENS AND LOOSENS
NECK. TIGHTENS AND LOOSENS SHOULDERS,
TIGHTENS AND LOOSENS ARMS, OTHER
BODY PARTS FITTING RUBEN V.O.

RUBEN
(V.O.)
So, here's what you gotta do. Figure out
which muscle area is hurting. Then,
tighten it some more, and release it. Start
with your neck, then your shoulders. Do
your arms and hands. Feel good all over.

SHIFT TO GRAPHIC WITH RUBEN V.O.

RUBEN
(V.O.)
Number three. Laugh at your mistakes.

INT. FAMILY ROOM–DAY

PARENT 4
(Sitting)
Can you do that? Can you laugh at your
mistakes?

(ANGLE CLOSE UP)
You need to. Mistakes are normal. Say to
yourself, "It's okay to goof; I'm only
human."

SHIFT TO TESTIMONIAL.

PARENT 5
When I admit I made a mistake, I take
the pressure off. And I don't feel angry
anymore. Because I have nothing to be
angry about.

INT. KITCHEN–DAY

PARENT 5 TALKS TO CHILD. CHILD REMAINS
SILENT.

PARENT 5
(Standing)
I'm sorry. I got angry when I shouldn't
have.

and down movements, and corrections needed. It's one or the other: either you concentrate on writing, or you concentrate on operating equipment. Both won't work. And thankfully, modern computer technology has come up with a solution.

Many scriptwriters now use efficient software programs for writing. On IBM, IBM-compatibles and Macintosh, programs automatically format camera angles, character directions, dialogue, scenes, pagination, and even will time the length of the screenplay. Other software programs are idea brainstormers, generating new plots, new character dimensions, and may troubleshoot your writer's block. Supplementary programs round out the scriptwriter's arsenal of tools to forge ahead under deadlines and not be disturbed by idea droughts and mechanical hang-ups.

Advantages thus are manifold; but the biggest problem with writing software is that these programs are in their infancy. Five years ago writing software was a dream. Today they've become a booming business advertised in all the Hollywood trades as the greatest thing since peanut butter. But the fanfare is for commercial propaganda, not because the program has years of test validity. That means you have to weigh the pros and cons of each tempting program. Table 11.1 lists the prominent software programs available to scriptwriters. Call or write to the company for free brochures and further information on computer requirements.

TABLE 11.1. Scriptwriting software programs

Software	Purpose	Requires	Price	Contact
InfoSelect	Organize notes	IBM XT, AT, PS/2, DOS 2.0	$149.95	Micrologic, PO Box 70 Hackensack, NJ 07602
Final Draft	Script processor	Macintosh	$349	Mac Toolkit 606 Willshire Blvd., Ste 604 Santa Monica, CA 90401
Ideafisher	Thesaurus of ideas	IBM PC/XT/AT, DOS 3.1; also Macintosh	Unavailable	Fisher Idea Systems, Inc. 18881 Von Karman Ave, Ste 100 Irving, CA 92715
StoryLine	Chart structure of story & plot	PC (640K), DOS3. or Macintosh (2MB)	$345 Demo-$10	US: 1-800-33-TRUBY CA: 310-575-3050
Superscript Pro	Scriptwriting	Wordperfect 5.1, IBM	$159	ITE Technologies 1800 S. Robertson Blvd., Ste 326-W Los Angeles, CA 90035
Scriptware	Script formatting	IBM PC/XT/AT, DOS 3.0	$299.95 Demo-$9.95	1-800-788-7090
Plots Unlimited	Generates story ideas	IBM (640 RAM), DOS 3.0 Macintosh (1-2 MB)	$399 Demo-$9.95	1-800-833-PLOT
WritePro	Writing tutorial program	IBM PC/XT/AT, DOS 3.0, Macintosh (1-2 MB)	IBM-$79.95 Mac-$99.95	1-800-755-1124
Script Perfection	Converts Wordperfect into Screenplay	IBM, Wordperfect 5.0	$95	1-212-855-8640
Movie Master	Screenplay & Teleplay	IBM PC/XT/AT, DOS 3.0	Unavailable	1-800-526-0242
Scriptor 4.0	Screenplay & Teleplay	IBM PC/XT/AT, DOS 3.0, Macintosh (1-2 MB)	Unavailable	Screenplay Systems 150 E. Olive Ave Ste 203 Burbank, CA 91591
Dramatica	Storyforming & Storytelling	IBM, Macintosh	Unavailable	Screenplay Systems 150 E. Olive Ave. Ste 203 Burbank, CA 91591 1-800-84-STORY
Script Thing	Script processor	Wordperfect, Microsoft Word, IBM-Windows, Macintosh	$149	ScriptPerfection Enterprises 3061 Massasoit San Diego, CA 92117-2522 619-270-7515

Chapter 12

Selling Yourself in the Movies

Does this whole idea of writing for the movies still boggle your mind? You still can't help wondering, "Why in the world would a Hollywood producer give two cents about my expertise or screenplay?" Here you are, some 2,000 miles away from California, and you know that out of 10,000 scripts sent annually to agents and production companies, only a handful get through the first cut. And less than a handful pass the second cut. Heaven only knows how few reach the magical step of preproduction. Of the nearly 600 movies made in 1993, several thousand times that number of aspiring screenwriters received rejection letters. So, at these odds, is your luck better at being hit by lightening? Maybe it is. But that's if you take a passive or wait-and-see approach to selling yourself in the movies.

There are more ways than one to skin a cat. And selling your expertise and screenplay is the same thing. Luring Hollywood to your talent involves a series of stepwise strategies, all aimed at beating the UCLA film school prodigies and the sons and daughters of actors and directors. If you *want in, you must push to get in; but push sensibly and through doors of opportunities that only you can get through.* Consider in this section many different strengths you have over competitors and how you might maximize them.

MEDIA PSYCHOLOGIST

What is a *media psychologist?* It is a script consultant able to analyze a character's motivation and actions for believability. In *Silence of the Lambs,* who do you think the writers consulted on Hannibal the Cannibal's dialogue? In the *Psycho*-thrillers, accuracy made up half the suspense. Scripts that are psychologically accurate are commercially more powerful. Take a social problem, such as that depicted in *Boyz 'N the Hood.* Who verified the writer's and director's gut feelings about how oppressed characters might rebel or overcome rebellious attitudes? The media psychologist (social worker or consultant) saves script researchers enormous time and effort digging for reasons to explain behavior. As consultant, you serve as advisor on TV and film productions and may work individually with actors, helping them identify with feelings and sensations for a role.

Media consulting is a wonderful way to expose your expertise *before* you embark on scriptwriting. Writers can get a behind-the-scenes look at movie making and the politics and personalities of actors and producers. Insider information abounds: who to talk to and who to stay away from–all of these pointers shape your perceptions of the industry. This awareness frequently desensitizes the self-defeating shyness of writing ambitions. It also lends insight into *what directors and companies want in the way of commercial scripts.* Better still, your credibility is instantly established in front of powerful decision makers who not only trust your opinion but may also trust your script proposals.

Who to Contact

Media consulting for mental health providers is a relatively new field. Some are California-and New York-based therapists who already were treating people in cinema and just expanded their practice to group consulting. Other therapists had HMO agreements with the Screen Actors Guild (SAG) and, again, broadened their contacts from actors to producers and directors. While psychologists always have been in the media, their specialized role as film consultants charts a new direction open for competition.

The first step to build a media consultant practice is asking yourself which types of movies or TV shows you want to work on: Educational/industrial, or feature length? If the former, send an inquiry letter to the production companies with intentions to follow up by telephone in two weeks. For feature-length movies, first read through the *Daily* (or weekly) *Variety* under the Film Production Chart. Note the films currently in progress and whether the titles intuitively fit your expertise. Send a letter to the name of the executive producer listed under each movie title. Address the letter to the production company; addresses are found in the *Hollywood Creative Directory* or other reliable movie industry resources (see below). For TV shows, get a copy of *The Journal of the Writer's Guild of America, West.* Flip to the pages of the TV Market List. Named are all the TV shows currently in production with contact names and telephone numbers.

Remember to pitch your idea strongly but succinctly, and get their permission to send follow-up credentials. In those credentials, offer the names of local, regional, or national TV, radio, or celebrity personalities with whom you've worked and can testify on behalf of your consulting services.

State Office

Is it too risky? Does it still feel like a long shot? Okay, try a shortcut. Did you know there is a film commission in every state, even in large cities who are a heartbeat away from Hollywood? Michigan, for instance, has two film offices. One is the Michigan Film Office in the capital city of Lansing; the other is inside the Detroit Mayor's office. Officials work hand-in-hand with producers who plan on filming in the state. Remember *Anatomy of a Murder?* How about the secret romance of *Somewhere in Time?* And the blockbusters *Beverly Hills Cop I & II?* Two years ago *Hoffa* finished its filming in Detroit. All of these movies set up production schedules and authorizations through city and state public offices. How can you work with these offices? Local contacts *always are easier than national contacts.*

First set up an appointment with the director of the film office. Indicate at the meeting your expertise at understanding the personality and culture of state residents and how valuable this knowledge can be to visiting productions. Suggest that the state office offer this service as a fringe benefit to lure new film business when, for example, they attend Hollywood conventions and exhibit their prospects (e.g., Association of Film Commissioners International).

SELLING THE MOTION PICTURE

You're never really *done* with a script. You're just temporarily finished with it. Scriptwriting is a continuous process from idea formation to revising multiple drafts in preproduction and during production. The working copy is a mess. Actors, directors, cinematographers, and other writers fuss over dialogue and stage direction, knowing that a quality movie requires healthy flexibility. Even on educational and industrial films, visualizing what really happens in proper sequence may require editing and re-editing. And so the job of scriptwriting is never over.

But early in the imperfect stages of the script you may consider sending feelers out to production companies. A positive reply is better than no oasis in the middle of the desert. But be patient. First finish your script and protect it. Then after it is WGA protected, send it off for review. This is the beginning of a new career and it involves the beginning of many new self-promotion strategies.

Protecting Your Screenplay

There are many forms of manuscript protection in the United States and abroad. Most original literary works published in standard print media have a copyright register with the Library Congress in Washington. But that's not the ordinary form of protection in the movie and TV industry. Television scripts, outlines, and treatments, ideas for game shows, and the like are protected by registration with the Writers Guild of America (WGA), or more specifically, the Writers Guild of America, West (WGAW). Guild registration is available to members and nonmembers of the guild.

Registering your manuscript and ideas is for two reasons. First, it times, dates, and identifies your creative effort as your own. That way, if there is ever any dispute as to the authorship of a work, or the time it was created, WGA officials simply look at the WGA registration to make the determination. That's what propelled columnist Art Buchwald to an unprecedented legal victory over Paramount on credit rights for the Eddie Murphy hit *Coming to America.* Second, WGA registration shows producers that you have the foresight to protect your property.

Send one 8 1/2″ x 11″ unbound (no brads, staples, etc.) copy of the script, treatment, outline, or other material for deposit in the Guild files, along with a cover sheet that includes the title of the material, your full legal name, and social security number, plus a check payable to WGAW for $20.00 (for nonmembers) or $10 (for

WGAW and WGAE (East) members) to WGA Registration, 8955 Beverly Blvd., West Hollywood, CA 90048-2456. Your material, when received, is sealed, dated, and recorded. A numbered receipt is documentation of registration. Registration is valid for five years. After that, WGAW automatically destroys the material unless the term of registration is renewed for another five-year or ten-year term at the current registration rate.

On documents sent to producers, use the wording: REGISTERED WGAW NO._____ . This wording appears on the front cover or on release forms.

Inquiries to Independent Producers

Now your screenplay is legitimate. But tougher terrain lies ahead. Sending out inquiry letters to independent producers is different from other inquiry letters. When pitching for radio, TV, and books, an electric opening and four to five paragraphs sufficiently conveyed your message. Now try conveying the message in fewer words, fewer paragraphs, and with bigger hooks. Debuting your name and screenplay is an art in semantics (Figure 12.1). First, open the letter with an inquiry. Ask whether producers are looking for your movie genre (comedy, drama, romance fiction, etc.). Enhance the genre by comparing your screenplay to box office hits within a two- to three-year period. The more recent, the better.

Begin the second paragraph briefly describing the story line or protagonist's dilemma. Boldface, capitalize, or italicize the character's name for added emphasis. The third paragraph is your megaphone. Write clearly but convincingly why your credentials are perfect for the screenplay. Use levity, if you can, to soften perceptions of arrogance and imply a humble personality. Prospective producers certainly want informed writers but also writers that are flexible, adaptable, and calm under pressure. Finally, ask the producer if you can send the script for "consideration."

For quicker transmission, resort to the fax approach. Alert producers specializing in your genre (e.g., features direct to video, commercial, infomercial, animation, motion picture, etc.) with a splashier headline and shorter description that is bound to feed their impulse-buying frenzy (Figure 12.2). West Coast producers, contrary to popular opinion, are always on the lookout for non-L.A.

FIGURE 12.1. Inquiry letter for screenplay submission

BEST IMPRESSIONS INTERNATIONAL INCORPORATED
4211 OKEMOS ROAD, SUITE 22, OKEMOS, MICHIGAN 48864, U.S.A.
PHONE OR FAX: 517-347-0944; TELEPHONE: 1-800-595-BEST

September 17, 1993

Raymond Zamora, Producer
Sunrise Pictures
1945 W. Commonwealth Ave.
Unit E
Fullerton, CA 92633

Dear Mr. Zamora:

Looking for a feature length comedy? Where a little truth never hurts? Welcome to the government. First came *9 to 5,* then *Working Girl*, then *Article 99.* Now it's ***UnCivil Service***.

What's so civil about service? Not much. That's what Samantha discovers. She's bright and eager. And the only one who is. But it's too late for her to quit and too soon to beat the system. So she'll get even *her own way.* That's ***UnCivil Service***. A comical look at who really works in government.

The authors know their subject well. One works in civil service—try nearly 20 yrs. And the other, well, he's a psychologist who treats civil servants. Together the authors have 30 books including self-help, fiction, and a screenplay. In fact, Doug Ruben recently was on DONAHUE.

Enclosed please find a synopsis for initial review.

May we send you the script for your consideration?

Cordially,

Douglas H. Ruben

FIGURE 12.2. Faxed inquiry letter for screenplay

BEST IMPRESSIONS INTERNATIONAL INCORPORATED

4211 OKEMOS ROAD, SUITE 22, OKEMOS, MICHIGAN 48864, U.S.A.
TELEPHONE or FAX: 517-347-0944, or 1-800-595-BEST

FAX COVER SHEET

DATE: 7-18-94
ATTENTION: Timothy Cogshell, MYTHIC IMAGE PRODS
FAX NUMBER: 818 766 6681
FROM: Paul Smith, Best Impressions International Inc
NOTES: For the best FEATURE DIRECT TO VIDEO, please consider–

SEDUCING SPIRITS

***Just published*–**a chilling horror about a missionary family caught in the web of satanic cults. Gripping like *The Unholy.* Filled with terrifying plot twists like *Serpent and the Rainbow.* Now available for screenplay adaptation.

Authors Osman & Ruben can write the screenplay. Ruben is author of over 31 books and two screenplays. Ruben just appeared on *Donahue.*

Authors Marilyn Osman and D. Ruben's book *Seducing Spirits* (Northwest Publishing) explores ancient lore of demonic assaults. Possession of the youngest son mysteriously coincides with an epidemic of pregnancies. But the offspring are growing too fast, and forming a strange empire out of control. Human sacrifice, murder, and mayhem result when good battles evil in a confrontation that shakes a small community.

For synopsis and info, call 1-800-595-BEST (mailbox-Ruben) or fax request at 517 347 0944

writers so they can break out of their comfortable nucleus of local talent. Especially for story editors or contacts on the road in between shootings, fax relays can bypass the sludge pile of over-the-transom submissions read through at a later time.

Inquiry letters sent ahead of the scripts are always advisable. Even ads specifically requesting the full screenplay (and SASE) should be initially answered with a letter. Receive approval for your idea, first, before running up a postage bill of expensive mailings. Second, an affirmative reply allows you to open your reply letter with "Thank you for requesting," which suggests an invitational status over an over-the-transom one (Figure 12.3). Invited screenplays get read or sent to script analysts faster because the producer *already showed interest in its prospects.*

Now, you may wonder, "Who do you actually send the script to?" Small companies listing only one or two producers and clerical staff are easy to figure out; address inquiries directly to the producer or executive producer. But larger companies list many varieties of administrative titles, from managers and development writers to production staff. Layers of administrative levels also appear: presidents, vice-presidents, and assistants. Key personnel, however, include story editors, writers, directors of creative affairs, and acquisitions of new properties. These role players create new ideas, new directions, and sift through the dense jungle of over-the-transom and invited screenplays, advancing commercially promising ones to the front office. Other prominent personnel may be gender-specific. If two story editors are listed–one male, one female–address your inquiry to the gender similar to your protagonist. It may seem a waste of postage, but realize that inquiries stand a 50-50 chance of being tossed for a basket in file 13; blocking this free throw will depend on whether the reader can *identify with what you're saying and who you're saying it about.* You will be surprised how many favorable replies come from the gender who says to himself or herself, "Yeah, now that's a story I can relate to."

Odds at inferring the right message play another role in your inquiry letter and later in the review of your screenplay. Who really reads the screenplay page by page? That's easy: Story editors and the other people to whom scripts are sent, right? No, not always. Readers are like Oscar voters. Revealed this year was the shocking truth that Oscar committee members gave their ballots to spouses and close friends.

FIGURE 12.3. Reply letter for screenplay submission

BEST IMPRESSIONS INTERNATIONAL INCORPORATED

4211 OKEMOS ROAD, SUITE 22, OKEMOS, MICHIGAN 48864, U.S.A.
TELEPHONE: 517-347-0944

November 30, 1990

Mr. Michael Stipanich
Writers and Artists Agency
11726 San Vicente Blvd.
Suite 300
Los Angeles, CA 90049

Dear Mr. Stipanich:

Thank you for requesting our screenplay, *UnCivil Service*.

UnCivil Service-It's like striking oil on a subject just waiting to be tapped.

Enclosed is the screenplay and release form.

We look forward to your reply and hopefully working together.

Very sincerely,

Douglas H. Ruben
Best Impressions International Inc.

They, themselves, did not cast the ballot. Likewise, script readers range from the producer's spouses, girlfriends, boyfriends, secretaries, even tailors and car repairmen. Why all these people? There are two reasons. First, there is no time available; hectic daily schedules in independent and heavyweight companies entirely squeeze out personal relaxing time to read screenplays. Second, does it really take special qualifications to figure out if a script has commercial possibility? No. Everybody goes to the movies. So, everybody can make a reasonably intuitive guess on good and bad screenplays. In fact, less technically minded readers are more impartial to screenplay quality. That means you never know who first liked your script. But it doesn't matter. Somebody liked it, and that's all that counts.

Synopsis, Treatments, and Outlines

Reading through every page of the screenplay is an arduous task–one that many producers do not have time for. They want a telegraphic overview of who the key characters are, plot development, technical or cinematographic requirements, and a market concept: Will the story sell? Frequently they can gauge these projections from a treatment, synopsis, or outline instead of from the screenplay itself. In fact, producers sold on the screenplay idea may offer to buy the screenplay entirely on speculation or *on spec,* meaning they retain the rights to the first drafted screenplay for a price. Prices vary from the standard $3,000 to outrageous five- and six-digit figures for screenplays bought on spec. Properties bought on spec may even be different from the material you sent in. Producers may dislike your one story line but feel your creative writing potential is worth investing in for another project under consideration.

Getting to that point begins with knowing what a synopsis, treatment, and outlines are. *Synopses* are one- to two-page summaries of major plots and subplots, describing pivotals in character development (Figure 12.4). *Treatments* are three- to five-page descriptions of the story idea in narrative form. Treatments include a broad brush of the key features of a story idea, containing a list of main characters described in 20 words or less. *Outlines* are when you get into multipaged, longer narratives. This detailed rendering of a story runs between 20 and 50 pages. Paragraphs are placed between what are called "master scenes," or overall settings of action. Although

FIGURE 12.4. Synopsis of screenplay

UnCivil Service
Screeplay by Douglas & Marilyn Ruben

Zealous female executive SAMANTHA (SAM) (35 yrs old) excited for her first day in a state rehabilitation office. Promised a high position, great career move. Her arrogant male counterpart JASON (30-ish) also will work there. Both shown getting ready in morning. She's immaculate, he's a slob.

SAM gets a ride with her best friend JENNY, JENNY's late and speeds through town. Car just misses collision with JASON's car. JASON stumbles out, shocked, and sarcastically greets them. He embarrasses SAM.

SAM and JENNY are late for work. Both are coworkers. SAM rushes into conference room to meet her new boss. She thinks it's the wrong room. But it's not. Greets 10 handicapped people sitting around an oval table. All of them doing peculiar things. One man in motorized wheelchair clicking it forward and backwards. Two people with prosthetic arms shaking them up and down. A blind man is listening to his talking watch announce the time followed by a John Sousa march. And worst, her boss HAROLD speaks doubletalk and makes no sense. SAM tries to leave but is trapped. She's told her job is to find jobs for these people. This blows her expectations. This isn't why she was hired. But, oh well, for now.

After meeting, SAM bumps into her secretary THELMA, who warns the office is chaotic and her boss is Freddy Kruger's worst nightmare. She says, "consider me your bodyguard." Both overhear loud fight between complaining employee GRACE and HAROLD.

HAROLD introduces SAM to her job partner. Guess who–JASON. His sarcasm and innuendos piss her off. SAM rebuffs it. He's in shock. Sets him straight for now.

SAM tells JENNY she hates her job, hates her life, hates her boss. She's in hell. JENNY corrects her–"No, you're in the civil service." SHIFT to blind client FRANK threatening to beat up rehab counselor BRAD with his cane unless BRAD gets him a real job. BRAD got him a job as a dishwasher. But FRANK has a masters and PhD–he's slightly pissed.

SAM meets JERRY–office sleaze and moocher. He tells sob story that SAM falls for and she lends him money. SHIFT to HAROLD asking JASON if he can handle the "employee placement" project. The one he's doing with SAM. Space-ranger JASON assures him. JASON then gets the inside scoop from co-worker TOM on how to pad the travelog.

SHIFT to THELMA telling GRACE that SAM's working too hard while JASON's loafing. JERRY bops in and tries to swindle THELMA. It backfires big-time. JERRY's humiliated. SAM hears from THELMA she's been suckered from JERRY. Told to beware of future scams.

Exhausted SAM stumbles into elevator onto wheelchair client NEAL. THELMA behind her. She apologizes for bumping him. Told he's paralyzed from waist down. Caring, she rubs what she thinks is his side she bruised. NEAL loves it. SAM figures he can't feel it. THELMA breaks the news. He can. It's not his thigh–it's his penis. SAM's embarrassed.

FIGURE 12.4. (continued)

SHIFT to montage of scenes of SAM getting jobs for rehab clients. SAM on the phone, in person, signing papers with, presenting flow charts for, shaking hands with store owners, factory VIPs. After each scene see her check off another client name on list. She finishes placement job in record time.

SAM confronts JASON on being lazy. She leaves office early. It's the weekend. JASON tricks SAM into letting him into her apartment. SAM resists his sexual advances. He promises to leave after using the bathroom. Comes out naked and gives SAM a bear hug. Disgusted, SAM kicks him out.

Monday SAM gets wind of lottery scam in office. Gambling in civil service is illegal, but oh well. Staff figure JERRY stole winning ticket they all paid for. Time for revenge. Coworker TOM tells JERRY police are after him. He better empty his desk belongings in TOM's bag and get out quick. JERRY panics. He does it. Staff recover the stolen ticket. Just then HAROLD calls SAM into office. Tells her she's a trooper, did great job, but no promotion. It's a guy thing. JASON gets promotion instead. SAM loses it. HAROLD gets pompous. SAM tells him "he has no balls." Proves it by grabbing him between the legs. HAROLD moans. SAM quips, "Harold, you do have balls!" She's suspended without pay.

SAM ends up in a bar. Drunk. Union man DEACON calms her down. Says he can turn things around and get her back to work. It happens. Time passes. Three weeks later JASON is screwing up the office. JENNY, SAM, DEACON plot against HAROLD and JASON. At mall SAM explains how they'll invite handicapped people to a conference that doesn't exist. State won't approve it but HAROLD and JASON won't know. They'll beef up egos of HAROLD and JASON by letting them be head honchos of the conference. SAM also tells JENNY she "lusts" for DEACON.

Plan gets into motion. JASON gets off on being conference director. HAROLD is high as a kite on being executive director of conference. Both fall into trap. Later that night DEACON meets SAM to talk strategy. Talk turns to lust as both make love.

One week later the sting is pulled off. SAM tricks JASON into inviting TV and radio stations to conference. SAM lets JASON brag to media that conference was all his idea. But just as things get going, SAM sees news headlines that DEACON was indicted for fraud. Learns he took the rap for a con artist. Con artist was HAROLD. Now SAM and DEACON go full force to retaliate. TV and radio stations converge on the lawn. Downtown near the Rehab building there's traffic jams. Eight thousand handicapped people crowding the streets, on front lawn of building, looking for conference. JASON and HAROLD cornered by media. They panic. DEACON slips in question about his embezzlement. HAROLD's exposed. Tries to run, but can't. That's when GOVERNOR enters. GOVERNOR fires HAROLD, fires JASON, and puts SAM in charge.

LAST SCENE is SAM interviewing zealous female executive BECKY for a job. Tells her to chill out. BECKY reminds SAM of herself. BECKY promises to be efficient. "Not here," says SAM, "not in the uncivil service." Both laugh and FADE OUT.

longer, outlines must still be clear and compelling to be taken seriously. As a rule of thumb, then, keep outlines short like a synopsis. Not only will it probably be read, but your brevity will show off your writing expertise and ability to "cut to the chase."

Rejections, Agreement, and Release Forms

Rejection letters come in all types and sizes. Many politely refuse your idea or screenplay because it doesn't fit the studio's direction; others state they are not accepting unsolicited screenplays at this time. Still others take a different angle; they refuse the idea or screenplay for "legal reasons." By "legal reasons" is meant the risk of liability of considering unsolicited properties that writers later claim were the groundwork for blockbuster hits. Historically, unemployed writers never were outspoken about their materials being stolen by studios. But mammoth out-of-court settlements in the last decade have prompted overprotective steps to assure that writers know beforehand that, *if their screenplay is reviewed, that review does not constitute an agreement and that producer is not entitled to any material related to the screenplay unless explicitly worded in a formal contract.* This stipulation is to prevent claims of plagiarism asserted against motion picture producers. As a result, studios make a hard and fast rule that their employees never read nor consider unsolicited literary material, musical compositions, lyrics, ideas, or suggestions of any nature whatsoever unless submitted through a recognized (WGA) literary agent.

One rejection letter from Twentieth-Century Fox Films, for example, warned that:

> I must advise you that it is the policy of Twentieth Century Fox Film Corporation ("Fox") not to consider or accept any unsolicited story ideas or other literary material unless it is submitted through an authorized literary agent who is a signatory with the Writer's Guild of America. In accordance with this policy, therefore, we return the enclosed material unread.
>
> Furthermore, although we have not read your submission we must advise you that to the extent, if any, that your submitted material is based upon or incorporates identical or substantially similar elements (e.g., characters, plot, etc.) of a property owned or controlled by Fox, your submitted material

is an unauthorized derivative work, and, as such, is an infringement of the copyright in Fox's property.

Please be advised that in such cases Fox reserves all of its rights and remedies, at law or in equity, with respect to any such unauthorized derivative work.

Imagine receiving this bulldog in your Friday mail. It insinuates that you're dishonest, a plagiarist, and are litigious. Well, so much for a happy weekend. Harsh legal threats are among the potpourri of strange replies. Each letter politely or impolitely disposes your hours of calculated mailings and may discourage subsequent attempts at inquiries. But don't despair. Like every rule, there are always the exceptions. And in showbiz, exceptions make up the rules.

Despite major studios' policies of no unsolicited readings, one out of four scripts considered in a day came from "unsolicited" sources. Remember, nothing is absolute in Hollywood. *Anything goes.* The reason for latitude is not due to lazy enforcement of good principles, but because *there are good properties out there that producers want to buy.* And they *will* get access to them. The main way of accessing synopses, treatments, outlines, and screenplays is by using a *submission agreement or a release form.* Release forms may be sent along with an affirmative studio letter, or the writer may send one without being asked for it.

It is customary to include release forms in all property submissions (Figure 12.5). The release essentially promises the producer that you won't turn around and sue him and stipulates a working understanding of the review and negotiation process should problems arise. Releases act as a legal document, but do not replace *legal advice* you may wish to consult before or during the studio-review process.

What Companies Buy

What studios buy depends on what they can afford and the risks they take on the property. Unknown writers stand a poor chance of selling a script for big money at the first corner. Of course, it always happens. More frequently, producers buy *on spec,* as mentioned earlier, or through performance agreements. In the first case, *on spec,* advance royalties are paid to retain the rights either to the first draft of the screenplay or another property by that writer. Producers who

FIGURE 12.5. Release form submitted along with properties to producers

RELEASE FORM

Date March 27, 1993
TITLE OF MATERIAL SUBMITTED:
"Uncivil Service"
Mr. Gary Troy, President
National Screen Artists, Inc.
211 No. Valley St., Ste 204
Toluca Lake, CA 91505
Mr. Troy:

I understand that legal propriety requires that you do not read unsolicited material submitted by a source other than an established agency except in accordance with the understanding, and subject to the conditions set forth herein. I am submitting herewith certain material described in Exhibit A (hereinafter referred to as the Material). I acknowledge that the Material was created and written by me without any suggestion or request from you that I write or create the material. I am executing and submitting this letter in consideration of your agreement to review the Material with the express understanding that my claim or right is limited to the features of the Material as specifically synopized or as attached hereto:

1. Except as otherwise specifically stated herein, I represent:

  (a) I am the author of the Material and that the material is original with me:

  (b) I have the exclusive rights to submit the Material to you on the terms and conditions set forth herine: and

  (c) I have the power and authority to grant to you all the rights in the Material.

2. You agree that in the event you elect to use the Material, you will pay me the applicable scale compensation required by the Writers Guild of America Theatrical and Television Basic Agreement.

3. I understand and agree that your use of material containing features and elements similar to or identical with those contained in the Material shall not entitle me to any compensation if you determine that you have an independent legal right to use such other material, either because such features or elements were not new or novel, were in the public domain, or were not originated by me, were independently conceived or because other persons (including your employees) may have submitted or may hereafter submit material containing similar or identical features and elements.

4. I agree that, should I bring any action against you for wrongful appropriation of the Material or any part thereof, such action shall be limited to an action at law for damages; that in no event shall I be entitled to an injunction or any other equitable relief. I further agree that, as a condition precedent to any such action, I will give you written notice by certified or registered mail, of my claim, stating the particulars in complete detail, within the time prescribed by the applicable statute of limitations, but in no event later than 90 days after I acquire knowledge sufficient to put me on notice of any such claim.

5. I have retained a copy of said Material, and I release you from any liability for loss or other damage to the copy or copies submitted to you.

6. I hereby acknowledge that I have read and understand this Agreement: That no oral representations of any kind have been made to me; that there are no prior or contemporaneous oral agreements in effect between us pertaining to said Material; and that this Agreement states our entire understanding. Any provisions or part of any provisions which is void or unenforceable shall be deemed omitted and this Agreement with such provision or part thereof omitted shall remain in full force and effect.

Sincerely,

NAME: Douglas H. Ruben

NAME:_____(signature)

ADDRESS: 4211 Okemos Road, Suite 22

CITY: Okemos

STATE: Michigan ZIP: 48864

TELEPHONE NO: 517-347-0944/517-349-1289

EXHIBIT A

TITLE OF MATERIAL: *Uncivil Service*
FORM OF MATERIAL (screenplay, treatment, etc.)
Sceenplay

WGA REGISTRATION NO. 43061

SIGNATURE

3-27-93
DATE

are eager beavers and strongly believe they have a screenplay winner may *option* the property. Here they pay a larger sum based on seeing the actual first draft and promise to purchase the screenplay if all the parts fall into place (e.g., money to produce the movie).

Spec-script and option purchases are on the rise. Recently, for example, Castle Rock Entertainment paid roughly $1 million in a deal with writer-director Frank Darabont and producer Niki Marvin for the screenplay adaptation of Stephen King's *Rita Hayworth and the Shawshank Redemption*. But Walt Disney studios lead the pack. They paid $650,000 against $850,000 for David Loughery's retelling of Alexander Dumas' classic *The Three Musketeers*. And Amy Brooke Baker's and Peter Osterlund's *Countermeasures* earned $500,000 against $750,000. Clearly, then, the spec-script recession is over.

Still, some producers are so emotionally sold on the screenplay they want to buy it outright, but pay nothing in advance. Here's how they accomplish it. They send a *performance agreement* that stipulates paying the screenwriter an advance sum ranging from a minimum amount to 5 percent of the total movie's budget, whichever is higher; plus, they pay a percentage of royalty on sales. Meaning, they may offer to pay, for example, either $50,000 (minimum) or 5 percent of, say, a low average movie budget of ten million dollars. That's a whopping one million dollars–or money paid before the screenplay ever goes to production. Of course, all the riches remain in limbo until the studio secures backers for a production budget and knows for certain the project "is a go." Scripts are held by performance agreements for a period of months until a deadline. Once that deadline expires, either there is an extension made or the offer dies. No money out, but a lot of money promised. Does that mean performance agreements are the best deals to negotiate? Not necessarily. Any deal, from spec to option and variations in between, hold enormous prospects for screenwriter stardom and should not be refused.

Living Outside of New York or California

Cries of alienation come from outside the worlds of Hollywood and New York. Writers living in other states believe their chances are slim to none unless they rub elbows with the movers and shakers of TV and film. But the irony is this: where are many movies being filmed? *Not in Los Angeles or even in California and New York.* Earlier we discussed how state commissions on film actively recruit producers to shoot movies in their own province. Filming not only has taken to the roads, but lately, in reaction to the smog, crime, and especially racial riots, Los Angeles filmmakers seriously are considering moving their industry to another location. Already Disney (MGM) and Universal Studios built working studios in Orlando, Florida, and Paramount is not far behind. Individual actors also have Everglades fever, opening studios from Jupiter (Burt Reynolds) to Southern Florida Coastline (Sylvester Stallone). But what about in Detroit, Chicago, and Arizona? Studio relocation and expansion outside L.A. is hot news and will probably result in *something happening.*

So, is it possible for nonresidents of movie town to be a part of the industry? Absolutely yes. Writers should keep tabs on where companies may move to or how many movies they produce on remote. *Daily* or *Weekly Variety, Hollywood Reporter,* and other trades will follow this wave of action in every detail.

Collaboration with an Established Writer

Teaming up with established writers is a double-edged sword. Benefits include connections with Hollywood insiders and facilitated studio deals. Those advantages sound incomparable. But teamwork is usually unilateral. Heavyweights take nearly all of the writing credit and consequently steal higher royalty percentages. It is much like doctoral chairmen who place their names on *your dissertation.* You end up doing the majority of work and receiving the least amount of credit. Still, collaborative efforts allow quantum leaps over the political and bureaucratic obstacles that usually stifle early writing ambitions. You can find a collaborator in several ways. First, collaborators solicit help through advertisements appearing in *The Hollywood Scriptwriter, The Hollywood Reporter,* and *Daily Variety.* Second, flip through pages of *The Writers Guild of America Directory.* Selectively pick a writer whose film or TV credits are familiar to you or parallel your interests. Write an inquiry letter briefly describing who you are and your willingness to apprentice this writer's next major project.

Using a Script Analyst

Frequently ads appear enticing new writers to get top advice before throwing their ideas to the lions. Advisors are script analysts hired by independents, larger companies, and agents to carefully *tear apart* story line, character formation, and other script dimensions including an analysis of commercial possibility. Script analysts usually may be experienced screenwriters turned consultant, or consultants waiting for their first big break in movies; being a script analyst certainly beats being a waiter. Insight they shed on your material is helpful but no more educational than might be gained from a strong screenwriting seminar or from collaboration. Plus, their opinion is still *their opinion.* And that's only one opinion. Remember, there is no such thing as unanimity in Hollywood; what one producer thinks is maudlin sentimentality, may appear as meaningful romance fiction to another producer. The script analyst cannot prepare your screenplay for all interpretations but may help polish your ideas and writing techniques.

WGA and nonWGA

Another obstacle ramming into your ventures is the union. Unions are good and unions are bad; that's not a new concept. In TV and film, the WGA is not just a puppet. It is a recognized proactive and powerful force policing the production industry by assuring equal pay and tracking payment of residuals to the membership. WGA writers receive a payment scale commensurate to writing credits and experience. But nonWGA members are not entitled to WGA salaries or may be refused writing assignments until they join the rank and file.

So, how do you join the rank and file of WGA? First, realize there are two organizations under the umbrella *Writers Guild of America.* Writers Guild of America, West is for writers who live West of the Mississippi. Writers Guild of America, East, is for writers residing east of the Mississippi. Second, requirements for membership owe little to your academic credentials; more important is your tally of writing credits. An aggregate of 12 units of credit as defined by a *Schedule of Units of Credit* must be verified. All employment or credit must be with a company or other entity that is signatory to the Guild's Collective Bargaining Agreement, and is within the jurisdiction of the Guild. The 12 units must be accumulated within the preceding two years of application. Here is the *Schedule of Units of Credit:*

2 units:

For each complete week of employment within the Guild's jurisdiction on a week-to-week or term basis.

3 units:

Story for radio play or television program of less than 30 minutes in duration shall be prorated in five-minute increments.

4 units:

Story for a short subject theatrical motion picture or for a radio play or television program of not less than 30 minutes nor more than 60 minutes in duration.

6 units:

Teleplay or radio play of less than 30 minutes in duration which shall be prorated in five minute increments. Or, television format or presentation for a new series; "Created by" credit given pursuant to the separation of rights provisions of the WGA Theatrical and Television Basic Agreement.

8 units:

Story for radio play or television program of more than one hour but not more than two hours in duration. Or, screenplay for a short subject theatrical motion picture. Or, radio play or teleplay of not less than 30 minutes but not more than 60 minutes in duration.

12 units:

Story for a feature-length theatrical motion picture or for a television program or radio play of more than two hours in duration. Or, screenplay for a feature-length theatrical motion picture. Or, teleplay for a television program or a radio play for a radio program of more than one hour in duration. Or, writing a "bible" (explains character and story line profile). Or, long-term story projection on an existing, five times per week non-prime time serial.

Additional Considerations:

A rewrite is entitled to one-half the number of units allotted to its particular category.

A polish is entitled to one-quarter the number of units allotted to its particular category.

Sale of an option earns one-half the number of units allotted to its particular category, subject to a maximum entitlement of four such units, per project in any one year.

Where writers collaborate on the same project, each shall be accorded the appropriate number of units, allotted to the category of the work.

Finally, membership fees are not like joining your local health club. They're a bit steeper. Initiation fee is $1,500 and the application must be accompanied by supportive documents such as copies of sales contracts, employment contracts, or other acceptable evidence of employment or sales.

Using an Agent

As with any writing endeavor, refinement and marketing can be left up to the experts. Your expertise is in mental health. Agents are experts in sizing up studio-interest prospects for motion picture, television, and radio story sales. They act as advocates and liaisons, pushing for the best deal earning the author maximal advances (from specs, options, performance agreements) and themselves a hefty commission of 10 to 15 percent. Like realtors, they dream of the big cash, but realize that frequent small deals will pay their mortgages. So, most agents are happy to make *any reasonable deal.*

Agents come in two types. First, there are WGA signatories whose services must comply with the WGA BASIC AGREEMENT. This agreement stipulates payment schedules, types of contracts and percentage splits allowable, and carefully defines the agent-writer relationship. Signatories, for example, cannot charge a reading fee just for considering your script for representation. Agencies that offer script critique services at a fee violate this agreement. WGA signatories may lose initial service fees but have open door policies into many major studios. By contrast, nonWGA agents are free to advertise any fee for service but struggle for studio recognition and may not be allowed to negotiate deals.

Still a third consideration is where agents are located. Does it matter if the agency resides outside of Los Angeles or New York? Reflecting on earlier optimism, with studio relocations in mind, agents outside the prime time area may be okay if they prove they have established networking ties with producers. Ask them to send you a list of their clients' screenplays, teleplays, or credits.

Where to Find an Agent

Shopping for an agent is a tough job. WGA and nonWGA signatories have their advantages and disadvantages, so where do you start? Several resources below direct you to names and addresses of agents and their expertise. Send an inquiry letter briefly describing the screenplay and yourself. The shotgun approach of mailing 50 inquiries hoping some will reply is inadvisable. Be selective; send five to ten inquiry letters only. Be careful of the come-ons such as "If you pay us to get your script into shape, we'll be happy to represent it for you." Reserve payment for actual services rendered toward promoting the screenplay, for example, in postage, telephone calls with producers, and in-person deal negotiations. The best arrangement, naturally, is paying only the 10 to 15 percent commission based on a screenplay sale; that will definitely mobilize agents into action.

A final word on agents is this: Don't always think the biggest is best. Giants such as The William Morris Agency, Creative Artists Agency, International Creative Management, and Triad Artists are virtually impossible for admission unless your credits wave like a Fourth of July flag. Mid-size firms such as the Christopher Nassif Agency, the Gersh Agency, InterTalent Agency, Lewis & Quinn, and The Kraft Agency accept unsolicited inquiries and readily work with unknown writers. Even agencies representing ten to 20 clients are worth considering. *It's not how big they are, but how effective they are at selling properties.* In recent years the top executive reps at William Morris, for example, left to create their own small agencies and are just as insider-smart as their William Morris counterparts. So, read through the agent listings and determine which agency can best handle your expertise and screenplay. Here are some resources for getting that list of agents:

Hollywood Scriptwriter (Annual Agency Review)
1626 N. Wilcox #385
Hollywood, CA 90028

Hollywood Agents Directory
3000 Olympic Blvd., Suite 2413
Santa Monica, CA 90404

Studio Blu-Book Directory
6715 Sunset Blvd.
Hollywood, CA 90028

Entertainment Industry Contracts:
Negotiating and Drafting Guide (4 volumes)
Matthew Bender
DM Department
1275 Broadway
Albany, NY 12204

Resources on General Information on Motion Pictures

Daily Variety
5700 Wilshire Blvd.
Los Angeles, CA 90036

Dramalogue
PO Box 38771
Los Angeles, CA 90038

Emmy: Magazine of Television Arts & Sciences
Subscription Dept.
5220 Lankershim Blvd.
North Hollywood, CA 91601

Feature Directors: Their Credits and Their Agents
3000 Olympic Blvd., Suite 2413
Santa Monica, CA 90404

Feature Writers: Their Credits and Their Agents
3000 Olympic Blvd., Suite 2413
Santa Monica, CA 90404

Hollywood Creative Directory
3000 Olympic Blvd., Suite 2413
Santa Monica, CA 90404

Hollywood Distributors Directory
3000 Olympic Blvd., Suite 2413
Santa Monica, CA 90404

The Hollywood Reporter
6715 Sunset Blvd.
Hollywood, CA 90028

Hollywood Scriptwriter
1626 N. Wilcox #385
Hollywood, CA 90028

International Motion Picture Almanac
Quigly Publishing Company, Inc.
159 West 53rd Street
New York, NY 10019

The Journal of the Writers Guild of America, West
8955 Beverly Blvd.
Los Angeles, CA 90048-2456

Writers Guild of America Directory
Directory
8955 Beverly Blvd.
Los Angeles, CA 90048

Just a final note: scripting movies ultimately depends on your emotional immune system. If you've got the stamina for sending many inquires and creatively alternating them between fax and mailed letters, something *will happen.* Be patient. Be professional. But most important, be *persistent.* Despising the weekly batch of rejections will only give you an ulcer unless you realize it's par for the course. All media undertakings are like that. Writing screenplays just takes a little tougher skin than other forms of media to weather it out. So, whether dabbling in movies, teleplays, or technical videos, do yourself a favor and realistically plan on it taking longer to break into the industry and making that first million. And if you don't make that million, believe me–you'll have the best time in your life trying for it.

PART IV:
REFERENCES AND SUGGESTED READINGS

Ballon, R. (1995). *Blueprint for Writing: A Writer's Guide to Creativity, Craft & Career.* San Francisco, CA: Extension Press.
Cannon, D. W. (1993). *Authorship: The Dynamic Principles of Writing Creatively.* Los Angeles, CA: Hannah House.
Field, S. (1979). *Screenplay: The Foundations of Screenwriting.* New York: Dell Publishing.
Field, S. (1984). *The Screenwriter's Workbook.* New York: Dell Publishing.
Helitzer, M. (1986). *Comedy Writing Secrets.* Cincinnati, OH: Writer's Digest Books.
Sautter, C. (1986). *How to Sell Your Screenplay: The Real Rules of Film and Television.* New York: New Chapter Press.
Seger, L. (1987). *Making a good script great.* Hollywood, CA: Samuel French.
Walter, R. (1988). *Screenwriting: The Art, Craft, and Business of Film and Television Writing.* New York: New American Library.
Wolff, J. & Cox, K. (1988). *Successful Scriptwriting.* Cincinnati, OH: Writer's Digest Books.

Index

Page numbers in italics indicate figures; page numbers followed by t indicate tables.

THIS CONFIDENT CHURCH

This Confident Church

Catholic Leadership and Life in Chicago, 1940–1965

Steven M. Avella

University of Notre Dame Press

Notre Dame　　　　　London

Photographs are by courtesy of the Archives of the Archdiocese of Chicago and the Archives of the Archdiocese of Milwaukee.

Portions of chapters 1 and 5 appeared in "Reynold Hillenbrand and Chicago Catholicism," *U.S. Catholic Historian* 9 (fall 1990): 353–370.

A version of chapter 4 appeared in "The Rise and Fall of Bernard Sheil," *Critic* 44 (spring 1990): 2–18.

The author is grateful for permission to use them in this work.

Library of Congress Cataloging-in-Publication Data

Avella, Steven M.
    This confident church: Catholic leadership and life in Chicago, 1940-1965/Steven M. Avella.
    p.   cm.
    Includes bibliographical references and index.
    ISBN 0-268-01879-0
    1. Catholic Church—Illinois—Chicago Region—History—20th century. 2. Catholic Church. Archdiocese of Chicago (Ill.)—History—20th century. 3. Chicago Region (Illinois—Church history. I. Title.
    BX1417.C46A83   1992   91-51121
                                                                     CIP

To Philip Gleason
Quid retribuam?

Contents

Foreword

For most of the twentieth century, Chicago has been the largest Catholic archdiocese in the United States. Yet more than large numbers have set Chicago Catholics apart from (and in their own eyes, above) their American co-religionists. Indeed Chicago Catholicism displays a distinctive style all its own.

Chicago-style Catholicism flows from at least four historical sources: ethnic diversity, able clerical and episcopal leadership, social and political liberalism, and soaring self-confidence.

Ethnic diversity harks back to the very beginnings of Chicago in the mid-nineteenth century. Whereas most other American dioceses were dominated by either the Irish or the Germans, Chicago welcomed large numbers of both. Then at the turn of the century, waves of Eastern and Southern Europeans churned the mix even more. By the early twentieth century, Chicago Catholics were organized into separate "ethnic leagues" that were virtually sub-dioceses in their own right. Roman authorities recognized Chicago's pluralism by alternating Irish and German archbishops at the head of the see throughout most of the twentieth century. Today, the city's archbishop is Italian and his auxiliary bishops are Irish, Polish, Mexican, and African-American.

The other keynotes of Catholicism Chicago-style do not date back so far. In the nineteenth century the city's Catholics were neither ably led, politically liberal, nor self-confident. In fact, Rome considered Chicago an ecclesiastical disaster area. The earliest bishops took one look at this muddy frontier town and started making plans to leave. One bishop literally went insane. At the turn of the century, a cabal of Irish-born pastors

mounted a challenge to Archbishop Patrick Feehan and his American-born advisers, resulting in a schism and excommunications that broke the archbishop's heart and hastened his death.

This turbulent history has had one consequence that lasts to this day. Rome has never entrusted the archdiocese to a native Chicagoan but has always brought in an outsider to serve as archbishop. This stands in sharp contrast to New York, where nearly all the ruling bishops have been natives and even a bishop from New Jersey is considered a foreigner.

One of the outsiders sent by Rome to clean up Chicago's clerical mess, George William Mundelein (1916–1939), finally turned around the city's reputation and established the tradition that has marked it throughout the rest of the century. A "consolidating bishop," Mundelein centralized the administration of the Chicago archdiocese, set it on a firm financial footing, and tied it more closely to headquarters in Rome. He also trumpeted his 100 percent Americanism and forged close political ties with local Democratic politicians and with President Franklin D. Roosevelt. In all these ways, Mundelein "put Chicago Catholicism on the map." He also chose inspired associates, such as auxiliary bishop Bernard J. Sheil, the founder of the Catholic Youth Organization, and seminary rector Monsignor Reynold Hillenbrand, who trained a generation of seminarians in social and political liberalism. When Mundelein died in 1939, he bequeathed to Chicago Catholics a sense of self-confidence that bordered on arrogance.

Steven Avella's book, *This Confident Church*, takes up the story of Chicago Catholicism after the death of Mundelein and brings it down to the days of the Second Vatican Council. Avella is well aware of Chicago's ethnic pluralism, but he emphasizes the other three aspects of Chicago's uniqueness: its outstanding clerical leadership, social and political liberalism, and self-confidence. He tells the story with great richness of detail, for he is the first scholar to use the full resources of the Chicago archdiocesan archives since they were reorganized a handful of years ago and put under the able professional management of John Treanor and his staff. He also ferreted out many other sources, such as the entertaining memoir of Monsignor John D.

Fitzgerald, and he has interviewed all the surviving principals.

The two archbishops who succeeded Mundelein in Chicago, Samuel A. Stritch (1940–1958) and Albert G. Meyer (1958–1965), were more typical products of midcentury Catholicism that their predecessor. Mundelein was a towering figure who would have risen to the top in any line of work. Indeed, his lay admirers used to tell him: "There was a great mistake in making you a bishop instead of a financier, for in the latter case Mr. Morgan would not be without a rival on Wall Street." No one would have said this to Stritch or Meyer. Indeed, as products of a narrow clerical culture, it is hard to imagine either as anything other than a priest or bishop. For this very reason, however, a close study of their careers reveals much about the contours of Chicago Catholicism before the Second Vatican Council.

Cardinal Stritch was a beloved figure, with a self-effacing smile and a pleasant southern lilt to his voice. He earned a reputation as the "bishop who said Yes," a permissive, tolerant figurehead who allowed "a thousand flowers to bloom" in Chicago. Albert Meyer, on the other hand, projected a forbidding Germanic image and the scholarly manner of the seminary rector he used to be. When I was a teenager I had the opportunity to serve as an altar boy at Holy Name Cathedral, and I used to think, and joke with my fellow altar servers, that Cardinal Meyer must suck on lemons before leaving the sacristy. I couldn't have been more wrong. Steven Avella demonstrates that the public images of Stritch and Meyer should be reversed. He comments astutely: "Stritch may have looked and acted more like kindly Pope John, but he was more ideologically attuned to Pius XII. Meyer, by contrast, looked more like Pius XII but came to feel more spiritual and intellectual kinship with John XXIII."

Non-Catholics who couldn't care less about episcopal politics will still find much of interest in this book, particularly the several chapters dealing with race relations and social action. Avella narrates the stormy history of racially changing neighborhoods, urban renewal, and the civil rights movement in Chicago. He doesn't slight the courageous leadership of social action priests such as John Egan and Daniel Cantwell, nor gloss

over the widespread racism that clung to many other priests
and lay Catholics in Chicago. Cardinal Meyer emerges as an
unlikely hero of the Catholic civil rights movement. He seemingly reasoned himself into a liberal in a thoroughly medieval,
syllogistic fashion: All people are equal in the sight of God,
Negroes are people, *ergo* Negroes must be treated equally. End
of argument.

　　This book also presents much more about Bishop Bernard J.
Sheil than I thought would ever make it into print. A fascinating
and enigmatic figure, Sheil would literally give a poor man the
coat off his back, but he also possessed a monumental ego and
spent money lavishly on his own rectory appointments. His
audacious social experiments and free-spending ways condemned him to remain an auxiliary bishop all his life. Before
Cardinal Cody sent him into retirement in 1965, Sheil apparently burned all his papers, and his associates have remained
closemouthed to this day. Yet somehow, Avella has dug up a
great deal of fascinating information about "the People's
Bishop," as he liked to be called in his more megalomaniacal
moments. The resulting chapter on Bishop Sheil is, therefore,
worth the price of this book all by itself.

　　Above all, Steven Avella emphasizes that Chicago
Catholicism was supremely self-confident at midcentury.
Catholics in Chicago carried themselves with an "easy arrogance" that infuriated their co-religionists elsewhere, say in
Boston or New York, but which accurately reflected their position in the Windy City. With a Catholic-dominated Democratic
machine ruling the city and the capable leadership of
Mundelein, Stritch, and Meyer at the episcopal helm, Chicago
Catholics had every reason to feel confident. The social action
experiments of Reynold Hillenbrand's disciples provided examples for the rest of the Catholic Church and foreshadowed the
changes of Vatican II. Finally, Cardinal Meyer played a crucial
role in passing the declaration on religious liberty at the ecumenical council. No wonder Chicagoans swelled with pride.

　　I don't mean to suggest that Avella is an uncritical booster
of Chicago Catholicism. Far from it. His account is balanced,
fair, and critical in the right places. Yet *This Confident Church* will
help correct the misimpression that nothing of value happened

in "the bad old days" before Vatican II. Too many modern-day, liberal Catholics seem ashamed of their ecclesiastical past and try to forget or deny it. Avella's work shows how misguided this historical myopia is.

Unfortunately, the soaring sense of self-confidence that Avella found in Chicago Catholicism in the first half of the twentieth century has been absent in recent years. Though confidence can lead to arrogance, it is also a prerequisite for reform and progress. Only self-confident Catholics can reach out to others in social action and ecumenism. With any luck, historical work such as Steven Avella's book will help Catholics discern the sources of self-confidence in the past and help them regain it in the near future.

Edward R. Kantowicz

Acknowledgments

The completion of this manuscript would have been impossible without the assistance of many people.

First and foremost, the rich treasures of the Archives of the Archdiocese of Chicago were first opened to me by His Eminence Cardinal Joseph Bernardin (with the help of a letter from Father Daniel J. Pakenham) and the late Father Menceslaus Madaj. Father Madaj's successors, John Treanor and Timothy Slavin, made possible an even wider scope for this study. Staff member David Deitz was most helpful to me, and Nancy Sandleback gave me access to the iconographic collection of the archives. Their courtesy, professional assistance, and genuine kindness (including an occasional free lunch from the archdiocesan food service) made possible the bulk of this work. Chicago's archdiocesan archives are among the best preserved and administered in the American Church. I am equally indebted to the Chicago Historical Society and especially Mr. Archibald Motley, who assisted me with unfailing patience as I worked my way through the papers of Daniel Cantwell, the Catholic Labor Alliance, and the Catholic Interracial Council of Chicago.

I am grateful as well to Archbishop Rembert G. Weakland, O.S.B., for giving me access to the Archives of the Archdiocese of Milwaukee. Its former director, Father Thomas Fait, was most helpful in some inquiries. The chancellor, Father Ralph Gross, and the associate chancellor, Dr. Barbara Ann Cusack, regularly allowed me access to the chancery vault. The present archivist, Mr. Timothy Cary, has already provided me with some iconographic materials.

The staff of St. Francis Seminary's Salzmann Library was supportive. I would especially like to thank its former director, Father Lawrence Miech, and the current director, Sister Colette Zirbes, O.S.F., for their assistance. Former staff member Noel McFarren was also helpful.

The Archives of the Diocese of Toledo were made accessible to me by Bishop James Hoffman. Father Kenneth Morman was my host and I was ably assisted by Sister Nora Klewicki, O.S.F., who was in the midst of organizing a very valuable collection of papers.

In the Archdiocese of Cincinnati, former archivist Father Jerry Hiland and his associate, Gail Arbino, couldn't have been more cooperative and helpful. Discussions with Father M. Edmund Hussey provided additional insights into Cincinnati's Catholic past and the character of John T. McNicholas, O.P.

At the Catholic University of America, archivist Anthony Zito and Sister Anne Crowley, S.N.D., gave me access to everything I wanted to see and were most helpful with suggestions for further avenues of research. To them both I am grateful. H. Warren Willis, archivist of the United States Catholic Conference, graciously provided me with many fine sources. So also the archivists of the University of Notre Dame were most gracious in their assistance with the Hillenbrand papers.

The staffs of the Franklin D. Roosevelt, Harry S Truman, and Dwight D. Eisenhower presidential libraries were of great help in tracking down the often thin threads of evidence concerning White House dealings with Chicago's Catholic leaders. Their professionalism and willingness to render assistance made the trips worth it. So also the staff of the Great Lakes Regional U.S. archival repository in Chicago, which holds the papers of Judge William Campbell. Judge Campbell gave me access to his personal papers just weeks before his death. They proved to be an important source of information on the Sheil career. My colleague, Dr. Athan Theoharis, introduced me to the vagaries of Freedom of Information Act requests and made possible the retrieval of FBI files on Cardinal Stritch.

Any number of people examined the manuscript at various stages and offered important suggestions for its improvement, correction, expansion, and contraction. I would like to thank Mr.

Thomas Stritch, nephew of Cardinal Stritch, for his assistance with this book. I am deeply indebted to my friend Father F. Paul Prucha, S.J., of the Marquette University history faculty for his careful reading and his constructive comments. Monsignors John Tracy Ellis and Harry Koenig read earlier versions of the draft and were most encouraging. Father Martin Zielinski, a historian on the faculty of the St. Mary of the Lake Seminary, read and commented on much of the text as did the Salvatorian Father Daniel Pekarske. Edward Kantowicz's study of the Mundelein Era was a source of inspiration to me and Ed's encouragement and help in writing this sequel to his work are much appreciated. I am grateful to him as well for writing the foreword. Historian Eileen McMahon read and offered helpful comments, as did Dr. Patrick Carey of Marquette University. Ann Rice, editor for Notre Dame Press, gave the text a thorough going-over and saved me from a lot of fatuous errors. Readers from the Cushwa Center for the Study of American Catholicism also offered important suggestions. I am grateful to them and to director Jay P. Dolan.

Technical assistance with the production of the text was given with great generosity by my dear friend Ms. Barbara Phelan. Without Barbara, computer technology would have completely eluded me. Mrs. Marelene Groff of office services at St. Francis Seminary patiently reproduced thousands and thousands of pages of drafts of this work. She is a gem. Jane Frances St. Peter collated and processed the reams of raw data I took out of parish reports and produced the graphs that appear in the appendix. Her married surname "St." is well merited.

In travels in Chicago I was often the beneficiary of much hospitality and kindness on the part of priests and lay people whom I interviewed. Rarely did I meet with a bad reception, virtually always was I given the courtesy of a fair, frank, and honest interview. In other parts of the country I imposed on the courtesy of relatives and friends for bed and board. In Washington, D.C. Rosemarie Schmidt and Jamie Bradshaw graciously allowed me to camp out at their Capitol Hill address during research trips. The faculty of Mount St. Mary's Seminary of the West in Cincinnati were my hosts during my stays in that city.

Above all I am grateful for the constant and steady encouragement of the friends and loved ones that God has blessed me with. First of all I offer gratitude to my parents and family, whom I love so dearly. I thank my friend and walking companion Father Gerald Hauser, raconteur extraordinaire, who has given me many fine insights. I cite also the support of my former and current department chairpersons, Sister Justine Peter, O.S.F., of Cardinal Stritch College and Dr. Thomas Hachey of Marquette University—scholars and gentlepersons of the first order. I am grateful as well for the encouragement and support of faculty and students at St. Francis Seminary in Milwaukee, especially Father Melvin Michalski and Mr. Brian Mason. The community of learning at Cardinal Stritch College, especially Presidents Camille Kliebhan, O.S.F., and Mary Lea Schneider, O.S.F., colleagues Robert Flahive, George Buessem, Florence Deacon, O.S.F., Marna Boyle, Linda Plagman, and Angelyn Dries, O.S.F., as well as my beloved "scholars" have meant the world to me. I thank them with all my heart. My circle of close friends in Milwaukee has done more for me than they could even know: Jane and Chris Andacht, John and Jane St. Peter, Casimir and Sue Mleczko, and of course, C.G.

I cannot conclude this list of thanks without an acknowledgment of Philip Gleason. From the moment I first met him, his clear, incisive, and sensible scholarship, as well as his encyclopedic grasp of American Catholic history and its sources, has never ceased to amaze me. Often at the cost of neglecting his own scholarly work, Phil Gleason always had quality time for his graduate students. A word of encouragement from him meant everything and when he administered correction, it was always in a manner that left dignity intact while challenging a person to do better. This good, decent, and kind scholar has befriended me and helped me every step of the way in my desire to be a good teacher and a professional historian. *Quid retribuam* ... what could I return to such a man? To him do I gratefully dedicate this work.

Steven M. Avella
Marquette University
March 7, 1992

Introduction

The photographer from the National Catholic News Service caught the poignancy of the moment: two Catholic prelates, Cardinal Samuel Stritch of Chicago and Archbishop Albert Meyer of Milwaukee, wrapped in an awkward embrace of farewell on the docks of New York. In the background, on the April day of 1958, the American Export Company's liner *Independence* was waiting to take Stritch to Rome to assume his new duties as pro-prefect of the Congregation of the Faith. The two had first met during the summer of 1925 when Albert Meyer was still a Milwaukee seminarian going to school in Rome and Stritch was the young "boy-bishop" of Toledo, visiting the Vatican on his first *ad limina*. From then on their respective paths would cross and recross, would parallel and converge.

In 1930, when Stritch was appointed archbishop of Milwaukee, he had asked Meyer to join the faculty of St. Francis Seminary and in 1937 appointed him rector. When Stritch left Milwaukee to become archbishop of Chicago in early 1940, Meyer was among those who escorted the new bishop to his installation. The older man watched Meyer's progress from afar, rejoicing in 1946 (the year Stritch himself was made a cardinal) as his young protégé was elevated to the episcopate. In 1953 only canons of ecclesiastical protocol (cardinals could not be present if the apostolic delegate presided at a liturgical function) kept the cardinal archbishop of Chicago away from St. John's Cathedral when Meyer was installed as archbishop of Milwaukee. On that occasion Meyer wrote to Stritch:

> It was just about twenty-three years ago this month that I returned to Milwaukee from Rome to receive an appointment as

1

assistant at St. Joseph's.... When Your Eminence came to Milwaukee shortly thereafter as our Archbishop it was not long before we learned to know you only to love you. Words fail me as I strive to express the tremendous influence for good made upon my youthful priesthood by Your Eminence. I am sure Your Eminence knows me well enough to understand that these words come from the heart, and are not meant to be idle flattery.[1]

Three years later, when Milwaukee's major seminary celebrated its centenary with the erection of new buildings, Meyer recalled how Stritch had originally planned the expansion in the thirties. Thoughtfully, he invited Stritch back to Milwaukee to dedicate and bless the new facilities.

Now, as he watched the *Independence* cast off, Meyer must have sensed Stritch's sadness as the liner carried the aging prelate to sure Roman oblivion in a job that he had neither asked for, nor wanted. The farewell embrace of these two men was highly symbolic of the shift taking place in the Catholic Church. At about the same time Stritch left Chicago, the long reign of Pope Pius XII would end. Indeed, Meyer's appointment to Chicago would be one of his last acts; a new pontiff, John XXIII, would stand on the balcony of St. Peter's to receive the triple tiara. John would usher a new era into the Church. Not quite the full flush of reform (that would happen in the sixties and seventies) but certainly different from the foregoing era. So, too, Meyer ushered in a transitional period for Chicago Catholicism. Indeed, the Archdiocese of Chicago from 1940 to 1965 was a microcosm of the flowering of Catholic life in one era and its transition to a new era. Pius XII and John XXIII would have a parallel in Stritch and Meyer.

Stritch, a short, pudgy man, had been born in Dixie and remained indelibly southern in his speech and life-style, despite his living for nearly forty years north of the Mason-Dixon line. He never lost his soft Tennessee accent or his easy-going, casual habits. Unfailingly genial and courteous, his manner resembled the courtly urbanity of an old-fashioned southern gentleman. His administrative style reflected the maxim he often repeated to new bishops: "Never run your diocese from behind a desk." Stritch loved the press of a crowd, an opportunity to preach or

speak, meetings of the National Catholic Welfare Conference (as well as the endless run of banquets and ceremonial occasions) that were part of his official duties. Desk work and tiresome administrative detail he gladly delegated to his subordinates. His years in Chicago (1940–1958) were a period of unparalleled growth as the centralizing and expansionist initiatives of his predecessor (Cardinal George Mundelein) reached fruition.

Stritch and his subordinates fortified and expanded the Catholic "presence" in Chicago. If Cardinal Mundelein put the Catholic Church on the map in Chicago, Stritch and his associates hoisted the map higher for all American Catholics to see. By 1955 *Life* magazine, that bellwether of American popular tastes, acknowledged this dynamic growth: "Today the Catholic Church is nowhere more active and prosperous than in the United States and few areas of the Church are more thriving than the Archdiocese of Chicago, the largest in the U.S.A."[2] Chicago's priests, sisters, brothers, and laity coped with the tremendous Catholic expansion into the suburbs. They built parishes, staffed overcrowded schools, and developed one of the most extensive Catholic high school networks in the nation. They reoriented mammoth Catholic Charities agencies to the needs of special children and the increasing number of elderly persons. Out of their ranks came the impulse of professionalization that revolutionized the cemetery system and provided capable administrators such as George J. Klupar, who completed the work of administrative centralization begun by Cardinal Mundelein.

But Chicago was also a diocese in transition. Mass migration of Catholics to the suburbs emptied the once prosperous urban churches and schools, and the preponderance of Catholic suburbanites altered the character of Chicago Catholicism. Changing neighborhoods, the growing black population of the city, and the need for a more professional and better-educated Catholic laity were issues on the front burner of the Stritch years. However there was no dearth of dedicated Chicago Catholics, clerical or lay, who wanted to take on the challenges. Encouraged by Stritch's episcopal "permissiveness," the problems of a changing Church were attacked with a confidence born of the theological verities of the time.

Chicago was the home base of Bishop Bernard J. Sheil (1886–1969), one of the most esteemed members of the American Catholic hierarchy. He was the founder of the Catholic Youth Organization, darling of organized labor, friend of Franklin D. Roosevelt and other New Dealers. In the 1940s he expanded the sports-minded Catholic Youth Organization (CYO) program to include an educational department that would study social issues. His public speeches (written by a well selected brain trust) reflected a new concern for social justice, democracy, racial tolerance, and world order. From labor halls to the halls of Congress, Sheil vigorously spoke out for racial justice, espoused public housing, and urged American society to extend the blessings of democracy and equal rights to a greater portion of its citizens. His knack for raising funds, his impresario's sense for the dramatic, and his consistent record for attracting the best and the brightest to his employ made the CYO Educational Division one of the most creative and efficacious organizations of the era.

The activities inspired by Monsignor Reynold Hillenbrand (1903–1979) and his clerical disciples were another feature of the Chicago Catholic landscape. Hillenbrand motivated the seminarians of the archdiocesan seminary as no other rector had done before or since to tackle the problems of urban and suburban Catholic life, especially through the liturgy and with an organizational methodology derived from Canon Cardijn's Specialized Catholic Action movements. He captivated students with his discussions on the Mass and the sacraments as the communication of divine life that would help humanity overcome the crippling individualism which made people selfish and heedless of the common good. Hillenbrand lived what he preached, devoting strenuous efforts to make the seminary responsive to the needs of the changing world, and he regularly went outside the seminary walls to do his part to change the society. Even after his firing in 1944 Hillenbrand's ardor did not cool, nor did his vision diminish, and he continued to affect the destinies of the liturgical and lay apostolate movements which he had helped create.

He was far from alone in this vision. He poured his spirit into the impressionable young seminarians and his own

classmates. He encouraged bright young priests to study sociology, ethics, education, and English literature, first, in order to effect even more changes in the seminary system and then in society at large. These included Fathers Daniel Cantwell, John Egan, William Quinn, William McManus, James Killgallon, John Hayes, William Boyd, all of whom became spokesmen for an aggressive Catholic response to social issues. Cantwell and Egan, perhaps the two brightest and most prominent of "Hilly's men," worked the lessons of their theological and graduate training into a variety of enterprises from public housing and race relations to marriage and family preparation. Indeed, both would rise to positions of prominence and become advisors to the Catholic archbishops of Chicago on pressing urban problems that beset Chicago Catholicism of the day. This remarkable group of priests and their lay disciples in the Young Christian Workers, Young Christian Students, the Christian Family Movement, the Cana Conference, Catholic Labor Alliance, and the Catholic Interracial Movement breathed the air of the social encyclicals and the liturgy, which they discussed endlessly at various forums, priests' meetings, in circulars, and in days of recollection and retreats at Johanna Doniat's Childerly Retreat House in suburban Wheeling, Illinois.

Although differences of style and organization sometimes built barriers between the bishops and their subordinates, "Hilly's men" and Sheil's minions, there really was a commonality of purpose: the reconstruction of the social order. Under the detached but benign Stritch they had ample leeway to implement their plans. But they yearned for more positive leadership—and this would soon come.

The transition would come abruptly, as Samuel Stritch's tenure (and life) ended in the early months of 1958. Since mid-January, Stritch had been at Hobe Sound on Jupiter Island, a pilgrimage he had taken every year but one during his tenure in Chicago. Not only did it restore his sagging spirits, it provided a break from the miserably cold weather that affected his sinuses. There, together with his friend Cardinal Mooney, and some of his official household, he could golf, sleep, and just do nothing. Florida was particularly cool that season. "This year,"

wrote Cardinal Stritch to editor Dan Herr, "one had more time to read than in other years."[3] But the leisure time to read did not extend to the piles of mail that his vicar general, George Casey, regularly sent down to him from the Chicago chancery. Stritch ignored the mail until February 5, when Casey received a telegram from Monsignor Angelo Dell'Acqua of the Vatican Secretariate of State politely inquiring, "Whether Your Eminence received my letter of January 17?"[4] Within the hour, the vicar general called Stritch and informed him of the message. Stritch pawed through his mail and found the letter. Opening it, he could not believe his eyes. The Pope had appointed him pro-prefect to the Congregation for the Propagation of the Faith.[5]

Stritch quickly cabled Dell'Acqua that he had received the message and promised a response. He then huddled with his housemates, Monsignors Patrick Hayes and Edward Burke, and called over to Cardinal Edward Mooney at nearby Stuart, Florida, for advice. Together, the three men concocted a letter to Dell'Acqua. Painfully hacked out by the cardinal himself on a portable typewriter, Stritch's letter informed Dell'Acqua, "I find I cannot take on the responsibility of accepting this important office with its far reaches in Holy Church unless the Holy Father commands me." Stritch defended his refusal, citing his lack of knowledge "of the procedures and practices of the Roman Curia," his inability to master "several modern languages," and his incapability to "rise above all nationalism which is so distinctive of the high officials of the Roman Curia." His penultimate reason was the most important: his health.

> I am in my seventy-first year of age. With the exception of a chronic nasal infection my health is fairly good for my age. I do have to take precautions. My personal physician constantly urges me to avoid overtaxing myself. My temperament is such that under heavy strain I become nervous and must take some rest. I know the problems of the Archdiocese of Chicago after seventeen years and I am able to do this work. The Archdiocese is large and demands the constant, immediate attention of the Archbishop. Honestly I fear that if I were to take on new unfamiliar, very important and exacting work at my age and in my condition, the strain would be too much for me.[6]

Dell'Acqua replied on February 13, sweeping away Stritch's protestations and insisted that he accept, lauding the Cardinal's "exemplary priestly and episcopal ministry," and assuring him that "English is the language most often used in reports." In response to Stritch's plea to remain in Chicago and occasionally visit Rome to take care of business, Dell'Acqua extolled the virtues of "the mild climate of the Eternal City."[7] Eventually, it became apparent that this was clearly a command of the Pope himself, and Stritch cabled his acceptance of the appointment on February 24.[8]

What was behind this mysterious appointment? Truly, it was strange for the pope to appoint a man in his seventies to head a sprawling Vatican bureaucracy (although seventy is young for Roman cardinals.) Moreover, to pluck Stritch from the leadership of one of the largest American archdioceses seemed doubly strange. Even the secular United Press International wondered about this in a lengthy article run over its wire services on March 18, 1958, suggesting that Pius XII might "clarify the status of the Archdiocese of Chicago" by appointing Bishop Martin O'Connor of the North American College to succeed Stritch.[9]

The real truth has died with the principals of this little drama, Pope Pius XII and Cardinal Stritch. We are left only with speculation of varying degrees of plausibility. One reason that can be dismissed at the outset was that the Holy See was punishing Stritch for a serious financial scandal that occurred in his chancery in late 1957. This scenario is rehearsed among many priests and lay persons to this day and seems logical, given the extent of the scandal (over a million dollars in theft) and Stritch's lackadaisical style of administration. However, those investigating the scandal, Bishop Cletus F. O'Donnell and Monsignor James Hardiman, discount it as a cause. The scandal was discovered in late 1957 and Stritch's appointment was dated January 17. It is hardly possible the Vatican could have even known of the problem, much less decided to handle it in such a drastic way. The proximity between the discovery of the theft and Stritch's appointment was purely coincidental.[10]

Another reason, advanced by a Roman insider, portrays Stritch as a sacrificial lamb in a bitter dispute between Francis

Cardinal Spellman and Bishop Fulton J. Sheen. The hatred and mistrust between these two men had been well known since Sheen had become auxiliary bishop of New York in 1951.[11] Sheen was an eloquent speaker and a popular orator around the nation, as well as in the pulpit of St. Patrick's Cathedral. By contrast, Spellman rarely preached and often was overshadowed by his more eloquent and sartorially elegant auxiliary. Moreover, Sheen's imperious ways did not set well with Spellman, and the simmering enmity between them erupted in a dispute over funds collected for the Propagation of the Faith, of which Sheen was the national director.

To increase the income of the national office of the Propagation of the Faith, Sheen wanted to add to his general collection all the specialized collections of individual religious communities in the United States. He offered his office as national clearinghouse for the distribution of the contributions, with the excess sent directly to Rome. This aroused a storm of opposition among many religious orders who depended on the collections gathered by their visiting parish missionary speakers to sustain their missions and sometimes elaborate building projects in the States as well. The Maryknoll Community was especially fearful of this prospect and sent a delegation to Cardinal Spellman to argue against Sheen's move. Spellman relished the opportunity to do battle with Sheen and used his position as the chairman of the Episcopal Committee for the Propagation of the Faith to interfere with the plan. Moreover, Spellman had long been uncomfortable with Sheen's financial autonomy and sought to bring the Propagation of the Faith under the direct jurisdiction of his episcopal committee. The ensuing battle between the two finally necessitated negotiation by the Curia and, ultimately, a decision by the pope. In Solomonic fashion, Pius XII attempted to split the difference between the two men. He permitted Sheen to retain the autonomy he insisted on as head of the Propagation of the Faith, but he rewarded Spellman by ending the controversial collection scheme and allowing him the right "to inspect all financial records."[12] Unfortunately, the quarrel became public, and after the affair was over there was a need to repair the public relations damage done. Moreover, the incumbent prefect of the Congregation of the Propagation of the Faith, Pietro

Fumasoni-Biondi, had been no help whatsoever to Spellman and Pius XII in resolving the matter. Pius XII had longed to be rid of the aging cardinal, a relic of the days of his predecessor, and this apparently led Spellman to suggest to Pius XII that Stritch, the head of the largest and wealthiest archdiocese in the United States, be appointed to this curial post.

Since the publication of John Cooney's critical biography of Cardinal Spellman, one may be inclined to believe the worst about the cardinal archbishop of New York. Indeed, there is one small reference in Stritch's letters that indicates that Spellman may have had some hand in his "promotion" when the prelate wrote to Spellman just before his departure from Chicago: "I am sure that you understand well the sacrifice which I must make...."[13]

However, there is a bit too much of the element of conspiracy in this conjecture to ring completely true. The most plausible explanation for Stritch's "boot upstairs" is related to the "sacrificial lamb" theory, but has less of the sinister and conspiratorial overtones of a Spellman plot. Indeed, Stritch was appointed to help Pius XII with a difficulty in his official household. The prefect of the Congregation Propaganda Fidei was the elderly and nearly blind Pietro Fumasoni-Biondi, once Apostolic Delegate to the United States. He had known Stritch as a student at the Propaganda and had been a close friend of Stritch's patron and shirttail relation, Bishop John B. Morris. Stritch had a genuine affection for the failing senior cardinal. Pius XII, it was reported, had no use for "Big Fu," as he was known, and engineered the Stritch appointment to help ease the old man out of an office he would not voluntarily resign. But he was also chosen in recognition of the importance of the American church as a source of strength for the burgeoning mission field. This was all the more urgent during the fifties, when Pius XII had encouraged a massive missionary effort on the part of American Catholics and such activities had picked up considerably. Pius XII, no doubt, saw in the appointment of the archbishop of Chicago the opportunity to tap into the sources of wealth among rich American Catholics, whose contributions would be more necessary than ever to sustain the ever-growing missionary efforts around the globe.

Whatever the case may be, Stritch promptly returned to Chicago and announced the sad news to select members of his household. On March 2, 1958, Stritch released the news of his new appointment to the press. His coworkers were dumbfounded. "What an atomic blast hit Chicago when the news about His Eminence arrived," wrote secretary Dan Ryan to Monsignor Ernest Primeau in Rome. "We are all shocked and 'all shook up.'"[14] Letters poured in from all sides, congratulating Stritch and offering their good wishes. In the midst of all this, Stritch noticed one omission which he commented on to his friend Judge Edward Tamm:

> It is strange that I have had messages from many foreign Governments and from many high officials in my own country and have not had even a word from the President of my own country. I have been and will always be a devoted citizen of my country, which I love with an abiding love, and I have sacrificed myself at times to comply with the President's wishes. It seems to me rather strange that the foreign Governments should express their satisfaction at this recognition of an American citizen and my own President should be silent.[15]

Ten days later, Eisenhower wrote a letter of congratulations and Vice-President Nixon sent one as well. On March 19, Senator Hubert Humphrey rose in the Senate to offer a commendation to Stritch and to read into the *Congressional Record* the notice of his appointment.[16] Yet, even these provided little consolation. He had shared his feelings about the whole matter with Monsignor J. Gerald Kealey: "At my age to leave Chicago and take up residence in Rome ... meant a sacrifice that had a touch of Gethsemane in it."[17]

In the midst of the numerous farewells and receptions, Stritch began to complain of stiffness and pain in his right arm. Attributing it to "writer's cramp," he ignored it until Holy Thursday. En route from his residence to Holy Name Cathedral for his last Mass of the Holy Oils, Stritch cried out in pain in the car, alarming his secretary.[18] The pain passed and Stritch bade farewell to Chicago on April 13, waving goodbye to a crowd of fifteen hundred who had gathered at Union Station to see him off. He and Hardiman took the crack Twentieth-Century Limited

to New York, where Spellman hosted an elaborate farewell banquet attended by numerous bishops and dignitaries. On April 17 Stritch boarded the *Independence* and set sail for Naples. On board the ship, the excruciating pain in Stritch's right arm eventually gave way to numbness. The doctor aboard the ship examined Stritch and discovered the blood clot in his arm that was causing him pain and was the first to suggest the possibility of amputation. Hardiman pleaded with Stritch to disembark the liner when it arrived for a port call at Algeciras, Spain, and fly back to the United States for treatment, but the cardinal refused. Upon arriving at Naples on April 27 his condition had deteriorated badly. Monsignor Joseph Emmenegger, an American priest from Milwaukee, was on hand to greet the prelate and wrote to his superior, Archbishop Meyer:

> The arrival of His Eminence at Naples was indeed sad. I went there with Bishop [Martin] O'Connor to meet him; it was evident that he was a very sick man, but held up most courageously in face of the confounded confusions at the port, withstood the rather hectic train trip to Rome; immediately upon his arrival, doctors were called and already at that time it seemed likely that the amputation of his arm would be necessary.[19]

Emmenegger had reported accurately. Stritch was rushed to Rome's Clinica Sanatrix and immediately was examined by Dr. Pietro Valdoni, a cardiovascular specialist. Hardiman also called for Stritch's longtime physician, Dr. Ralph Bergen, and a professor of surgery at Loyola Medical School, Dr. John Keeley. The arrival of the two American doctors was facilitated by Judge Edward Tamm and the FBI, who moved Keeley and Bergen through passport procedures and facilitated their hasty journey to Rome.[20] They concurred in Valdoni's diagnosis, and on April 28 the Italian physician performed the amputation of Stritch's right arm in a forty-five-minute operation.

For a whole month after the surgery hopes rose that he would be able to recover adequately to assume his duties. On May 18 he was able to offer Mass for the first time since the amputation. Pathetic scenes of the one-armed cardinal offering Mass, aided by the faithful Hardiman, were plastered all over the *New World*. But that Mass was to be his last. The very next

day, he suffered a serious stroke that paralyzed his right side. The combination of thrombosis, amputation, and stroke, in addition to the psychological sadness and weariness, left him with little capacity to resist. Surrounded by his close friends, Monsignor Patrick Hayes, Bishop Roman Atkielski, and Hardiman, Stritch died on May 27. After embalming at the North American College, his body was shipped to Chicago for official obsequies. On June 3 a Solemn Pontifical Requiem Mass was offered by Cicognani, and Stritch was laid to rest in Chicago's Mount Carmel Cemetery. Pius XII had never visited Stritch in the hospital, nor had there been any hint as to who Stritch's successor would be. Symbolically, the filling of this post would be one of the last acts of Pope Pius XII, who himself died in October of the same year. The passing of Pius XII and the accession of John XXIII represented the close of an era of Catholic life that had begun with the condemnation of modernism and ended with the convocation of Vatican II. It was mirrored in Chicago with the death of Stritch and the accession of Albert G. Meyer. At the solemn Mass of Requiem in Chicago's Holy Name Cathedral, Archbishop Albert Meyer stood by the bier of his former patron to pronounce the ritual absolution. Within a few months Meyer was named Stritch's successor. The two paths that had crossed and paralleled each other now converged in the administration of the largest American archdiocese: Chicago.

Meyer was a tall, heavily built man with none of Stritch's Southern charm and garrulity. Rather, his priests knew Meyer as a shy and highly formal prelate with a reserve that resisted easy familiarity and small talk. His talks lacked the easy-going eloquence of the southern bishop and resembled the more scholarly and staid presentations of a classroom teacher, heavily larded with quotations from papal speeches and encyclicals. But he was a conscientious administrator, good for every detail, and faithfully at his chancery desk presenting himself to the problems and duties of the archdiocese. Moreover, he was far more curious about the changing conditions around him and much more open to new data and new approaches than was his predecessor. Stritch may have looked and acted more like kindly Pope John, but he was more ideologically attuned to Pius XII. Meyer,

by contrast, looked more like Pius XII but came to feel more spiritual and intellectual kinship with John XXIII.

Meyer continued to provide for the ongoing Catholic move to suburbia and also fine-tuned the administrative structures of the huge archdiocese to match its rapid growth and his engaged style of leadership. But he clearly had a different approach to solving social issues than his more conservative predecessor. He accurately tracked the first gales of the national civil rights movement which were now blowing northward and touching the consciences of the large urban churches of the north. Unlike Stritch, who hesitated and vacillated in these matters, Meyer swung the prestige of his office behind a forceful policy of inter-racial justice. His words and actions brought an end to an era of timidity in racial matters. Under Meyer as well, urban issues, inextricably linked with racial matters, also began to receive the full-time, professional attention that they deserved from such a large institution as the Catholic church of Chicago—an institution that had a vital stake in Chicago's future.

Unfortunately Meyer's "domestic policies" did not have much time to be felt, since the convocation of Vatican II in 1962 quickly shifted the epicenter of Catholic life to Rome. A cardinal by the time of the council's opening, Meyer was compelled to put his huge diocese on automatic pilot in order to give full attention to the absorbing theological issues debated in those historic years. At the council Meyer would soar to international prominence, outdistancing the paladins of a previous era, Francis Spellman and Fulton J. Sheen. His unimpeachable integrity and his careful consultation with respectable scholars made him what theologian Yves Congar called "the peritus of the bishops." When Meyer took the floor at Vatican II the bishops were attentive. They listened not only to the clarity of his ecclesiastical Latin, or because of his cardinalitial rank, but because he spoke so effectively for ideas whose time had come: modern biblical scholarship, a richer ecclesiology, and religious liberty. Meyer had always been a man of clear convictions and principles, and it would be simplistic to ascribe any one reason for his significant role at the council. But, without a doubt, the years spent in Chicago with its nearly intractable problems, its

burgeoning growth, and its confident optimism flavored his stance on the Church's relationship with the world. Although his work on religious liberty received the most publicity, his close friend Bishop John Grellinger firmly insisted that Meyer's real interests at Vatican II were the documents on the Church, *Lumen Gentium* and *Gaudium et Spes*. It would have been interesting to see the directions of Chicago Catholic life if one so intimately linked with the direction of the Council, and so in tune with its inner dynamism, had lived to see it implemented. Instead, he died before the last session and the baton of leadership was passed to the unsteady hands of John Patrick Cody. An era of Catholic life in America that civil rights activist John McDermott aptly called "this confident Church" ended with Meyer's episcopate, as the hopefulness of the conciliar era gave way to the tumult of the sixties and seventies, when again Chicago would be a microcosm of events that would characterize the American Church at large.

1

"This Is Chicago"

The long yellow coaches of the Milwaukee Road railroad moved at a rapid clip on the cold morning of March 6, 1940, filled with civic and ecclesiastical dignitaries. Along the Milwaukee-Chicago line crowds gathered to wave and shout their greetings to the passengers. At Techny, Illinois, black-cassocked priests and novices of the Society of the Divine Word stood, as one reporter described them, "in solemn ranks, their heads bare."[1] As the train pulled into Union Station a crowd of 12,000 waited to catch a glimpse of the man who would lead Chicago's nearly one and a half million Catholics, Samuel Alphonsus Stritch. Thousands of CYO members were on hand to cheer the new prelate as Mayor Edward Kelly silenced the crowd to announce the city's greetings to the new archbishop: "We know no religion on such an occasion as this. We know only Americanism. This is Chicago where all races, creeds, and colors are welcome."[2] From the rail station Stritch proceeded to Holy Name Cathedral. Lining the streets were over 300,000 Chicagoans, including some 45,000 Catholic schoolchildren having a free day to welcome their new bishop. In rites resplendent with "the medieval splendor of Roman Catholic ritual" Stritch was enthroned as the fourth archbishop of Chicago on March 7, 1940, and began a reign that would span eighteen years.

Stritch was born August 17, 1887, the fifth son of Irish-born schoolmaster Garrett Stritch and the American-born Katherine (Katie) Malley. Garrett Stritch passed away when "Sammy" was barely eight and Stritch later testified: "My mother was of

15

course, the greatest influence in my life."[3] Under the watchful eye of Katie Malley Stritch, Sammy grew up a delicate, bookish lad, imitating the voracious reading habits of his parents. This was evident even in grade school at nearby Assumption parish, where the young lad was soon leaping over schoolwork, taking the grades two at a time. At the age of ten he was ready for high school.

As older brothers married and moved out Stritch found a strong male image in the priest whose Mass he served daily, Father John B. Morris. Born in 1866 and ordained in 1892, Morris had been trained for the priesthood in Rome and was the rector of St. Mary's Cathedral in the city of Nashville. Later he would become the bishop of Little Rock, Arkansas, and also indirectly linked to the Stritch family by the marriage of his sister Ellen to Stritch's older brother Thomas. When the young Samuel Stritch declared his interest in the priesthood, Morris took him under his wing and urged him to attend the Cathedral grade school and later introduced him to Thomas Sebastian Byrne, the bishop of Nashville.

Bishop Byrne was a native of Ohio and former rector of St. Gregory's Seminary in Cincinnati. Eager to build up a well-educated and respectable native clergy for the far-flung diocese (it then encompassed the whole state of Tennessee), he too encouraged the vocational aspirations of young Stritch and sent him to St. Gregory's Seminary. When Stritch completed his classical course in 1904, Byrne sent him to the North American College in Rome to attend classes at the Urban College of the Propaganda. Only sixteen years old, Stritch arrived in the Eternal City in the late summer of 1904 and began his studies for the priesthood that October. Stritch was gifted with a keen mind, a facility with foreign languages, and his parents' love for reading and study. In one of the most accurate depictions in Marie Cecile Buerhle's adoring biography of Stritch, she describes the diminutive seminarian as happily curled up under a tree reading Ludwig Von Pastor's massive *History of the Popes* while the other boys of the North American played ball and other games.[4] Stritch was bright and probably would have loved a career as a seminary or college professor. Indeed, all his life Stritch demonstrated a fondness for the speculative and especially for the categories of

neo-scholastic thought, which he fondly referred to as "the great underlying truths which are perennial and independent of the flux in human events."[5] Aloisius Muench remarked in his diary what many felt about Stritch when he was archbishop of Milwaukee: "Comment is that a good scholar and historian were lost when he was made a bishop."[6]

By the age of twenty-two he was ready for ordination and a special rescript was procured allowing him to be ordained under the canonical age of twenty-five. On May 21, 1910, Stritch was raised to the priesthood in the Lateran Basilica by Cardinal Pietro Respighi. After his ordination and completion of his studies Stritch was on his way back to Nashville, where he accepted a temporary assignment at Assumption parish. He was then dispatched to St. Patrick's parish, one of the largest in the city of Memphis, where he soon became pastor. He had been there only six years when Byrne called him back to Nashville in 1916 to serve as his secretary. Later, when the bishop's health began to fail, Stritch assumed more and more *de facto* control of the affairs of the diocese. In addition to keeping the excitable Byrne quiet, so as not to aggravate a chronic heart ailment, Stritch had jobs heaped on him, one after another, including those of rector of the cathedral, superintendent of schools, and chancellor of the diocese.

On August 10, 1921, at the age of thirty-four, Stritch was named the second bishop of Toledo and became the youngest member of the American hierarchy. The ceremonies of consecration took place on November 30, 1921, in Toledo's St. Francis de Sales Cathedral. Officiating was Archbishop Henry Moeller of Cincinnati, assisted by then Bishop Morris of Little Rock and classmate Bishop Thomas Edmund Molloy of Brooklyn. Stritch's predecessor, Bishop Joseph Schrembs, preached the sermon.

Stritch's nine years in Toledo (1921–1929) coincided with the relatively prosperous 1920s and were happy and busy years. Even though the newspapers contrasted him to Schrembs, "[who] was particularly active in community affairs," by noting that Stritch "is retiring [and] a student of history and a reader,"[7] the 'boy-bishop' embarked on an energetic program of expansion and institutional reform. On August 26, 1930, Stritch was

appointed to succeed the late Sebastian G. Messmer as archbishop of Milwaukee and Karl J. Alter succeeded to the see of
Toledo.

Milwaukee was a territorially smaller jurisdiction than
Toledo, comprising seventeen counties of southeastern
Wisconsin. Yet it had over 300,000 Catholics (nearly twice as
many as Toledo), 533 diocesan and religious priests, and 323
parishes. In the late fall of 1930 Milwaukee was a diocese sliding
into the abyss of the Great Depression. Weeks after Stritch's
arrival the main bonding house of the archdiocese collapsed and
several parishes faced bankruptcy. Money was scarce even for
important social services subsidized by the archdiocese. Stritch
was forced to retrench and cut back on expenses and consequently his ten years in Milwaukee were not as happy or productive as the ones spent in Toledo. His fiscal woes were
exacerbated by some serious shortcomings as an administrator
that became apparent against the backdrop of serious financial
difficulties.[8]

All his life Stritch simply could never adjust his working
habits to the tempo of the urban-industrial world in which his
episcopal ministry took place. His nephew Thomas Stritch
attests that many of the Stritch family seemed to lack the kind of
energy, the "get-up-and-go" of many successful people. His personal secretary, Monsignor James Hardiman, believed that
Stritch's poor eating habits and his heavy smoking also may
have contributed to his slow manner and unhurried pace. Even
though it often irritated his more task-oriented coworkers,
Stritch consistently refused to emulate the dawn to dusk patterns of executives in the North. He often slept late, paid little
attention to bureaucratic problems, answered his own door,
rolled his own cigarettes, and was consistently indifferent to his
personal appearance.

Dealing with "difficult" people was especially onerous to
him. He imposed punitive measures with reluctance. When confronted by troublesome decisions or "problem" priests, he frequently temporized, hoping that "masterly inactivity" would
bring a solution.[9] Sometimes he just went to bed and hoped that
the next morning would bring a new outlook or a solution to a
problem. Stritch's administrative failings became a topic of

conversation among the clergy and were recorded in the diary of the rector of St. Francis Seminary, Monsignor Aloisius Muench.

> The Archbishop was not present this year. He was confined to his room with a bad cold. His is not a robust vigorous constitution. Yet he undertakes the tasks of a giant. There is no letting up in his activities. Fr. Barbian [archdiocesan superintendent of schools] told me he goes down "into the dumbs" [sic] easily. I have noticed that he is easily depressed by adverse news. He "can't take it" in the phrase of the day. In public he does not show his spells of melancholy. He successfully hides the inner man by smiles and pleasantry.[10]

Later in 1934 he wrote:

> He does not get letters out in time despite assurances and promises. New appointments should have gone out a month ago—they have not yet been made. An important letter on assessments has not yet been written.[11]

Moreover, his tendency to make high-flown promises and never follow through on them also disappointed the clergy. Muench complained:

> The Archbishop is spending a good deal of his time in keeping his ear to the ground to find out what people might think or say. Priests are beginning to mutter that he knows how to say nice things but does not do anything. It is true that his lack of making decisions is becoming more and more apparent.

Among those unfulfilled promises were pledges to convene an archdiocesan synod, rebuild St. John's Cathedral, build a new theologate, and send priests to Oxford and other prestigious European universities. One priest, taking a disdainful view of Stritch's promises, remarked bitterly of him, "He was a perfectly integrated fake, he believed his own bullshit." Stritch may have suffered from some form of clinical depression as this pathetic description seems to indicate:

> Not long ago, the A[rchbishop] sat in his room, darkened, brooding about something, and when Msgr. Traudt [the vicar general

of the diocese] tried to cheer him up, he left his study and went into his bedroom. The Sister told Msgr. that she found the A. crying in his bedroom. We feel that his nerves are worn down, hence his melancholy, his diffidence and lack of power of decision.[12]

But the same priests who criticized the archbishop often perceived a positive side to Stritch's penchant for "temporizing" and procrastination. Whatever his failings, he did possess enough acumen to surround himself with strong managerial types and gave them virtually free rein in their respective tasks. Moreover, he did not attempt to "micro-manage" the work of his subordinates. This permissiveness, as his priests called it, probably accounts for most of the successes he enjoyed in his years of church administration.

In October 1939 Cardinal George Mundelein of Chicago died in his sleep. On Christmas Eve of that same year, as Stritch was preparing to celebrate the pontifical Mass at midnight, he received a telegram from the apostolic delegation announcing his appointment to the see of Chicago. The Archdiocese of Chicago that Stritch inherited in the early months of 1940 had just come through a dynamic epoch in its history. Institutionally, the Chicago Catholic community had evolved from a maze of immigrant communities into a highly centralized and visible public institution.[13]

The Mundelein era was characterized by vigorous institutional expansion, beginning with the addition of a number of new parishes during Chicago's first suburban boom in the prosperous twenties. The growing size and complexity of the archdiocese required the centralization of administrative services under the direction of Mundelein himself and trusted subordinates like Monsignors George Casey and Edward Burke. The need for a stable supply of loyal, obedient, and docile clergy led to the establishment of a mammoth seminary system. The crown jewel of this program was St. Mary of the Lake Seminary, a veritable city of buildings in far-off Lake County which housed the newly established major seminary. Mundelein himself lived on the seminary grounds and kept a close eye on developments there. Mundelein swathed himself in the trappings of ecclesiastical grandeur, winning the coveted cardinal's

hat in 1924 and hosting a stupendous gathering of national Catholics at the Eucharistic Congress of 1926. By cultivating highly public contacts with the Roosevelt administration, Mundelein further enhanced his standing as a major player in national life and the prestige of his growing community of Catholics in northeastern Illinois. When he died in 1939 even the isolationist *Chicago Tribune*, which certainly disagreed with his pro-Roosevelt politics, eulogized him as one of Chicago's most enthusiastic boosters.[14]

In the year of Stritch's accession there were 422 parishes in the Archdiocese of Chicago, serving 1.4 million Catholics in the northeastern Illinois counties Cook, Lake, Will, Kankakee, Du Page, and Grundy. Catholics comprised one-third of the total population of these six counties. The elementary school programs of these parishes enrolled over 150,000 pupils, while the high schools registered another 27,949 students. Social institutions such as homes for the aged, orphanages, and hospitals were also an important part of Stritch's jurisdiction, although often under the direction of semiautonomous religious communities of men and women. These institutions served the multiple needs of Chicago's Catholic community, providing essential social welfare programs in an era before large government agencies became the major carriers of these services.

But statistics tell only a portion of the story. The practice of their religion was for many Chicagoans a thoroughly integrated part of their urban life, and Chicago Catholicism in 1940 was still a neighborhood faith where neighborhoods and communities were identified by the names of the parish churches in their areas. Eileen McMahon found this in her study of St. Sabina's parish on Chicago's South Side. "St. Sabina's parishioners," she wrote, "saw the parish as a place to foster religious devotion, to shelter their families from secular society, and a means by which to Christianize the rest of the world. Its devotional life, the school, its recreational activities, all combined to reinforce the parish community."[15] St. Sabina's was indeed a microcosm of Chicago Catholic life. Parish celebrations, devotional societies, mutual aid associations, and "novena Catholicism" were part of the fabric of life of Chicago's Catholics as the new decade dawned.[16] Around the infrastructure of the parishes, other

Catholic institutions took their place. Catholic schools, colleges, and volunteer programs drew many of Chicago's youth in the corporate culture of Catholic life. Added to all these was a still vibrant collection of ethnic communities including Poles, Italians, Germans, and others from central Europe.

Two important actors of the Mundelein era remained on the scene when Stritch arrived, Bishop Bernard J. Sheil, auxiliary bishop and disappointed candidate for the Chicago see and Monsignor Reynold Hillenbrand, the young and charismatic rector of St. Mary of the Lake Seminary. Both men contributed significantly to the conditions of Chicago Catholic life that Stritch found in 1940.

Bernard Sheil was born February 18, 1886, the son of James and Roselia Barclay Sheil.[17] Although poor, Sheil's family managed in time to acquire a good deal of money in the coal business. Indeed, Sheil apparently used a large portion of his $100,000 inheritance in the early years of the CYO. He attended St. Columbkille School on the Northwest Side and St. Viator College in Bourbannais, where he demonstrated above average skills in debating and sports.[18] As a pitcher for the St. Viator baseball team Sheil maintained that in 1906 he had pitched a no-hitter in a game against Big Ten champs, the University of Illinois, and attracted the attention of scouts from the Cincinnati Reds and the Chicago White Sox. The story was only half true; there were hits in the game, but the offers were real.[19] Nonetheless, he turned them down to attend St. Viator Seminary. He was ordained for the Archdiocese of Chicago in 1910 and served his first years of priestly ministry at St. Mel's Church, a large Irish parish on the West Side. There his interests in youth work were first piqued by his association with a short-lived Catholic Athletic League program as well as by his association with Father Raphael Ashenden, a fellow curate who would later work with him in the formation of the Catholic Youth Organization.[20] At the outbreak of World War I Sheil was transferred to the Great Lakes Naval Training Center for a year. After the war, he was assigned to Holy Name Cathedral with additional duties at the Cook County Jail on Illinois Street. At the jail he came into contact with numerous youthful offenders and vowed to do something about their plight.

In 1924 Mundelein promoted Sheil to chancellor of the archdiocese after the resignation of Father Dennis J. Dunne. Sheil cemented his relationship to Mundelein by playing an important role in organizing the Chicago Eucharistic Congress of 1926. His next promotion came in 1928 when he accompanied Mundelein to Rome on the quinquennial *ad limina* visit. Mundelein had recently lost his auxiliary, Edward Hoban, who was appointed bishop of Rockford, Illinois. When officials of the Consistorial Congregation urged the Chicago cardinal to name a replacement, he offhandedly waved toward Sheil and said, "name him." Certainly there was more than sheer caprice in Mundelein's choice, but the circumstances make the story seem plausible. On May 1, 1928, Sheil was consecrated auxiliary to the archbishop of Chicago.[21]

Sheil's interest in Catholic youth work was a response to the intractable problem of juvenile delinquency and crime that was so much a part of the Chicago urban scene. Sheil was also concerned with the ability of anti-Christian philosophies to make inroads among Chicago's youth and the poor. Largely in an attempt to appeal to the young toughs prone to lives of crime or to Communist agitation, Sheil sponsored the numerous athletic events that dominated the work of the CYO. The most popular and highly profiled of the CYO programs were the boxing tournaments that enthralled thousands of Chicago youths. Although not everybody was pleased with this emphasis on pugilism, the CYO was a great success, not only because of its popular athletic program but also its racial, religious, and ethnic inclusiveness.

Sheil's closest lay advisor was his personal attorney, William Campbell.[22] He was a devout Catholic and loyal parishioner at Holy Name Cathedral, very active in the Holy Name Society, and favored the cause of Catholic youth work, especially the Boy Scouts. Their mutual interest in scouting brought Sheil and Campbell together and the two became life-long friends, a relationship that would work to the advantage of both. Campbell began working with Sheil when asked to serve on the board of the Catholic Salvage Bureau. He later became an assistant director of the CYO as well as its corporate attorney, which meant he was also Bishop Sheil's personal attorney.

Campbell faithfully tended to the internal affairs of the CYO and often found himself cleaning up Sheil's erratic financial matters, rescuing him from threatened lawsuits over non-payment of rent for his Lake Shore Drive apartments, and constantly negotiating difficulties over rent for the Congress Street building that the CYO rented as its headquarters in the thirties.[23] In turn, Sheil was a great help to the bright and courteous young attorney, introducing him to Cardinal Mundelein and encouraging him in his participation in ward politics of the Chicago Democratic machine. The patronage of Sheil, and later Mundelein, as well as Campbell's own natural affinity for the political scene led to his first big break in 1935, when Harry Hopkins appointed him director of the National Youth Administration for the Chicago area. The NYA was an important stepping-stone for many up-and-coming young politicians, including men like Lyndon Johnson of Texas. By clever manipulation Campbell managed to incorporate the all-important work project operations into his office and ladled out patronage to his own benefit and that of his Democratic bosses. Campbell's appointment to the NYA post directly benefited Sheil and the Chicago Catholic community. Campbell was able to channel large sums of money to Catholic institutions in the form of government-salaried clerical and secretarial staff. This largesse not only benefited schools and youth programs but even organizations like the Chicago Interstudent Catholic Action movements (CISCA).[24] Campbell also smoothed the way for CYO activities to win support of other sources of public funding, such as the Chicago Community Chest and the Social Services Board. He also was helpful in securing federal recognition for the Holy Name Aeronautical School in Lockport, another of Sheil's enterprises.

The indirect effects of Campbell's favor were even more important than providing secretarial staff for Catholic agencies or legal counsel. Because of his contacts with Sheil and Mundelein, Campbell became an important intermediate between the Chicago Catholic leadership and the Roosevelt administration. This redounded to Campbell's benefit, for as the importance of these Catholic figures grew, Campbell's influence in the administration grew accordingly. Campbell's mounting

prestige within the Roosevelt administration put him in contact with a wide array of influential government and private figures, whom he in turn introduced to Sheil. These included well-known characters such as Thomas G. Corcoran, NYA administrator Aubrey Williams, and the *Washington Post* publisher, Eugene Meyer, and his wife, Agnes. Agnes Meyer was one of Sheil's most devoted admirers and generously aided any cause the bishop deemed worthy. It was she who regularly campaigned for Sheil's promotion to higher office.[25] Campbell also introduced Sheil to lesser-known figures like Undersecretary of the Treasury Edward Foley and others who would later become famous, like Attorney General Francis Biddle, Attorney General and later Supreme Court Justice Robert Jackson, and Adlai Stevenson. By 1937 Campbell had staked his turf as a go-between for Mundelein and Roosevelt so effectively that he could insist in a memo to Aubrey Williams about an official who made Catholic contacts on his own: "I understood that he was to have all further dealing with the officials of the Catholic Church at Chicago through me."[26]

Campbell's usefulness to the administration and to the Chicago hierarchy did not lack its reward. In 1938 he was strongly recommended for a federal judgeship by Sheil and Mundelein, though he received only the consolation prize of district attorney for northern Illinois. *Time* caustically commented on his appointment to the D.A.'s post, "NYA Director William Campbell ... couldn't wangle the district judgeship despite his friendship with Franklin Roosevelt's good friend George William Cardinal Mundelein."[27] However, Campbell made good use of the D.A.'s job, taking charge of a major investigation of gambling rings in the Midwest, successfully prosecuting racing-sheet mogul Moses Annenburg for tax evasion in 1939, and playing a role in the tax-evasion case that eventually sent mobster Al Capone to federal prison. The Annenburg and Capone convictions finally won Campbell a federal judgeship in 1940. Campbell's association with Sheil's enterprises (and legal problems) became more circumspect after his appointment to the bench. Yet his personal friendship with a host of wealthy and influential Chicagoans, especially in the Jewish community, would be significant in Sheil's fund-raising endeavors.

Campbell was Bishop Sheil's most important booster in the political arena. But any impression Sheil made with the power brokers in the Roosevelt administration was largely because of his proximity to Cardinal Mundelein. Sheil was able to arrange for extensive newsreel coverage of a visit to Chicago of the president's son James Roosevelt. Sheil managed to have the newsreels distributed to theaters in the East and pressed the Chicago *New World* to print extensive coverage of the event.[28]

Sheil's association with New Deal politicians grew even more frequent once Campbell introduced him to Roosevelt's close advisor Thomas ("Tommy the Cork") Corcoran. Both men were fun-loving, garrulous Irish types who thoroughly enjoyed one another's company. Sheil for his part became a kind of unofficial chaplain to the Corcoran family, baptizing their children and spending holidays with them. In 1937 Corcoran pressed federal authorities to build an airport near Lockport, Illinois, the site of Sheil's Holy Name Flying School. The following year, when Sheil was awarded the Order of the Purple Heart for his work at the Great Lakes Naval Station during World War I, Roosevelt sent warm words of commendation.[29] Sheil responded in kind by adding his voice to those who recommended Corcoran for the post of solicitor general in 1938.[30] Throughout 1938 Sheil emerged more and more from his role as an understudy for the aging, and sometimes ill, Cardinal Mundelein to an outright stand-in for the prelate.

In early December 1938 Mundelein asked Sheil to deliver a short disclaimer of Father Charles Coughlin's right to speak for the Catholic Church in the United States. Timed to follow Coughlin's recently resumed Sunday afternoon broadcasts, Sheil's speech was designed to have maximum impact on the Catholic audience. Sheil read:

> His Eminence George Cardinal Mundelein of Chicago, having been importuned by news commentators and correspondence from every section of the country in reference to the broadcasts of Father Coughlin of Detroit makes the following statement: "As an American citizen, Father Coughlin has the right to express his personal views on current events, but he is not authorized to speak for the Catholic Church nor does he represent the doctrine or sentiments of the Church."[31]

The brief statement hit the front page of the *New York Times*, and Tommy Corcoran, who had helped to write it, was quick to disseminate the news to White House staffers, who reported in a memo: "Tom Corcoran says that Bishop Bernard J. Sheil is Auxiliary Bishop of Chicago; he is the individual who publicly raked Coughlin over the coals for Cardinal Mundelein. Tom thinks this information ought to leak out to the Press so that they will know who Sheil is."[32]

Sheil moved into the limelight again when he threw his support behind the organizing activities of the CIO. Sheil's endorsement was linked to his support for the work of Chicago community organizer Saul Alinsky, who had begun organizing the neighborhood in the area of the stockyards known as "Back-of-the-Yards." The efforts to organize the Back-of-the-Yards worked in tandem with the plans of CIO to organize packing-house workers. Sheil's support for the CIO initiative came at a time he was seeking to repair his bad press from involvement in another Chicago labor controversy. That dispute centered on a series of articles on youth that Sheil had written for the Hearst-owned *Chicago Daily American* in the summer of 1938. In early 1939 the Chicago Newspaper Guild had struck the Hearst paper. As a ploy to demoralize Catholic workers the paper's management had run the Sheil columns to imply that Sheil supported management's side in the dispute. When the columns appeared in late January, Newspaper Guild spokesmen reviled Sheil as a scab. Sheil was stung by the accusations and met with the union leaders in late February 1939, where he decried "the preposterous and totally false impression ... that the appearance of the articles at this particular time was in effect a public rebuff on the part of a Catholic Bishop to the courageous Catholic members of the Newspaper Guild...."[33]

Still smarting from the humiliation of being called a "scab," Sheil dramatically signaled his support for the CIO by appearing on the dais with John L. Lewis at a huge rally at the Chicago Coliseum in July 1939. At this famous rally Sheil delivered a ringing invocation in support of the workers and their cause. This established his reputation as a friend of organized labor and cemented his standing with the White House by his mention of the name of Roosevelt before John L. Lewis and the

excited workers. Campbell was quick to report this to Corcoran, who telephoned FDR's personal secretary, Missy.LeHand (another informal Catholic liaison in the White House), "Campbell, Chicago District Attorney telephoned today to say that the Cardinal had expressed the wish that Bishop Shiel [sic], auxiliary Bishop of Chicago, might have a few moments audience tomorrow. The Bishop who made the invocation introducing the President's name at John Lewis' Stockyards workers meeting last week, is in Washington ... en route ... to Rome."[34] One week after the speech, Sheil met with Corcoran and was soon ushered into the presence of Roosevelt.

Sheil's finest hour, as far as the Roosevelt people were concerned, came just after the cardinal died in 1939. Hitler had invaded Poland in September of that year, and Roosevelt took advantage of the international crisis to press for changes in American neutrality legislation to allow for a renewal of the expired cash-and-carry provisions for purchasing weapons in the 1937 law. As a tense debate opened in the United States Senate, Campbell and Corcoran prepared a radio speech for Sheil strongly supporting Roosevelt's policies. It was scheduled for delivery at a CYO convention in Cincinnati, Ohio. On October 2, the evening before Sheil was scheduled to deliver the speech, Mundelein died unexpectedly and Sheil was appointed administrator of the archdiocese. After weighing the pros and cons, the decision was made to go on the air with an addendum to the text eulogizing the recently deceased Mundelein. The president was delighted with the address and commented in a letter to *Chicago Daily News* publisher (and later secretary of the navy) Frank Knox: "Things seem to be getting better and, incidentally, Bishop Sheil's speech on Monday night last was grand."[35] That same day Senator Scott Lucas of Illinois had the entire text of the speech entered into the *Congressional Record*. Soon after his radio address Sheil met with Roosevelt, who effusively thanked the bishop. All of this had a purpose: to get Sheil the Chicago post or one of equivalent prestige.

Indeed, FDR did make some half-hearted attempts to have Sheil promoted. After his meeting with Sheil, Roosevelt dispatched Postmaster General Frank Walker and Secretary of the Interior Harold Ickes (both strong supporters of Sheil) to

Archbishop Francis Spellman to press for Sheil's appointment to Chicago. Spellman, who already regarded the Chicago auxiliary with suspicion, remained impassive and claimed to have no influence on the decision. Ickes in particular, according to his diary, lobbied Roosevelt to press for Sheil's appointment directly with the Vatican. Ickes had first come to know Sheil in 1923 when then Father Sheil had presided at the marriage of his stepson, Wilmarth, to Betty Dahlman of Milwaukee in Ickes's Winnetka, Illinois, home.[36] Ickes's own son, Raymond, had participated in Sheil's CYO boxing program. The Ickes-Sheil relationship was not close, but the Progressive-minded Ickes admired the liberal principles of both Mundelein and Sheil. But FDR refused to press further for Sheil's appointment to Chicago. Ickes and Corcoran urged Roosevelt to lobby Vatican officials for Sheil's appointment to the soon-to-be-created Archdiocese of Washington. According to the agenda Roosevelt drew up for Myron Taylor, his special emissary to the Vatican, the issue of Sheil's promotion to Washington was listed.[37] Taylor did bring up the issue of Sheil's promotion with Cardinal Secretary of State Luigi Maglione, but, like Spellman, Maglione brushed aside the request, informing Taylor that such matters were handled by the Consistorial Congregation.[38]

How heavily Roosevelt wanted to lean on Vatican officials is unknown. Clearly he had been willing to exert pressure to neutralize his clerical nemesis, Coughlin. It appears from the Ickes diary notations that he wanted to save his political capital with the Vatican for other battles and did not consider the Sheil appointment to Chicago or Washington as politically advantageous or necessary once Coughlin was out of the picture and Spellman was providing necessary information and support with Rome. Nevertheless, Sheil was a welcome visitor in Washington and often made his way to the White House during the annual meetings of bishops for off-the-record chats with Roosevelt.

During the war Sheil was recruited as part of the government war-bond drive and worked especially with bond sales among the ranks of organized labor. His friends in high places regularly appeared at lectures and testimonial banquets and occasionally expedited a customs case or provided air transport

for one or the other of the bishop's trips. But none of them, from Roosevelt on down, were able to pull the kinds of levers with ecclesiastical officials that would have gotten him a diocese of his own. To achieve this Sheil himself would have had to work more effectively with Stritch, and this he was unable to do. Another holdover from the Mundelein era, Reynold Hillenbrand, would have difficulties with Stritch as well.

Reynold (or Reinhold) Henry Hillenbrand was born in Chicago July 19, 1904, the second of George and Eleanor Schmitt Hillenbrand's nine children. Reynold entered Quigley Preparatory Seminary in the fall of 1920, just two years after his older brother Frederick. At Quigley, Reynold was a bright pupil showing a particular love for English literature and writing. In his final years he served as editor of the seminary annual *Petite Seminaire*. He also edited the school newspaper, *The Candle*, which included a witty column called "From the Crow's Nest."

The new major seminary of the Archdiocese of Chicago was still in its formative stages when Reynold arrived in 1924, and adjusting to the new environment was a bit of a task for the city-bred Hillenbrand boys. Reynold wrote to his Uncle Henry Schmitt, a priest of the Archdiocese of Milwaukee:

> I imagined at first that I wouldn't 'fancy' the drastic change from the city mode; but I got accustomed to it.... Some one could ask me for a biretta and I don't think I would bring him "a board," or an altar card. In fact, when we got back to the city, it seemed odd at first to see so many people at one time and that they weren't wearing cassocks, zimaras, et al."[39]

The seminary was indeed a world unto itself. Cardinal Mundelein closely monitored every aspect of the seminary's life in order to assure himself of a stable supply of obedient and docile clergy. Moreover, St. Mary of the Lake opened just as Rome was tightening up on the requirements and regulations for clerical formation. Classes were in Latin and discipline was strict. Few visitors were permitted on the seminary grounds, and the seminarians went home rarely.

As part of Mundelein's penchant for "going first class," he procured the services of the Jesuits of the Missouri Province to serve as the academic faculty, while he retained a small corps of

diocesan priests to serve as administrators and disciplinarians. Hillenbrand, who later clashed with the sons of Loyola, was at first quite enamored of them, writing to his parents in 1924: "As has always been repeated in the past, the Jesuits are THE teachers. There is not a single one whom not everybody liked at first and continued to do so."[40] The effects of seminary study and formation on Hillenbrand could scarcely be overstated. Hillenbrand especially liked the more speculative and thought-provoking courses in the seminary curriculum. To his parents he commented: "The philosophy will hold no terrors in about a week, after one gets used to having the professor 'spout' it for an hour or two each day."[41]

During his two-year philosophy course, he managed to keep alive his interest in literature, constantly requesting classics from his collection of books at home and squeezing in reading periods whenever the crowded seminary schedule allowed. "The time is apportioned so well," he wrote, "that one finds time to do only what he is supposed to at that particular moment."[42] His master's thesis was a flattering study of Jesuit educational methods. His membership in the seminary's Bellarmine Society sharpened his abilities at public speaking and his literary tastes.

His spiritual formation blended with the rigorous intellectual training of the cycle of dogma classes required of every candidate for the priesthood. Nightly, according to Jesuit practice, Hillenbrand made points of meditation to be considered the next day. His preserved notes reveal an introspective and intense seminarian, highly idealistic, who focused his energies on a single goal with determination and purpose. Like most perfectionists, he suffered: "I can be disillusioned," he wrote in his diary, "I can become suspicious, become cynical, can let these things work on my morale so I cannot see the hundred good qualities and possibilities." He urged himself: "Be overlooking, be understanding, sympathetic; kindly, gentle and so teach and lead [youth] to higher things."[43] One passage was a paean of devotion to the Holy Father, Pius XI:

Thank God for our Holy Father and for the blessings He has given Him. He is a great man in many ways: Pope of the

Missions; he has settled the Roman Question which vexed the Church until now. He depends on the prayers of the faith [*sic*]. My Catholic sense has been blunted and my Catholic growth stunted if I do not pray for him everyday and for his many projects, especially for the missions. He needs God's grace and blessing.[44]

His attachment to the papacy was more than a passing phase of a youthful and idealistic young seminarian. The words of the Holy Father were for him the "living voice of Christ" in the present time. Writing an obituary for Hillenbrand in 1979, Robert McClory described this "literal cleaving to papal documents as the unquestionable word" as the chief characteristic of Hillenbrand's career.[45] What was true of him at his death was also in evidence from his youth. But more than anything else it was the apostolic thrust of Pius XI's pontificate that sent Hillenbrand's spirit soaring. In one telling passage, he laid down a challenge to himself, a challenge that bore a prophetic note for his future career:

> Pray.... Especially for the Church in this country—that it may be a power in this country—not in any political sense, but that its principles and ideals may enliven the people and solve their problems. We wonder about the destiny of this great nation. Consider the resources of the nation, the immense territory, the multitudes flocked to it from all nations, filling its coasts, cities, and countrysides—surely it has a destiny. No nation since Greece and Rome has so much power to influence. Cardinal Cerretti said all nations look to it. How much, therefore, she can do not in a political but in a religious and lasting way.[46]

Hillenbrand excelled at his studies and by the end of his second year was selected for graduate work at the seminary. Because of this he was ordained a year early on September 21, 1929, with five other classmates. After ordination he remained at the seminary to complete doctoral work in theology, writing a thesis on the subject which would be the theological underpinning of his later endeavors: the indwelling of the Holy Spirit.[47] Years before the encyclical *Mystici Corporis* was written, theologians were expanding their notions of the activity of grace in the

human soul from a static "possession" to a dynamic activity which perpetuated the saving work of God in the historical order.[48] This notion of divine indwelling was at the heart of Hillenbrand's efforts for liturgical and social reform. Indeed, Hillenbrand did not even use the term "grace" as much as he used the more dynamic "Divine Life."

When Hillenbrand completed doctoral studies in June 1931, Mundelein sent him on a special year of study and travel in Rome. After touring France, Switzerland, and Northern Italy with four classmates he arrived at the French-Canadian College. In this cold, damp building he lived with other graduate priests and took lessons in Latin and Greek from Father Pietro Parente. That very year saw the publication of the encyclical *Quadragesimo Anno* by Pius XI, and Hillenbrand had the opportunity to read and discuss it with the graduate students in the residence. He was especially interested in the stories of many of the French-speaking priests who had taken their seminary studies at Louvain and spoke of the efforts of Canon Joseph Cardijn to reclaim disaffected workers for Christianity. The Roman year sharpened an interest Hillenbrand was developing for what was then called "the social question."

Hillenbrand took maximum advantage of the time spent in Rome, familiarizing himself with the city. He even visited the stigmatic Theresa Neumann at her home in Konnersrueth as well as some of the great Benedictine abbeys to observe the first stirring of the liturgical movement. Moreover, he made a trip to the Holy Land before he returned to Chicago and his new duties.[49] Upon his return in 1932, he moved into the rectory of Holy Name Cathedral and was appointed to teach English at nearby Quigley Seminary. Young students like George Higgins recalled Hillenbrand's love for English literature and his knack for enticing the young men to read the classics by simply leaving them on his desk and urging them to borrow the books.[50]

The decade of the thirties continued to be years of intense learning for Hillenbrand, especially in regard to the conditions of life in a modern industrial city. Walking back and forth to Quigley or strolling in the Loop, Hillenbrand came face to face with the effects of the Great Depression, which was descending on the once thriving metropolis like a shroud. Chicago was hit

particularly hard by the economic slump as its once booming industrial economy ground to a standstill. Thousands were thrown out of work. Even worse, as the nation's transportation hub, Chicago became a mecca for thousands of transients who swelled the throngs of indigents and unemployed. By 1930 a "Hooverville" had appeared at the edge of the Loop on Randolph Street. Historian Roger Biles reports that by May 1932 Chicago's unemployment rolls included 700,000 people, fully 40 percent of its work force. Some 130,000 families received over $2 million in relief funds.[51]

Of all the places to live in the city of Chicago, the Cathedral rectory was perhaps the best for a priest of Hillenbrand's social interests, for it was an ideal location for reflection on the causes of and solutions to this great upheaval. The rector of Holy Name Cathedral, the wide-girthed Monsignor Joseph Morrison, was one of the truly outstanding pastors of the Chicago clergy and provided an ambience for discussion and action. Morrison was anything but an intellectual, but he had a practical pastoral sense which made him a natural patron of anyone who wanted to tackle the wretched social conditions of the times. The dinner table and parlors of Holy Name rectory were places of provocative discussion, and Morrison generously provided meeting rooms, sandwiches, and beer to social activists and charities of all types. Moreover, as Mundelein's master of ceremonies, he had a sharp interest in the correct performance of the liturgical rites. This interest was further stimulated by the Chicago Eucharistic Congress of 1926 and by his regular attendance at other congresses around the world. Moreover, it brought him into contact with the work of Virgil Michel, O.S.B., of St. John's Abbey in Collegeville, Minnesota. Hillenbrand benefited from this interest as well.

In 1933 Cardinal Mundelein proclaimed a celebration of the famous double jubilee—the ninetieth anniversary of the establishment of the diocese and the twenty-fifth anniversary of his own consecration as bishop. Conveniently the whole celebration dovetailed with Chicago's Century of Progress Exposition. A mission band of diocesan priests was established to commemorate the event and, as an obvious show of his pleasure, Mundelein appointed Hillenbrand its head. For the next

three years Hillenbrand traversed the diocese giving missions to virtually every parish in the archdiocese, seeing firsthand the difficult conditions of the parishioners and the exigencies of parish life in typical Chicago rectories. As a side interest Hillenbrand began giving instructions to the young women preparing for street preaching with the Catholic Evidence Guild at Rosary College. He remained at the mission work until 1936, when Mundelein appointed him second rector of St. Mary of the Lake Seminary. In introducing him to the students, Mundelein is reported to have said: "I know the seminary can be a dull place, so I've given you a man with imagination."[52]

The eight years Hillenbrand spent as rector of the major seminary (1936–1944) were perhaps the most innovative period of that institution's history. Hillenbrand's infectious enthusiasm for social and liturgical issues captured the imagination of the seminarians and caused one of them to eulogize the Hillenbrand era as a time when the seminary was "a Jerusalem place."[53] By the time he was dismissed in 1944, more than five hundred priests of the Archdiocese of Chicago had some exposure to the charismatic rector who called them by their first names.

Hillenbrand's primary impact was felt in the liturgical life at St. Mary of the Lake. The liturgical movement had begun in Europe in the past century, but it had been carried most effectively to the United States through the work of Benedictine Virgil Michel. In the mid-twenties Michel had met with two like-minded liturgical activists, Father Martin Hellreigel and Reverend Mr. Gerard Ellard, S.J. Together they launched a periodical called *Orate Fratres*, which explained the meaning of liturgical reform and disseminated the latest liturgical research. Until his untimely death in 1938, Michel was the guiding light of the movement. He summed up the basic purposes of the liturgical movement in a little syllogism that he often repeated:

> Pius X tells us that the liturgy is the indispensable source of the true Christian spirit. Pius XI says that the true Christian spirit is indispensable for social regeneration. Hence the conclusion: The liturgy is the indispensable basis of Christian social regeneration.[54]

Hillenbrand enthusiastically seized on Michel's ideas. The quality of seminary liturgical life had not been high on the list of

priorities of teachers and authorities at the seminary. Two daily Masses were celebrated for each class. One was in the house chapels, where the students did not receive Communion. The other was held in the large seminary chapel. Hillenbrand soon introduced occasional dialogue Masses with the students and common recitation or chanting of the Divine Office.

As part of the rector's responsibilities, Hillenbrand had regular meetings with deacons. He used these sessions to acquaint them with some of the realities of priestly life but even more to instill in them the basic principles of liturgical reform and Church teaching on social questions. He also made important changes in the seminary worship schedule which reinforced classroom learning. *Missa recitata* (Mass wherein the whole congregation rather than only the acolytes responded to the prayers) became a regular practice in the Sunday and feast-day schedule of the seminary. Hillenbrand was usually the celebrant and preached a homily on the readings of the Mass. Other liturgical speakers who augmented the lessons given by Hillenbrand included Jesuit Gerard Ellard, who preached two retreats; Donald Attwater, an associate editor of *Orate Fratres* and a leader of the liturgical movement in England; and Maurice Lavanoux, a liturgical architect.

An added dimension of the movement corresponded with Hillenbrand's own interests in changing the social order. Largely because of Virgil Michel, an important stress of the liturgical movement in the United States had been the restoration of an organic society. In particular, the notion of the Mystical Body of Christ appealed to these reformers as the ultimate paradigm for the new social order. Michel had begun to elaborate the strong interrelationship between the work of liturgical renewal and the work of social regeneration.[55]

Hillenbrand saw to it that the seminarians began to hear more and more of the Church's social teaching and, above all, of the connection between social action and the liturgy. During his years as rector a steady stream of the most important figures associated with social and liturgical issues came to speak to the isolated seminarians at Mundelein. As one example, while on a vacation with Hayes in 1936 or 1937, Hillenbrand had visited Dorothy Day in New York. In February 1938 Dorothy Day made

her way to the seminary to speak about the work of the Houses of Hospitality. The seminarian chronicler recorded the event in momentous tones:

> Tonight the seminarians were treated to something different. For the first time in the history of the seminary, they heard an address in the auditorium by a woman. She was none other than the well-known leader of the Catholic Workers [sic] movement which has spread from New York through the United States, Miss Dorothy Day. She impressed the seminarians with what she said and in how she said it, particularly when they were told she had left a sick bed to speak to them.[56]

Day had already opened her first House of Hospitality in Chicago on Blue Island Avenue. At Hillenbrand's insistence, seminarians devoted time to the new enterprise, and two enterprising Chicago Catholics, John Cogley and Edward Marciniak, became part of the first staff of the house. Other speakers in the 1936–1944 period included Father John Gilliard, S.S.J., who spoke of his work among blacks; Baroness Catherine de Hueck (whom Hillenbrand later considered eccentric); Australian Jocist Paul McGuire; Edward Skillin of *Commonweal*; Hispanic and labor advocate Bishop Robert Lucey of Amarillo; interracial activist Father John LaFarge, S.J.; and labor arbitrator Monsignor Francis Haas. Hillenbrand was grateful to them all and expressed to Haas: "They [the seminarians] know so little of the social action of the Church that anything you tell them would be of great interest and profit."[57]

Not only did Hillenbrand promote the social teaching of the Church, he was intent on putting that teaching into action. In 1937 the Social Action Department of the National Catholic Welfare Conference hosted a Summer School of Catholic Action for priests at St. Francis Seminary in Milwaukee. There were three goals for these schools: to study the social encyclicals; to gain knowledge of actual labor conditions in the United States; to review techniques of priestly involvement in economic problems.[58] Hillenbrand and his friend Father John Hayes attended the Summer School and heard talks by well-known Catholic social activists such as John A. Ryan, Francis Haas, Wilfrid Parsons, S.J., and Bishop Robert Lucey.

Returning to Chicago, Hillenbrand replicated the study-club technique recommended at the conference and, with Hayes and another priest-friend, Father William Boyd, immediately began to organize a support group of like-minded priests which met at the Cathedral rectory. This small study group of priests grew rapidly and eventually came under the chairmanship of Father Bernard Burns, who came to the Cathedral as an assistant in 1939. In 1938, Hayes and Hillenbrand offered a series of Lenten sermons entitled "A Catholic Slant on Economics," lavishly advertised on the front pages of the *New World*. Hillenbrand and Hayes liberally invoked the support of Cardinal Mundelein by quoting an address he gave at a Holy Name rally in February:

> Our place is beside the poor and behind the working man. They are our people, they build our churches, they occupy our pews, their children crowd our schools, and our priests come from their sons. They look to us for leadership, but they look to us, too, for support.[59]

Every Wednesday and Saturday a different theme or topic was addressed, beginning with "The Rotten Roots of Capitalism—Five Centuries of Decay" and concluding with "Shall We Try the Catholic Solution—the Occupational Group System."[60] Meanwhile, the study group began to grow in numbers, and the gathering steam of CIO organizing pushed the social activists into open advocacy of the rights of the unskilled. On two occasions in 1938 Hillenbrand delivered a plea for the organization of unskilled labor in the printing trades, first at the National Catholic Conference on Social Problems held in Milwaukee in May and at a similar gathering in Cleveland a few months later.

In Chicago in the late 1930s labor organizing began to take a hold on Chicago's biggest industries: steel and meat-packing.[61] Smaller groups of unorganized workers who had been scorned by the American Federation of Labor seized the moment and also began to mobilize. Since a large number of these unskilled laborers were Catholics, Hillenbrand, Hayes, and Boyd began a series of labor schools in 1938 throughout the diocese. Using outlines drawn up by Hillenbrand and Hayes, workers were schooled in labor history and parliamentary

procedure. Above all, workers were given a strong dose of the social encyclicals, which assured them that the Holy Father wanted them to organize and encouraged them to resist Communist efforts to subvert the labor movement. By 1940 there were eleven labor schools around the Archdiocese of Chicago.[62]

But as diligent as his efforts were in the study clubs and labor schools, Hillenbrand was looking for something that would bring about a more thoroughgoing change in the hearts and actions of individual Catholics—something that would issue in action. His friend Hayes would express it best in a talk entitled "Work of the Priest." "While priest's study groups are very valuable as preparation they do not really tackle the job assigned to us by the Pope—to make Catholic social teaching known to the people and eventually operative."[63] Hillenbrand soon found his methodology.

In 1938 Hillenbrand secured Mundelein's consent to host a Summer School of Catholic Action for priests at St. Mary of the Lake Seminary. Even though the format and speakers were much the same as in Milwaukee, the summer session at Mundelein highlighted the role of the laity in the work of social reconstruction. In the course of the proceedings, Hillenbrand was struck by the talk of a young priest of the Oklahoma City diocese, Father Donald Kanaly. Kanaly had just returned from seminary studies at Louvain and made a dynamic presentation about the Specialized Catholic Action movements associated with Canon Joseph Cardijn. Jocism had developed in the Low Countries and France, and it had taken firm root in Canada and even in some of the French-Canadian areas of New England. Cardijn's vision was to recapture the lost workers of Europe for Christianity.

His method was a distillation of St. Thomas Aquinas's teaching on the virtue of prudence. His program of intensive Christianization involved the organization of small groups of Christian workers and students called study circles (*circles d'etude*), which gathered to plan for the rechristianization of their schools or workplaces. Stress was placed on the notion of like-to-like: workers had to work with workers, students with students, and the study circles had to be composed of members

of the same sex. Action always proceeded from inquiry. A young militant (as the leaders of Cardijn's cells were called) would learn how to observe, judge, and then act. Kanaly told the assembled priests the story of Cardijn and the zeal he had for the salvation of the working classes. He spoke movingly of the priest's rejection by Cardinal Desire Mercier and of his ultimate vindication by Pius XI. He then went on to describe the technique that Cardijn formulated:

> It is quite different from the ordinary study club ... it is only the worker, the typical worker who will ever be able to win back the other workers. For the "cell" the priest should choose two, three, four or five, not more than seven workers who are representative of the parish. [Cardijn] insists that this should not be made up of boys or girls of the "goodie" type ... this cell will have to be composed of *typical* workers.... For six months try to form leaders. Then send them back among the other workers. They will be able to attract the other workers.[64]

Kanaly's speech electrified Hillenbrand. Jocism was not unfamiliar to the seminary rector, but he had never understood it as clearly as he did after Kanaly explained it. The small, like-to-like characteristics of the Jocists seemed to Hillenbrand a much better and more thorough way to change the minds and hearts of men than the widely diffused Catholic Action study groups or industrial conferences, which seemed to focus heavily on information and clerical direction. Hillenbrand immediately entered into discussions with Kanaly and the members of the priest's study group about the possibilities and ideals of Jocist methodology for his local Catholic community.[65] With an intensity only Hillenbrand could muster, he adopted the small group techniques of the Jocists as his own and blended them with his interest in the liturgy. For the remainder of his life, Hillenbrand would immerse himself in the work of founding small groups that would work to rechristianize the social order by an intensive program of education, prayer, and action.

A point of access to the "layperson market" occurred in 1939 with the appearance of Paul McGuire. Paul McGuire was an Australian layman who had made a name for himself as a commentator on the Spanish Civil War, a topic of great concern

to American Catholics in the late thirties. He was a strong supporter of Franco and his powerful anti-Communist message resonated well Pius XI's 1937 encyclical *Divini Redemptoris*—a forceful statement against communism. McGuire had also been a witness to the activities of the Jocists in France in the late thirties and recognized in Jocism a potent Catholic response to the intense organizing of the Communists. He introduced these ideas to American Catholics in a series of articles written for the Knights of Columbus monthly, *Columbia*, and also in some speaking engagements in various cities during 1938. In 1939 the Knights of Columbus sponsored McGuire on a major speaking tour around the country to share the message of Jocism.[66] In May 1939 he was invited by the Servites to the Basilica of Our Lady of Sorrows on the West Side of Chicago. The Basilica was one of the most popular devotional locations in the nation.[67] Its novena to the Sorrowful Mother had become a hardy staple of Chicago Catholic life and attracted thousands weekly. At the Basilica, McGuire spoke to enthusiastic groups of young people about Jocism and succeeded in forming twenty Catholic Action cells which met in the huge meeting hall of the church.

McGuire's work opened up the work of Jocism to the vast multitude of Chicago Catholic laity. Scattered cells from around Chicago, some begun by Hillenbrand's seminarians and others led by priests who had been at Kanaly's talk in Mundelein, soon joined forces with the McGuire-founded groups. From 1939 on, cells were formed throughout the Chicago area. Hillenbrand himself organized one for the students of Senn High School on the North Side of the city, coming into contact with Johanna Doniat, a teacher at the school and later director of Childerly, a retreat house for Catholic Actionists of all types, and with George "Red" Sullivan, who would become an important force in the Young Christian Workers.

The period 1940–1946 was a time of organizing and building for Catholic Action cells in Chicago, and Hillenbrand's interest in this work knew no bounds. He read voraciously all the material he could get on the movements and made contact with others promoting the work in other areas. The two natural leaders of the movements, Kanaly and McGuire, were unable to muster the resources or time to give the kind of direction the

groups needed. In 1940 Hillenbrand was introduced to Father Louis Putz, C.S.C., of the University of Notre Dame, a man who would later work closely with him to provide some structure and direction to the rapidly growing movement in Chicago and elsewhere. Putz had been a teacher in France and had served as a chaplain to the movements in Europe. Together Hillenbrand and Putz drew up guidelines for Catholic Action cells and laid plans for the coordination and ideological purity of the work in Chicago and elsewhere.

The activities of Hillenbrand and Sheil were emblematic of the vivacious and ebullient spirit of Chicago Catholicism in 1940. Chicago Catholic life was vibrant, active, and poised for significant growth when Samuel Stritch arrived in the early months of 1940. Stritch would step into this moving stream and would change and be changed by the challenging events of the next eighteen years.

2

Chicago in War and Cold War

Amid the celebration and general rejoicing surrounding Stritch's installation, the prelate's first formal address sounded an ominous note. Referring to Pius XII's recently issued *Summi Pontificatus*, Stritch told the assembled multitude: "As we look out over the world about us with Pope Pius XII, the sorry fact is forced on us that what happened on Good Friday ... has happened again—'There was darkness over the whole earth.'"[1]

In the early days of September 1939 Germany had attacked and conquered Poland, and a state of war existed. Although the fighting had temporarily abated in the winter of 1939 and the early months of 1940, the belligerent powers were crouched and ready to resume combat at any time. Preparations for war were already beginning in the officially neutral United States, especially in the city of Chicago, whose massive steel mills and machine shops were steadily building up production. Chicago was also in the center of a major debate about America's role in the unfolding developments overseas. As Chicago Catholics served in the armed forces and Chicago priests went in record numbers to serve as chaplains in every theater of the war, the war years and their aftermath would significantly affect Catholic life.

CHICAGO CATHOLICS AND THE NEUTRALITY DEBATE

Throughout the thirties, Chicago had been at the center of an important national debate regarding American intervention

43

in Europe and Asia.[2] As militarism and totalitarianism made a strong comeback during the Depression era, many Americans and in particular many Chicagoans, goaded by Colonel Robert McCormick's *Chicago Tribune*, determined that anything remotely resembling war preparations had to be stoutly resisted.

Given all this, it was no small matter that one of Roosevelt's staunchest Catholic supporters was none other than the cardinal archbishop of Chicago, George Mundelein. Mundelein had forged a friendship with the president in the early thirties and had given him crucial public support in 1935 when Charles Coughlin's violent public attacks had seemed to jeopardize the Catholic vote. Mundelein was also prepared to serve an important role in marshaling public opinion behind FDR's plans for a more interventionist foreign policy. Of the Mundelein-Roosevelt relationship, Edward Kantowicz has cautioned that people "must be careful not to exaggerate the cardinal's importance to the president," but added that "the consistent support of a German bishop from the conservative, isolationist Midwest for both foreign and domestic policies ... was a genuine asset to FDR."[3]

Mundelein's value to Roosevelt is intimated in Roosevelt's comments to Secretary of the Interior Harold Ickes as recorded in Ickes's diary citation on the day of Stritch's appointment: "Well, you and I have had a pretty severe blow today."[4] He was lamenting the appointment of Stritch rather than the administration's hopeful, Bernard J. Sheil. In losing Mundelein, the Roosevelt administration had not only lost a powerful ally in the battle for public opinion but still worse, found him replaced by someone they considered ideologically hostile, even fascist.[5] In the weeks before his installation, the White House had been informed of Stritch's toleration of pro-Coughlin material in the Catholic newspaper of the Archdiocese of Milwaukee and his general grousing about New Deal "statism."[6] There had even been a rumor that Stritch actively opposed neutrality law revisions, a claim he was compelled to explicitly deny in an announcement in the Catholic press.[7] Specifically, Roosevelt's concerns that Stritch "was favorable to Father Coughlin and that he was not in sympathy with some of their [own] measures" were conveyed to Postmaster General Frank Walker, who took

them up with Archbishop Francis Spellman of New York.[8] Spellman later related to FDR that he had phoned Stritch and asked "Archbishop Stritch the precise question whether or not he was favorable to [your] administration."[9] Stritch heatedly denied that he was a Roosevelt opponent. When Spellman later questioned him about unfavorable articles in the *Catholic Herald-Citizen*, Stritch wrote a lengthy letter (which Spellman forwarded to FDR) defending his policy on ecclesiastical intervention in political matters:

> My policy has been to support in every possible way civil authority and to inculcate respect for it. In my statements and activities I have tried to keep within the Mandate of my Sacred Office and carefully avoid entering the file of the purely political or purely economic. Indeed, it has pained me when ecclesiastics, claiming to speak merely as citizens, have conducted crusades of vituperation, supported by appeals to sentiment, half-truths and downright misrepresentations in fields which are surely not within the compass of their sacred calling.[10]

Alluding directly to the rumors that put him at odds with the administration he said:

> It is true that I refused to ask a Senator to vote for the President's proposal on the changes in the number of Justices on the Supreme Court, but my reason was that such an action was outside the Mandate of my Sacred Office.[11]

Roosevelt felt satisfied with Stritch's apologia and wrote to Spellman that Stritch "will prove a great success in the Chicago Diocese, not only along spiritual lines but also in pushing forward with the splendid social policies of the late Cardinal."[12] Nonetheless, Roosevelt privately continued to be suspicious of Stritch. By late 1940 the Washington/Chicago axis that both Mundelein and Roosevelt had so carefully cultivated fell by the wayside, assisted by a carefully placed wedge from the archbishop of New York. Roosevelt and Francis Spellman had already begun to cultivate a mutually beneficial relationship and the New York prelate became FDR's chief liaison with the Catholic hierarchy.

For his part Stritch did not seem to lament or regret the lack of official favor or special honors bestowed on his predecessor. Indeed, until Pearl Harbor, Stritch attempted to hew publicly to the line about his neutrality on political matters and often used the argument, repeated in his letter to Spellman, that he avoided all public comment on nonecclesiastical matters. One of his policy changes for the diocesan weekly, the *New World*, was to prohibit political advertising and pictures of politicians three months before an election.[13] When his friend Bishop John B. Morris of Little Rock wrote expressing confusion about the efforts of an isolationist group in New York to recruit him to their cause, Stritch counseled him: "I do not think it prudent or dignified for us to take cognizance of any of these committees. In present disturbed conditions we shall do well to keep on praying for a peace of justice and charity.... The Bishops must hold calmly to the norm of reason."[14]

When a leading isolationist group, the Citizens to Keep America Out of the War, directly asked for his participation in a public demonstration, Stritch politely declined, saying: "My duties constrain me to decline all invitations to take part in the programs of secular organizations."[15] Evenhandedly he discouraged those who took negative positions on England— positions with which he probably agreed. Such was the case of Monsignor William Cahill, pastor of Our Lady of Mercy on the North Side, who issued regular bulletin diatribes attacking the English. Stritch wrote the pastor a stern letter ordering him to desist from "introducing matters of a political kind."[16] To an Oblate of Mary Immaculate invited to address an isolationist group meeting in a city hotel, the chancellor of the diocese wrote: "We would prefer that you do not accept this engagement ... our policy in the archdiocese has been not to permit any of our priests to speak at such rallies."[17] Indeed, so frustrated did Stritch grow with the efforts to drag him into the debate, he wrote to Morris, "You are lucky to be in Little Rock and quite away from the pressure groups who want us to turn the Church into a political forum...."[18] Privately, Stritch did have serious reservations about American intervention in the war. But it is important to distinguish that Stritch's reluctance to embrace an interventionist foreign policy stemmed more from

Irish-American feelings of anglophobia than the pro-German isolationism of other Catholic opponents of Roosevelt, such as Charles Coughlin or Francis Beckman of Dubuque. Stritch expressed his reluctance to support American assistance to Britain as late as the summer of 1941, when he wrote to Archbishop John J. Cantwell of Los Angeles. After pointing out the flaws of nazism he summarized his feelings: "And yet, there are purely secular matters involved which prevent my conclud-ing that I must look upon England's war as a defense of Christianity."[19] Although he would patriotically rally round the colors after Pearl Harbor, Stritch was less than enthusiastic about the prospect of an alliance with England and wrote to Archbishop John T. McNicholas of Cincinnati, who was prepar-ing an NCWC statement on the war: "We ought to frankly rec-ognize the power, influence, and determination of the English imperialists."[20] If fears of perpetuating British imperialism fed Stritch's isolationist feelings, his anxiety over the willingness of the Roosevelt administration to embrace an alliance with Soviet Russia would play a larger role in his ambivalence about American entry into the war. Even while admitting the need for the alliance during the war, Stritch, in best scholastic fashion, explained to neighboring Bishop John F. Noll: "We must keep in mind always that we are cooperating today with Russia only on the basis of the moral principle of double effect."[21]

THE WAR COMES

When Japanese forces launched a surprise raid on the American naval forces at Pearl Harbor, Stritch patriotically ral-lied his people:

> Last Sunday afternoon, there broke upon us suddenly the news of the treacherous attack upon our country.... Disregarding the law of nations, a long previously planned surprise attack was made upon us.... Patriotism dictates the answer which should be made to this aggressor, the answer of a united people, the answer of free men whose courage and strength are not less than their determination.[22]

Chicago was now at war. Yet long before the actual out-break of hostilities, Mayor Edward Kelly had planned for this

contingency. Kelly's lobbying with the Roosevelt administration had secured Chicago a pivotal role in defense operations. Chicago's industrial might retooled and swung behind the war effort, adding laborers and extra shifts to meet the tremendous demands of wartime production. To the south, the massive steel mills of Gary and South Chicago stoked up to produce the vast quantities of steel and other metals needed. To the west and north of the city, defense contractors expanded production. Melrose Park's Buick plant added scores of workers, while Cicero's Western Electric plant turned out war orders around the clock. Farther to the northwest, in an area known as Orchard Place, Douglas Aircraft began manufacturing the huge C-54 transport planes, while to the southwest Pratt and Whitney made airplane engines.

These new jobs gave an added boost to the city's depression-scarred economy, as did the presence of thousands of military men and women stationed at Great Lakes Naval Base in Lake County or Fort Sheridan on the North Shore. City technical colleges and universities were overrun by GIs and naval personnel learning the technical skills necessary to master complex communications equipment and weaponry for the fight. The Kelly administration did everything it could to make Chicago run harmoniously for the duration. Using his authority as the head of civil defense operations for the city, Kelly mediated labor disputes, led massive war bond drives and salvage collections, and provided the often bored and homesick military personnel with entertainment and free transportation to the city's business and theater districts. A former Elks Club at 1766 W. Washington was converted into a recreation center for the military. The enormous Stevens Hotel on Michigan and Balbo became a military training facility and the luxurious Chicago Beach Hotel became a hospital.[23]

Chicago's Catholic community threw itself wholeheartedly into the defense efforts. Stritch endorsed the war efforts by committing surplus archdiocesan funds to government bond drives and urging parishes to do likewise. Even before the outbreak of hostilities an important priority had been the care of the increasing number of servicemen who were appearing in the city's military installations and posing challenges to the city's recreational

facilities. In Chicago the first Catholic efforts to provide recreational and spiritual services for the young servicemen had come at the direction of Bishop Bernard Sheil and the CYO. Beginning in March 1941 Sheil sponsored the first in a series of weekly entertainments and social programs at the 31 E. Congress headquarters of the CYO for the benefit of draftees stationed near Chicago.[24] The growing need for full-time recreational facilities required an expansion of Sheil's efforts. But in time Sheil's operations would be superseded by the United Service Organization (USO), which had been chartered by the government in February 1941, and the National Catholic Community Services (NCCS), created by the NCWC to represent Catholic interests in the care of military men and women.

Stritch quickly formed a local NCCS committee under the direction of Catholic Charities director Father William A. O'Connor and launched a fund appeal throughout the diocese for the support of the USO. In August 1941 O'Connor made provisions for a Catholic serviceman's center in Waukegan near Fort Sheridan and the Great Lakes naval facility. Later that month O'Connor secured the use of a second building for a center at 1112 South Wabash in the Loop—a building formerly occupied by the Paulist Settlement project.[25] Stritch took an active interest in the welfare of the servicemen flooding his diocese and wrote to NCWC General Secretary, Michael Ready:

> We have one bad spot in the archdiocese, Highwood. It is a small town just near Ft. Sheridan and is full of occasions of sin. Our building at Waukegan does take care of some of these boys for at my request, the North Shore Railroad has given soldiers a 7 cent fare from Fort Sheridan to Waukegan. Still many go to Highwood ... we ought to get busy and put up a building at once. Too long a delay will mean the ruin of many boys.[26]

By the next summer a facility in Highwood was opened. There the men could dance, play cards or billiards, use darkroom facilities, write letters, and if necessary speak with a priest. Later in 1942 the downtown NCCS center was taken over directly by the USO.[27] No doubt many a lonely Catholic serviceman found his future bride at the NCCS centers. The centers continued to operate until 1947, when the Highwood program finally closed.

Concern for the morals of the servicemen also led Stritch to lodge a vigorous protest with Navy Department Secretary (and Chicagoan) Frank Knox over the policy of distributing condoms to prevent the spread of venereal disease.[28] Knox was sympathetic but the high incidence of venereal disease among sailors caused him to cast aside Stritch's objections.

The war's effects were felt directly by many Catholic parishes which watched their sons and daughters march off to war. For example, St. Peter Canisius parish on the West Side sent 739 young men to the armed forces. Nineteen of them never returned.[29] Statistics like this were repeated all over the diocese and helped stimulate a win-the-war effort among Chicago's Catholics. Children in Catholic schools bought bonds, held blood drives, and collected scrap for salvage drives. By 1943 Chicago's Catholic community had subscribed to over $14 million in war bonds and given over $24,000 to Red Cross drives.[30] Representatives of local Catholic women's groups sat on the Chicago Commission on National Defense, while nearly 10,000 Polish women in Chicago devoted one or two days each week in war relief work under the direction of the Polish Civilian War Relief Unit.[31] The diocesan newspaper, *New World,* faithfully ran stories highlighting the work of Chicago servicemen and chaplains at Camp Forrest in Tullahoma, Tennessee, as well as weekly profiles of Chicagoans in service.[32]

The religious response of the Catholics of Chicago represented substantial support for the successful outcome of the war. Parishes adjusted their Mass schedules to accommodate the needs of around-the-clock defense workers in neighborhoods where the plants hummed twenty-four hours. Such was the case of St. Camillus parish on the Southwest Side, which inaugurated a 2:30 A.M. Mass for defense workers at the nearby Studebaker and Ford plants.[33] Spiritual support for the war effort took other forms as well. Beginning in September 1941 and continuing on through the remainder of the war, the Archdiocesan Union of Holy Name Societies of Chicago staged successive holy hours at Chicago's Soldier Field. These prayer gatherings, usually held at night by candlelight, attracted thousands of Chicago's Catholics who prayed the rosary for world peace and held candles aloft during the Benediction of the

Blessed Sacrament. Around the city there was a general quickening of devotional life as novenas for world peace attracted countless adherents. The most popular was the novena to the Sorrowful Mother, sponsored by the Servite Fathers in their huge Basilica of Our Lady of Sorrows on Jackson Boulevard. The novena, according to its historian, had conveniently shifted gears from its emphasis on spiritual and temporal help during the depression to prayers for the welfare and well-being of servicemen in combat overseas.[34] Similar acts of piety were recorded in a large report compiled by Chancellor George Casey. One parish reported: "On the tenth of this month, the men of the Holy Name received Holy Communion in a group of about 400 men and spent a Day of Recollection for the intention of the members of the parish in service." Another group of high school youth wrote: "To help maintain the morale of the men in service, our high school of over four hundred students, has made it its business to offer daily prayers, ejaculations, mortifications and offer little sacrifices for both the active servicemen and for the sick and deceased boys."[35] During the war years even the annual reports of Superintendent of Schools Monsignor Daniel Cunningham portrayed pictures of fighter planes and war material that Catholic schoolchildren had helped finance with their nickels and dimes.[36]

Other aspects of wartime life touched the Chicago Catholic community. The need to ration the nation's resources led to a virtual end to any kind of building projects, thus creating a large backlog of institutional needs that would have to be taken care of after the war. Chancellor George Casey was the main font of knowledge regarding government regulations, especially rationing. Casey's winning ways with federal rationing administrators could occasionally win exemptions—for example, securing materials to build Holy Redeemer Church in Evergreen Park by having it declared a priority building in 1942. In other instances he was not as successful, as in the case of St. Raphael's Church, a newly built church and school that had an oil burning power plant rather than the government-mandated coal furnace. St. Raphael parishioners and schoolchildren shivered through the winters with decreased fuel supplies. Stritch himself alluded to the effects of wartime restrictions in a letter to a

chaplain: "Here at home we are busy trying to get used to gasoline rationing. You would be surprised to see how many cars are off the streets."[37] At the urging of the NCCS, Casey compiled a large report of Catholic wartime activities in 1943, giving numbers of bonds sold and chronicling the main efforts of Catholics to support the war.

THE CHAPLAINS

Stritch encouraged the manifold wartime activities of his Chicago flock but had particular solicitude for the activities of the 112 priests whom he had released for chaplain duties in various branches of the armed services. Chicago's considerable loan of chaplains resulted not only from the size of its presbyterate but also because Stritch had promised lawmakers a generous share of clergy in exchange for the exemptions of seminarians and brothers in the 1940 conscription law.[38] Indeed, so many priests entered the service that the bon-vivant vice chancellor, Monsignor Edward Burke, complained good-naturedly "Chicago is getting to be a ghost-town as far as priests are concerned. One formerly could always arrange a get-to-gether and feel convinced of having a quorum. Now it is an utter impossibility to find any of your friends who have not left for the army or the navy."[39]

Since the military ordinariate insisted that chaplains report monthly to their Ordinary, Stritch's files were filled with the standard forms which recorded numbers of communions, confessions, and anointings as well as chatty letters of their experiences. These letters offer a fascinating insight into the life and experiences of chaplains and their charges. Most of them wrote of their admiration for the young recruits and commented frequently on their efforts to assuage homesickness, fear, and frustration with military life. A constant worry was the morals of the men. Chaplain Donald Kelly, aboard the USS *Independence*, wrote to Stritch:

> The lads have been flocking to Mass and communion much to the surprise and bewilderment of the "agnostic" officers. As long as I have them afloat, they live like seminarians, but when they

hit the beach ... oh boy! Catholic boys are usually leaders in everything. They play hard, they pray hard, and they sin hard.[40]

Stritch responded to Kelly:

> I think you are quite right in trying to provide recreational environments which will save them from temptations and occasions of sin. Poor human nature is so weak that in the face of temptation and danger it has a hard struggle.[41]

While struggling for the souls of the young men, many chaplains also had to deal with impatience of many servicemen with Catholic practices. One wrote: "Twice in a week two of my boys are getting married by a Justice of the Peace. I tried to talk both of them into doing it right, but they are too much in a hurry and doing things the Catholic way is just too much red tape." With an air of resignation he concluded "sometimes though, I really feel as though it might be just as well. A lot of those marriages won't last anyway, and when they do break up the Catholic party isn't stuck for life."[42]

Living with people of other denominations and faiths was a real eye-opener for many of the chaplains. Some immediately became suspicious and hostile toward Protestant rivals. Other saw in their counterparts real companions in the ministry. Chaplain Joseph M. Lynch attested:

> Living with so many ministers was a bit strange at first; however most of them are very decent fellows and we get along very well together. Many of them from the deep south have never seen a priest; they are gradually becoming accustomed to us.[43]

Stritch believed the interaction with Protestants in the service would offer a good occasion for convert making. "These experiences are very good" he wrote one chaplain who had just met some men from Southern Methodist University. "I have had many of them in my life. The humiliating thing for us is that in them we find out how easy it is to set the mind right when we have to have contact."[44]

As novel as the contacts with Protestants and Jews may have been, the circumstances of war also mandated changes in liturgical practice that also seemed foreign to the chaplains. "I

have been fortunate," wrote Father Bernard E. Burns, stationed in Italy, "I have never found it necessary to interrupt my Mass yet.... The front of my jeep serves as an altar, a little space of scrub is our church." He concluded "I have gained such control of my nerves that the whistle of enemy shells no longer is an external distraction."[45] Other innovations in liturgical practice were recorded in letters home. Stritch wrote to one man, who spoke favorably of his experience with evening Masses: "It is interesting how the men respond to evening Mass.... From it may come in the future great changes."[46] Another chaplain wrote home: "Mass in the afternoon is something entirely new to me, but it certainly does afford the armed forces a better chance to hear daily Mass."[47]

Some chaplains recounted wartime atrocities and tragedies they experienced. One wrote of viewing the bodies of Italian civilians gunned down by the retreating Germans:

> When we got into the town, we were greeted by a noisy crowd of citizens who took us to the spot. Along a wall lay the bodies of about seventy men and women, ranging in age from twenty to seventy. Three of them were women, two a mother and daughter and the other about sixty five.[48]

Others wrote of their homesickness. One chaplain writing from an "island paradise" in the distant Solomon Islands yearned to be home: "I must confess that the dark canyons of the Chicago Loop, the densely populated tenement houses, the noise and the filth and poverty and crime of the Windy City, will provide for me a bit of heaven on earth."[49] Perhaps Father Bernard Burns best articulated the feelings of most Chicago priests who served as chaplains when he wrote:

> I have read the New World with its description of the Holy Hour. It made me quite homesick for Chicago to look at the pictures. One has to be so careful here to keep from becoming depressed. The closer the end seems, the more impatient one becomes for the end. This business is teaching me many things; but the frightfulness of it all is indescribable.... There are moments of depression and loneliness that are only minimized by the fact that a priest here in the army shares it with his men.... The big mystery to me is how the men here who do not know God can stand it.[50]

HELPING THE POLES

If Father Burns and the other chaplains yearned to be home on the streets of Chicago, many Chicagoans of Eastern European descent were probably filled with thoughts of conditions overseas. The city's largest single group of Eastern Europeans were of course the Poles. Despite a lack of political clout, Chicago's Polonia did enjoy a strong group identity that made them a powerful force within the Chicago Church.[51] The Poles had bested the redoubtable Cardinal George Mundelein in contests over national parishes and clerical patronage. Samuel Stritch was less temperamentally inclined to challenge them and even curried their favor because he believed Poles had been excluded from the mainstream of American Catholic life.

There were various Polish relief organizations but the largest was the Polish Alliance, a group not directly linked to the Catholic Church but 90 percent Catholic in its membership. Its leader, Francis Xavier Swietlik, was the dean of the Marquette University Law School and well-known to Stritch. Under his sponsorship the Polish Council for Relief was established in 1939 which brought together the representatives of the principal Polish organizations to coordinate fund raising and relief operations. Stritch was also well acquainted with John Oleniczak, the president of the Polish Roman Catholic Union, another important source of information about Polish concerns. Consequently, when Polish community leaders brought Stritch their concerns about relief to war victims and controversial political decisions regarding Poland's boundaries, Stritch not only listened but was the most important non-Polish voice in the hierarchy to press these issues before his brother bishops and the United States government.

Stritch had first become aware of the plight of refugees during his service on a special bishops' committee on German Catholic refugees formed in 1936. Serving with New Orleans Archbishop Joseph Rummell and Fort Wayne Bishop John Noll, Stritch collected money for the refugees and tried in vain to secure modifications in American immigration laws to allow many of them to settle in the United States.[52] With the onset of war in 1939, the American bishops, one of the last free hierar-

chies left, were increasingly besieged with requests for relief funds. To better coordinate the collection and distribution of funds, Stritch proposed at an April 1939 meeting of the NCWC Administrative Board: "that we establish [a] general committee and make other committees sub-committees under it. There [would] be one general collection and this collection would be distributed through these committees, through any other sub-committees which might be set up, and also directly by the Committee itself."[53] This motion was tentatively approved. Under this plan a subcommittee on Polish relief was established, chaired by Bishop Hugh Boyle of Pittsburgh and included Stritch's auxiliary William David O'Brien, executive director of the Chicago-based Church Extension Society. Later the structure was formalized and a new committee was established known as the Bishop's War Emergency and Relief Committee. To comply with government regulations imposed to coordinate fund raising and the delivery of relief, the bishops changed this committee into a freestanding relief organization known as War Relief Services. For the support of these multiple demands a single collection was taken up annually on Laetare Sunday, the fourth Sunday of Lent.

In addition to his efforts to collect funds for Polish relief, Stritch did other things that signaled his concern for the plight of the Poles. To one Polish correspondent he wrote in 1941: "Here in Chicago, we have already given hospitality to six diocesan priest refugees from Poland and the religious of the archdiocese have taken in religious priest refugees."[54]

Soon after the establishment of War Relief Services, Dean Swietlik met with its executive director, Monsignor Patrick O'Boyle, and worked out a program of cooperation. German and later Soviet domination of Poland made direct relief virtually impossible. As a result the War Relief Services made a strong effort to supply Polish refugees huddled in camps all over the world. Stritch assigned one of his young priests, Father Aloysius Wycislo, to work with the organization to assist in the care of the large numbers of Polish refugees who were escaping their war-torn nation.[55]

Wycislo, a native of Cicero, who had pursued graduate study in social work at the Catholic University and had taught

courses in International Social Work, was then serving as an assistant to Monsignor William O'Connor of Catholic Charities. Upon arriving in New York for his appointment to War Relief Services, he became an assistant to Monsignor Patrick O'Boyle. Fleeing Polish bishops had informed their American counterparts that large numbers of Polish refugees were streaming into the Middle East via Russia and they needed attention and care. To respond to this need Wycislo was dispatched to that region in late 1943, where he began to track down the Polish refugees in Egypt. He discovered large numbers moving into the Holy Land through Iran and Iraq and there being conscripted into the British Eighth Army. Wycislo set up refugee camps for these wandering aliens not only in the Holy Land but also in Bombay, India, and in British East Africa. Moreover, at the request of Pope Pius XII, he undertook a mission to the forty thousand Italians interned in Egypt by the British. As the war moved up into Europe, Wycislo followed the armies to help with relief work. He moved into France and finally Germany itself, conveying food and serving as an effective agent of relief for the American bishops. When the war ended in 1945, he expanded his efforts into Poland, Czechoslovakia, and Hungary, where, at the request of the Polish American Relief Organization, he was able to start some programs for shipments of relief supplies. Wycislo's work with the War Relief Services would continue until the late fifties when a new archbishop, Albert Meyer, called him home and consecrated him one of his auxiliaries.

PEACE PLAN

Concern for the plight of his coreligionists in Eastern Europe and Italy was spurred not only by Stritch's humanitarianism but also by his activities on an important NCWC committee to publicize the papal peace plan. Stritch pondered the reasons for the collapse of international order and the awful implications for the peace of the world. Like many Americans he faulted the peace process that had ended World War I. Even more deeply, however, Stritch perceived the international crisis as just one more symptom of the growing secularism of the

world and the abandonment of the irreformable moral truths that undergirded true social order. "Without a doubt," Stritch wrote in the name of the bishops in 1943, "the maladies which afflict modern society and have brought on the catastrophe of world war is [sic] the social forgetfulness and even rejection of the sovereignty of God and the moral law."[56] The years 1940 to 1944 were years of intense involvement by Stritch in the work of understanding and publicizing Catholic principles of peace, especially those articulated by Pope Pius XII in a series of Christmas messages. To underscore his dream of disseminating Christian principles of peace a collection of papal statements on peace assembled by Yves de la Briere was translated and augmented by church history professor Father Harry C. Koenig of St. Mary of the Lake Seminary. Working under constant pressure from Stritch, who was eager to have the volume done before the war was over, Koenig published a massive nine-hundred-page volume that contained every papal utterance on peace from Leo XIII through Pius XII.[57] With the assistance of Chicago millionaire John Cuneo, the volume was printed and distributed by the Bruce Publishing Company of Milwaukee to all the bishops and to persons in high public office. One recipient was President Roosevelt, who thanked Stritch for the volume. Another was FDR's speech writer William D. Hasset, whom Ready described as "a stalwart Catholic."[58]

By the following year, the first spin-off of *Principles of Peace* emerged in the form of a commentary on the papal peace points by Professor Guido Gonella of Vatican City. Gonella, an expert on international law and an editor of the Vatican newspaper, had studied the statements of Pius XII and offered a lengthy commentary on them in a series of articles that appeared in the Vatican newspaper, *L'Osservatore Romano*. Gonella's commentaries were translated into English by Jesuit canonist T. Lincoln Bouscaren under the title *A World to Reconstruct*. In his introduction to the English edition of Gonella's book Stritch wrote: "The victory before us is a challenge to all good men to unite and conspire in reconstructing on the ruins of war a better social, political and economic culture in which the changed and the changing will be integrated happily with the eternal inescapable truths."[59] Later plans called for the expansion of the collection of

papal peace statements, the formation of peace committees in every diocese, and a series of study-club booklets for discussion of these matters on the popular level. However, the war ended before these plans could be implemented.

POSTWAR MATTERS

After the conclusion of the war, Stritch's concerns were focused on potential Communist subversion of Western Europe, especially in prostrate Germany and Italy. With the accession of Harry S Truman to the White House in 1945, Stritch's relationship with the White House was much happier than his experiences with Franklin Roosevelt. Part of this was because Stritch did not have to labor under the cloud of not being Mundelein or Sheil or of having "fascist" or pro-Coughlin sympathies. Even more, once the new president got his bearings, he often turned to people that his predecessor had kept at a distance or shunned.[60] Stritch's first contact with the new president had come soon after Truman's accession to office, when Stritch urged the president to lift wartime restrictions on building materials for much-needed churches and schools.[61] Truman responded quickly and sympathetically to the request. According to the memoir of his secretary, Monsignor John Fitzgerald, Stritch became a good friend of President Truman,[62] much to the chagrin of Cardinal Spellman, who later embraced one of Truman's arch foes, Senator Joseph R. McCarthy of Wisconsin. The year after he left the White House, Truman remarked in a letter to Bishop Bernard J. Sheil: "I am a very great admirer of Cardinal Stritch."[63] It was with the Truman White House that Stritch had some connections, particularly through two men that Fitzgerald had introduced to him: Gael Sullivan and Edward Tamm.

Edward Gael Sullivan (he dropped the first name later in life) was a native of Rhode Island and a graduate of Providence College. After his graduation in 1928, he entered the Dominican Order and was given the name Bede. Upon completion of his novitiate he was sent for studies at the newly opened Studium of the Dominican Order in River Forest, Illinois. Just prior to his

solemn profession, he left the community and taught school for a time at DePaul University. Sometime after his egress from the Dominicans he met Monsignor John D. Fitzgerald, a member of Cardinal Mundelein's household who was already cultivating a wide circle of friends in high places. Fitzgerald secured the young man a position with the 1933 Chicago Century of Progress Exposition. Fitzgerald was also instrumental in having Sullivan made associate director of the Federal Housing Administration for Illinois. He won the attention of Mayor Edward Kelly, who hired him as a speech writer in 1939 and two years later had the young man appointed head of the Federal Housing Administration in Illinois.[64] Monsignor Fitzgerald introduced Sullivan to Stritch, who took an instant liking to the man. Sullivan further ingratiated himself to Stritch when he secured a position in the Chicago FHA for Stritch's younger brother, Emmett, who had come on hard times in Memphis. When Sullivan resigned his FHA post to join the armed forces in 1943, he wrote Stritch an affectionate letter of farewell.[65]

Holding a series of important desk jobs, including deputy quartermaster general, Sullivan soon attained the rank of major and returned from the war as one of the rising young stars of the Democratic party. He won the attention of party boss Robert Hannegan and was soon given a patronage job as second assistant postmaster general, where he actually did some work improving airmail delivery. Sullivan's access to trans-Atlantic mail flights became the reason for Stritch's introducing him to Apostolic Delegate Cicognani. Sullivan was used as a faithful courier for Stritch and the apostolic delegate. From the postmaster's job Sullivan became an assistant chairman of the national Democratic party and worked assiduously with the party in the Midwest. When Hannegan resigned the chairmanship in 1947, Sullivan believed the job would go to him, but he was passed over for a fellow Rhode Islander, J. Howard McGrath. Sullivan remained at his post until April 1948, when he took a high paying job with the Theater Owners Guild. Because of his access to the White House and his practical ability to deliver, Stritch and other Chicago priests called on Sullivan often. As a reward for his service, Stritch had Sullivan created a Knight Commander of the Order of St. Gregory.

Another Fitzgerald protégé was FBI agent Edward Tamm. Tamm was born in 1906 in St. Paul, Minnesota, and received an advanced degree from Georgetown University. In 1930 he went to work with the FBI and soon rose to become a high-ranking assistant to J. Edgar Hoover. Tamm had become Hoover's liaison with the Roman Catholic hierarchy and had met Stritch in 1945 through Monsignor Fitzgerald. Hoover's cultivation of Stritch had begun in 1937 when the director sent the archbishop information on work he was doing to prevent internal subversion. At that time Stritch said to Hoover: "I have followed closely your work and I think it has been a great service to the Country."[66] Hoover took care, through Tamm's urging, to keep in contact with Stritch and did everything he could to maintain Stritch's goodwill. Tamm's first task was to escort Fitzgerald to the founding conference of the United Nations at San Francisco that year, dramatically sweeping bugs from the hotel room and tailing Fitzgerald. Fitzgerald's glowing reports of Tamm's solicitude deeply impressed Stritch, who struck up a warm friendship with Tamm as he had with Gael Sullivan. Stritch regularly called on Tamm for assistance with problems that came to his attention as chairman of the Administrative Board of the NCWC and as part of his own interests in a Catholic presence in the national government. For example, when Bishop Duane Hunt of Salt Lake City complained that the government was going to close down the much-needed Bushnell Veteran's Hospital in Brigham City, Stritch brought the matter to Tamm.[67] Stritch also used Tamm to run brief personnel checks on Francis P. Matthews, Joseph P. Kennan, and Edward P. Murphy, whom he was proposing to the Truman Administration as ambassadors to Brazil, Cuba, and governor general of Puerto Rico respectively.[68] Tamm also kept Stritch, via Fitzgerald, abreast of conditions in Yugoslavia. In the summer of 1946, Stritch used Tamm to influence positive action on a bill granting a loan to Britain (a remarkable turn of events for the anglophobic churchman). Tamm wrote Stritch: "The present outlook for the passage by Congress of the British loan is a most favorable one. I feel that your interest in affirmative action upon this proposed legislation has undoubtedly influenced the serious thought of a number of persons who have previously regarded the loan as

a definite stopgap against Soviet domination of Western Europe."[69]

When Tamm grew tired of FBI work, Stritch unsuccessfully attempted to fix him up with a job in McNicholas's Institutum Divi Thomae, a graduate school of applied science run by Dr. George Speri Sperti, the inventor of a popular ointment known as Biodyne.[70] But Tamm coveted a federal judgeship and Stritch used his Washington contacts to influence Truman to appoint him to the federal bench of the District of Columbia. Tamm acknowledged Stritch's influence in a letter soon after his nomination: "Were it not for your confidence in me, I know that I would not have been selected for this high office, and I, consequently, acknowledge my deep and lasting obligation to you."[71] Tamm's nomination ran into difficulties when it was revealed in late February that he had participated in a vote fraud investigation case in Missouri's fifth congressional district that had prematurely exonerated those accused. The contested 1946 election pitted a Democratic incumbent hostile to Truman against an administration-backed challenger. The challenger won the primary election with the help of the notorious Pendergast machine of Kansas City, but later lost the general election. Charges of vote fraud brought the intervention of the FBI. An investigative team headed by Tamm had exonerated the Pendergast machine. However, both Tamm and the Bureau were covered with embarassment when an independent group subsequently discovered that vote fraud had indeed taken place. Even worse, the district court appointment appeared to be a payoff for Tamm's (and Hoover's) services and was consequently held up in the Judiciary Committee. When Congress went into summer recess the nomination lapsed. In what was a grueling ordeal for Tamm and his family Stritch provided constant support and consolation to Tamm, who remarked to him: "I am deeply obligated to you for your wonderful support of me and for your kindly interest in my welfare."[72] Truman later appointed Tamm *ad interim* and in the next session of Congress formal approval was given to the nomination. After his appointment to the federal judiciary, Tamm continued to be a special link between the Bureau and Stritch.

The cardinal proved a good source of information on the

activities of the Catholic Eastern European groups whose causes he championed. In 1956 Stritch was considered to speak for the commencement exercises of the FBI National Academy. A background check reported: "Bufiles [*sic* Bureau Files] reflect cordial relations with Cardinal Stritch." At Stritch's invitation Hoover had willingly come to speak at the commencement of DePaul University in 1951. Indeed, Hoover had said to his associates "I ... had been making no commitments or speeches in view of the pressure of work, but this was one invitation I would like to accept if possible to do so."[73] Hoover and Tamm would render their last assistance to Stritch in 1958 when the cardinal lay dying in Rome, by expediting the flying visits of Stritch's personal physician, Dr. Ralph Bergen (whose passport had expired) and his closest friend, Bishop Roman Atkielski. Both Tamm and Sullivan demonstrated again and again their gratitude to Fitzgerald and Stritch for boosting their careers at critical moments by working conscientiously for Catholic issues.

DISPLACED PERSONS

The problems of displaced persons was another issue Chicago's Catholics dealt with during the Cold War era. If Stritch had been somewhat passive in the wake of the refugee problems of the thirties, he was a mover and a shaker on the matter during and after the war. While in Rome to receive the red hat in 1946, he had learned from Vatican sources that the War Department mandated the closing of a number of displaced persons camps for gentiles in the American zones of Germany and Austria by September 1. Since these camps contained thousands of Poles and others who were anxious to escape Soviet domination, the result would be to compel these persons to return to their homes in Soviet-occupied territory. Stritch was spurred to action.

He met with President Truman on March 27, 1946, and urged that the camps remain open. What he told the president must have been close to what he reported to Bishop Karl J. Alter of Toledo: "To close these camps would be nothing less than a subtle attempt to force these people back to Russian tyranny.

They have good reasons for not wanting to go back to the countries of their origins."[74] As in his lobbying for exemptions to the draft law, Stritch began again to orchestrate a campaign of public pressure to keep open the camps, filled with around 400,000 souls (mostly Catholic Poles, Lithuanians, Ukrainians, Slovenians, and Croatians). On the same day of his meeting with Truman and Secretary of State James F. Byrnes, Stritch wrote Casey urging pressure on Mayor Edward Kelly: "We have made it clear," he wrote with uncharacteristic bluntness, "that if these camps are closed on September 1st, there is going to be a great deal of public protest in the Dioceses of the United States.... It is necessary that we have certain powers in our political life back up our protests and back up our requests with our authorities." He directed Casey to contact Mayor Kelly "quietly" so "that the Mayor will see that for him there is the responsibility of a strong protest against closing these camps with the Washington authorities."[75] Casey was direct with Mayor Kelly, cautioning that lack of support for keeping the camps open might mean that "repercussions here will be great. Here in Chicago there are about 800,000 citizens of the national origins of these poor refugees."[76] Kelly dutifully sent the protest to Truman. The results were evident. In a letter to Stritch, Truman announced that he had reversed the closure order, and the camps remained open.[77]

The campaign to keep open the camps was only the opening round in Stritch's fight for displaced persons. He lobbied the bishops to urge the Holy See to set up an international commission on displaced persons. Working with a private Citizens Committee on Displaced Persons, Stritch lent his voice to initially unsuccessful efforts to relax American immigration laws to admit some of the displaced to the United States. In 1947 the prospects for liberalized immigration laws seemed better and the NCWC prepared to play a role in assuring foreign Catholics a new life in the United States. At the November 1947 meeting, the Administrative Board of the NCWC placed the matter under the War Relief Services and appointed a special "Bishop's Resettlement Committee" with Archbishop Joseph Ritter as chairman. A "National Resettlement Council" under the direction of Monsignor Edward Swanstrom of War Relief Services

was also established. It was "purely advisory in character" but brought together many groups such as the Rural Life Conference, Charity Directors, and representatives of foreign groups to assist in the placement of the refugees. Stritch recruited the services of New Dealer Leo Crowley for the board and accelerated his own efforts to accept the displaced into his diocese by appointing Father James Doyle to oversee efforts to place priests and religious in the Archdiocese of Chicago. These efforts opened the doors of Chicago's numerous motherhouses and parishes to clerical and religious refugees. This was especially true for a large number of Lithuanians who found a home in the Marquette Park area of Chicago, thus adding another vibrant subgroup to the already healthy ethnic mix in the archdiocese. A Lithuanian bishop, Vincent Brizgys, exiled auxiliary bishop of Kaunas, took up residence at Maria Hospital, run by the Sisters of St. Casimir. Brizgys and other Lithuanian priests from the Marianist order tended to the highly visible Lithuanian community, who were palpable reminders of the dislocation precipitated by the cold war. In all, the Archdiocese of Chicago aided in finding homes and jobs for close to two thousand European displaced persons.[78]

The admission of the displaced, accomplished by the relaxation of the national origins formula of the twenties, built pressure for a major rewriting of American immigration law in the early fifties. But what emerged was the McCarran Bill, which changed little of the controversial and discriminatory national origins formula. NCWC strategists led by Bruce Mohler of the Immigration Department and Monsignor Paul Tanner, assistant executive secretary, were inclined to accept the McCarran Bill with some minor modifications that permitted "pooling" of unused quotas. This acquiescence to the quotas formula was vigorously opposed by Monsignor John O'Grady, executive secretary of the National Catholic Charities.[79] No one was more pleased than O'Grady when President Truman vetoed the legislation in 1952. When McCarran and his allies worked to override the presidential veto, O'Grady scurried around the country talking to bishops urging them to pressure lawmakers to sustain the veto. He visited Stritch in October 1952, who wholly sided with him. After the meeting Stritch wrote:

> I do not want to be in any way misunderstood. I am and always
> have been against the National Origins Quota System in our
> immigration law. This principle has been embodied in the
> McCarran-Walter Immigration and Nationality Act. It is unfair,
> unjust and not in the interest of our country. I have always
> looked upon its reincorporation in our immigration law as being
> an unfortunate and tragic continuance of a bad policy.[80]

New York Cardinal Spellman took Mohler and Tanner's
side and protested vigorously to Stritch when the CISCA publication *Today* published an article criticizing McCarran. Stritch
promised to look into the matter but again voiced his support
for an alteration in the quota system:

> The difficulty of course in our immigration legislation is basic.
> When this legislation was first proposed we were against the
> National Origins Formula which was incorporated into it. Our
> reasons for convincing got scant consideration. When the
> Congressional Commitee undertook what they said was codify-
> ing the existing legislation they actually made important addi-
> tions and changes in the legislation but retained the National
> Origins Formula. I think that we are justified in opposing this
> legislation and criticising it but we ought to be objective and level
> our opposition and criticism at the Bill and not at persons.[81]

Despite the efforts of O'Grady and others, Truman's veto was
overriden and the McCarran-Walters Bill became law.

ANTICOMMUNISM

The anticommunist mood which characterized the
American Catholic community in the thirties had gone under-
ground during the period of the East-West alliance against
Hitler in the forties. Yet fears about Soviet expansionism and the
threat of internal subversion resurfaced during the Cold War.
Stritch's anticommunist credentials were certainly well-estab-
lished long before he arrived in Chicago. Along with many
American Catholic bishops he too decried Roosevelt's decision
to recognize the Soviet Union ("by recognizing Russia, we contributed to the stability of the continuance of the Communist

regime"),[82] and had protested Roosevelt's tolerance of anticleri-calism in Mexico and "of the plain sovietic expressions of the Mexican political dictators."[83] Stritch's dire warnings about Soviet intentions in Eastern Europe certainly reconfirmed his antipathy to communism.

In 1944, Stritch readily cooperated with the work of an NCWC commissioned study on communism undertaken by Father John Cronin, S.S., under the direction of Bishop Alter of the Social Action Department. Cronin began his research with a questionnaire sent to all the dioceses. Chicago's responses, prob-ably drafted by Casey, were relatively terse. Regarding the cur-rent state of public opinion on communism, the respondent wrote: "Communist sympathy in Chicago has been limited mostly to the Jews and the Poles." Moreover, the report ex-pressed some concern that "The CIO was in its birth the child of Russia. Lewis was selected as its leader through Russian influ-ence because he was of the revolutionary type."[84] But this fear was being dispelled "because of the tendency on the part of the CIO to get rid of all communistic sympathizers." Stritch did keep a wary eye on Communistic activity among labor unions and asked Monsignor George Higgins in Washington to report to him on the status of the CIO.)[85] Stritch followed Cronin's work carefully. "I did see Father Cronin when he was in Chicago," he wrote to Alter in July 1945. "We opened to him several sources of information. I think he spent a good deal of his time here with the F.B.I."[86]

However with all of Stritch's ideological opposition to communism and the large numbers of Eastern Europeans living in the archdiocese, Stritch never became publicly associated with the Red-baiting activities of the second Red scare of the fifties. In fact, according to his nephew, Stritch personally dis-dained the leading anticommunist of the era, Senator Joseph McCarthy.[87] Perhaps Stritch even secretly cheered when his aux-iliary Bernard Sheil leveled a blast against the Wisconsin Senator before a convention of the CIO. It was ironic that Stritch would later be accused of "firing" the controversial prelate, who resigned dramatically after he attacked McCarthy.

Chicago's Catholic community felt the prevailing winds and were treated to their share of sermons, editorials, and news

items in the *New World*, which informed them about the tragedies of communist subversion in Eastern Europe. Blunt cartoons appeared almost weekly which regularly portrayed Josef Stalin and other communist leaders as drooling beasts and fiends who menaced not only Christianity but civilization itself. For the great numbers of Eastern Europeans in Chicago this was a welcome emphasis. Large play was given to the trials of Aloysius Stepinac and Joseph Mindszenty. Indeed, like most American cardinals, Stritch personally intervened with President Eisenhower to have a physician at the bed of Stepinac.

At that time the bellwether of Chicago piety, the devotion to the Sorrowful Mother, reflected a shift in emphasis from prayers for the safe return of a family member in the service to public prayers to convert communist Russia or to bring world peace. Devotion to Our Lady of Fatima developed during the forties, a form of piety warmly encouraged by the pope and a host of Marian religious orders and pious groups intent on battling communism with the rosary. Fear of atomic destruction prompted other acts of piety, such as a crusade of prayer for peace by Father James T. Farrell at a parish in suburban Hinsdale. Farrell announced the crusade in his parish bulletin: "Only through a faithful return to Christ can the world be saved from a holocaust that defies the imagination and would definitely end our civilization as developed since the time of Christ."[88] Even the socially enlightened Bishop Bernard Sheil, who had been occasionally accused in the thirties and afterwards of having communist sympathies himself, gave an occasional speech lambasting communist influence in the city and elsewhere. Chicago Catholics in general never had the fanatical anticommunist feelings that characterized dioceses like New York, Brooklyn, or some of the cities of the East. Evidence of this is found in an interesting public discussion on the pages of the *New World* over columns written by archconservative columnist Paulist Father James Gillis. In his weekly column *"Sursum Corda"* Gillis had become an outspoken advocate of Joseph McCarthy and Douglas MacArthur. In 1953 a spirited debate was waged on the editorial pages of the *New World* consisting of letters both supporting and attacking Gillis's strong stands.[89]

In all of Stritch's World War II and cold war activities he tried valiantly to influence national policy to embrace Catholic norms of social justice and appealed for the use of the natural law as a standard for a just world order. When the *realpolitik* of the postwar world smashed these hopes, he returned to his own backyard in Chicago and attempted to cope with the rapidly changing social and economic conditions of Catholics in the postwar era.

3

Riding the Whirlwind:
Managing Postwar Growth

"The victory for which we have prayed and fought has come to our arms," Stritch announced in his V-E Day address on WGN radio, "Now is the time for right thinking and right action. We owe it to our heroes, we owe it to ourselves, we owe it to all the world."[1] A few months later the surrender of Japan was noted by the Dominican Sisters at the Visitation Convent on the South Side:

> The end of the war, V-J Day was received with prayers of gratitude by the sisters. There was no hilarity shown in the neighborhood. Those who heard Toscanini conduct the Eroica Symphony of Beethoven will long remember the somber, triumphant music with its undertone of sadness and melancholy. It somehow symbolized the struggle won but the greater struggle of the peace yet to be won.[2]

Stritch and the Dominicans expressed the concerns of many Americans in the aftermath of World War II. Filled with fears about Soviet domination in Eastern Europe and growing concern for Communist fifth-column subversion even in Chicago, Stritch was deeply preoccupied with ideas of social reconstruction. His hopes for a just and sane social order based on objective norms of international law collapsed in the *realpolitik* of the postwar era. As he gradually withdrew from commenting on the international scene, his interests were turned more and more

71

toward the area of the world he could reasonably affect—the Archdiocese of Chicago. The war had changed America in many ways; and, with those changes, the role and place of Catholics in Chicago were visibly and materially altered. The remaining years of Stritch's term and all of Albert Meyer's were spent coping with a Catholic community in transition. Clearest signs of these shifts were evident in archdiocesan financial policy, suburban expansion, education, and administrative reforms.

FINANCIAL CHANGES

The first noticeable change in Chicago in general, and among Catholics in particular, was a steady increase in numbers. Once the war was over, the return of the GIs and the almost immediate bulge in the birthrate began to be felt. Over 137,000 GIs returned to Chicago, many of whom claimed new brides or began families. The birthrate in the Chicago metropolitan area shot up dramatically from prewar levels. All social institutions in Chicago felt the effects, especially churches and schools, which were soon filled to capacity. The Catholic leadership of Chicago sounded an uncertain trumpet in the face of this dramatic increase in population.

Fears that depression conditions would resume once the wartime mobilization ended were accentuated by the unsettled nature of the economy in the immediate aftermath of hostilities. High interest rates, labor unrest, and a fiscal conservatism born of the depression era held Stritch back from immediately undertaking necessary and long-delayed building projects. He expressed this hesitance in a letter to Mother Mary Samuel Coughlin of the Sinsinawa Dominicans regarding a proposed expansion of science laboratories at Rosary College in River Forest: "Our experience just at the moment in building is not very happy. Things are unsettled and costs are very high. We are getting many plans drawn but are deferring our decision as to actual building until the spring. It seems we are going to be in a period of lower purchasing price dollar."[3]

When he came to Chicago in 1940, Stritch had been shocked to find the archdiocese some thirty-three million dollars in

debt—the largest part of it for the huge seminary that Mundelein had built in Lake County. Stritch was determined to reduce this massive indebtedness; consequently, soon after his installation he met with Charles Kerwin of the archdiocesan investment firm of Halsey and Stuart to study the debt structure of the archdiocese and offer suggestions concerning its retirement. With Kerwin's assistance, Stritch refinanced the most pressing part of the debt with the help of a $1.5 million loan offered at the fantastic rate of 2 percent interest by Chicago's Continental Bank.[4] Aided by the wartime revival of the city's economy and the loan from the Continental, Stritch had cut the enormous debt in half by 1945.

Stritch's conservative financial policies extended even to the upkeep of St. Mary of the Lake Seminary, the pride and joy of his predecessor. Mundelein's seminary had been built on the principle, "Nothing is too good for God's future priests." Stritch, on the other hand, was not as indulgent with the seminary, rarely staying in the palatial mansion on the grounds and appearing only for ordinations or to escort important out-of-town visitors. Typical of Stritch's refusal to lavish attention on the seminary was his reaction when informed that one of the piers on the seminary lake was in need of repairs. "Let it sink" was his laconic reply.[5] Although the rotting piers were later repaired (with help from the Hines Lumber Company) Stritch was glad to be rid of the seminary debt, writing Archbishop John T. McNicholas of Cincinnati in 1944, "Here we have paid off enormous amounts and are in a very good condition. With the seminary debt off my books I am much more comfortable."[6]

Stritch also reduced the sales of the Catholic Bishop of Chicago bonds that had been such successful fund-raisers for the archdiocese. The bonds had been successful for two reasons. Parishes were mandated to invest in them whatever surplus funds they had and scores of individual investors and religious communities bought the bonds, which retained a solid rating even during the worst of the depression. Wartime conditions and the flush of prosperity made outside borrowing less of a necessity, as Chancellor George Casey explained to the head of the Adrian Dominicans: "Due to present strange times we find ourselves in a very favorable financial condition. We are not

borrowing any new money; in fact we experience a difficulty trying to find existing obligations to pay off with surplus money we have on hand."[7]

Even parishes were encouraged to invest in government securities to support the war effort. For a long time Stritch had been uncomfortable with Mundelein's revenue raising and expenditure policies. He remarked to Aloysius Muench after a lavish Chicago celebration in 1934 (paid for by assessing the priests): "No bishop can in conscience put a priest on the black list for not contributing what is asked of him."[8] For the most part Stritch rejected these extortionist methods and insisted that the members of his administration do likewise. For example, he denied Auxiliary Bishop Sheil the right to assess blocks of tickets to parishes for CYO events. As in Milwaukee, he followed a conservative line regarding archdiocesan finances. But Casey convinced him not to completely dismantle Mundelein's effective fiscal apparatus. Fearing that tightening the sales of bonds, offering low interest rates, and holding some bonds off the market altogether might cause difficulties later on, Casey urged the archbishop to approve the issuance of a twenty-three-year issue for half a million and used the money to buy Victory bonds.

> In this way we would: help the government use up idle money of private persons ... we would get credit with the government for patriotic cooperation with the War Effort; most importantly, we can thus maintain for future use our market of private investors.

"Almost certainly," he wrote, urging the sales of the bonds, "we will have to use this means of financing when the war is over, for there will be considerable borrowing necessary for postponed construction, etc."[9] Even the sharp-minded Casey did not realize what his "etc." would mean in the postwar years.

SUBURBANIZATION

Once the hostilities ceased and the unstable conditions of the postwar economy righted themselves, countless Chicagoans moved outside the city's perimeters to suburbs that were springing up at the developer's touch. Since many of these emigrants

were Catholics, their reconstitution of Church life on the new suburban frontier would reshape the character of Chicago Catholic life.

When a large number of the 137,000 Chicago veterans returned from the armed services to their homes, pressures for growth and expansion were enormous. These demands would make the years 1946 to 1965 some of the most hectic and fast-paced in Chicago Catholic history. The growth in and around Chicago was most dramatic. Even when the Diocese of Joliet was formed in 1949 by removing four western counties (including fifty-six parishes and thirty-nine elementary schools) from the Chicago archdiocese, the growing city and metropolitan area still claimed the allegiance of more than one and a half million Catholics, 2,300 priests, and 393 parishes. Moreover, the numbers of schoolchildren continued to increase sharply, soaring over 100,000 in grade school and over 37,000 in the high schools. The locus of this growth was not the venerable city parishes founded in the heyday of the immigrant church.[10] Instead the Catholic population of Chicago shifted to former frontiers of the city, the older suburbs and, eventually, to the new tracts of single-family dwellings in parts of Cook and Lake counties that had heretofore been only prairies. Stritch wrote of this shift to a chaplain in the Korean War, "Chicago is emptying out into its suburbs. Thousands and thousands are going out into little homes in the suburban areas." He wrote further, "New parishes are needed, new schools are needed and of course priests are needed."[11]

Suburban growth had been a feature of Chicago life virtually since the inception of the city. Like many cities of great size Chicago had grown by annexing little suburbs that had sprung up in the path of its expansion. The advent of commuter rail lines had opened up a band of industrial suburbs, including Cicero, Blue Island, and Joliet. West of the city was the charming old suburb of Oak Park, a favorite haven of architect Frank Lloyd Wright; while to the north, the city of Evanston was home to prestigious Northwestern University. To the south were the steel communities of Chicago Ridge and old company towns like Pullman. Beyond the perimeter of the city were large tracts of prairie and farmland broken up by small farming villages like

South Holland, Oak Lawn, Mount Prospect, and Arlington Heights. Many of these small villages had incorporated and retained the semblance of small-town life.

During the twenties there had been a land boom and a large-scale exodus to the extremities of the city, facilitated in part by good economic times and the increasing mobility provided by affordable automobiles. Even though the depression stymied suburban expansion in Chicago, automobile ownership held steady, and even increased, during the thirties. Already city planners were looking forward to the day when they would need new roads to hold the increased volume of traffic, and in 1937 and 1939 Mayor Edward Kelly commissioned studies of how these new roads would look. The plans of the thirties would be the blueprint for the changes of the postwar era. The war did slow building and expansion, but the pent-up growth and rising affluence of Chicago's citizens made the postwar years a marvelous period of sustained expansion. After a brief period of postwar uncertainty Chicagoans resumed their steady march toward the city's borders and into newer undeveloped areas advertised by ambitious developers. Unlike the earlier suburban boom of the twenties which saw its largest increases in multifamily dwellings, the movement of the forties and fifties was largely toward single family dwellings.[12] Three factors merged which accounted for this boom: racial succession, increased automobility, and government housing policies.

The racial situation in Chicago was a significant factor prompting whites to move to the suburbs. In large measure, the expansion of Chicago's suburbs, especially those to the south and southwest, was the result of white flight from the rapidly changing neighborhoods of the south and west of the city. Black migration to the city had been fairly steady since early in the twentieth century, with only a brief pause during the worst of the depression. Easy transportation to the city and the promise of wartime work brought thousands of southern blacks to Chicago where they crowded into the tiny ghetto south of the main business district, into dilapidated housing and poor neighborhoods. The resulting overcrowding pushed the boundaries of that ghetto steadily south and west, spilling into previously all-white neighborhoods. Within a short time, sometimes months, a

given neighborhood could be all black. Occasionally, white communities would attempt to stanch the movement by restrictive covenants and even crimes of violence against "pioneer" black settlers. But, in 1948, the Supreme Court (*Shelley* v. *Kraemer*) forbade the use of restrictive covenants. Racial violence proved counterproductive, and mounting public opinion against such overt displays of racism eventually ended much (not all) white resistance. Instead of staying in the neighborhood, white homeowners fled to the suburbs that were beyond the means of the average black person. This began an accelerated movement of whites out of areas of the city that they or their families had lived in for several generations.[13]

The shift of many white families to the extremities of the city and to the newly created suburbs was also made possible by a new transportation revolution in Chicago. Automobile ownership steadily increased, and rail, bus and rapid transit lines were extended to accommodate commuters. The new transportation routes not only shuttled workers from the outlying areas to the city, they also stimulated the development of business and industries in the newly developed suburbs. Major employers, like Zenith, relocated their central offices in unencumbered areas outside the city. Shopping centers and service facilities sprang up, giving employment and additional incentives for people to move out of the city.

Perhaps the greatest magnet of the new expansion was O'Hare International Airport, built on the site of an old orchard northwest of the city. The new facility set off a tremendous cycle of business relocation and employee resettlement which accelerated suburban growth. O'Hare itself would soon become the single busiest air terminal in the United States and employ over 40,000 persons. With the building of the expressway system and the addition of spurs leading directly into the airport, the dominance of the site was cemented.[14]

CATHOLIC INSTITUTIONAL GROWTH

The dream of owning one's own home—long the prerogative of the very rich—materialized for many Americans after

World War II, when prosperity blessed the land and crucial government assistance became available.[15] Clearly, there was a need for more housing. The years during and after the war witnessed the worst housing shortage in Chicago since the Great Fire of 1871. Apartments and other multifamily dwellings were at a premium. Living in these cramped flats was all the more uncomfortable once children began arriving. The single-family dwelling became a necessity as much as a dream. With generous federal financing and better job opportunities, one of the greatest building campaigns since the Great Fire took off in the Chicago metropolitan area.

Like the ubiquitous land developers who had first developed Chicago in the 1830s, modern real estate developers, freed from wartime restrictions and hardships, began purchasing large tracts of land on the city's perimeter and building unattractive but affordable single-family dwellings that would fill the rapidly expanding market. The number of permits issued after 1950 for single-family dwellings in the unincorporated areas and suburbs skyrocketed. Lured by promises of easy credit and pushed by fears of black incursions into urban neighborhoods, middle-class Chicagoans heeded eager entrepreneurs who were willing to sell them homes with very small down payments. Almost overnight new suburbs sprang into existence in the metropolitan area and older ones were rejuvenated.

The change in Catholic demographics in this period is reflected in the burgeoning growth of parishes and schools in the outlying and suburban areas and the corresponding decline of the parishes and schools of the city. The launching pad for this stupendous postwar growth was sixty-three parishes founded by Cardinal Mundelein between 1920 and his death in 1939. The pace of parochial growth had been particularly dynamic during the prosperous twenties, reaching a high in 1927 when eleven new parishes had been created. The growth had been in all directions—northwest, southwest, and into the older suburbs, most new parishes being in the extremities of the city. Despite the depression, virtually all of these parishes included a school. Although all slowed their rate of increase during the thirties, they resumed a strong pattern of growth and physical expansion after the war. The southwestern areas of the

city provided the greatest evidence of change. St. George parish in Tinley Park offers a splendid example of how this growth occurred. Founded in 1934 southwest of the city, the site had only recently been farms and vegetable gardens. After World War II the area began to explode with single-family dwellings, By 1950 over two thousand families claimed membership in the parish. By 1960 the number was over six thousand. So rapidly did the numbers increase that a parochial school was opened in 1949 by transporting old Civilian Conservation Corps buildings to the parish site and reassembling them. A convent and new church followed soon after.[16]

Because the war had checked parochial formation and the postwar growth in population was so great, the boom in parish building had little precedent. In 1947 seven new parishes were erected, and in the following year, eight. From 1948 to 1958 an average of six to eight parishes were erected or missions raised to parochial status per year. All included schools and large plants that required expansion within a short time. In his first year Meyer approved the formation of eight parishes; in 1961, four; in 1962, eight; in 1963, four; and before he died in 1965, one more parish. Within twenty-five years between 1940 and 1965, one-fourth of Chicago's parishes serving close to half of Chicago's Catholic population were formed. Seventy-two were in the suburbs and twenty-eight on the fringes of the city. Of the seventy parishes Stritch founded, only twenty-four were in the city. Of the thirty parishes Meyer formed only four were in the city limits of Chicago.

The racially troubled South Side of Chicago experienced the first growth—over fifty new parishes blanketed the increasingly Catholic population south and west of the city. Typical was the osmosis that occurred from St. Gerald parish in Oak Lawn. Founded in 1934 by Mundelein, it grew so rapidly that seven parishes were carved out of its original boundaries. Its only rival as a parent parish would come later from St. James parish in Arlington Heights.[17]

Suburban development in the southwest resulted in the creation of one of Chicago's most famous suburbs, Park Forest. The suburb had sprung into existence in 1946 as the brainchild of developer Philip Klutznick, whose newly formed corporation,

American Community Builders, bought 2,400 acres of cornfields thirty miles south of the city and created "one of the first and largest of the planned communities of the country."[18] As in most of the southwestern suburbs, the availability of the Illinois Central railroad provided Park Forest with the necessary commuter transportation. Klutznick's plans included provisions for a Catholic church, and land near the popular Park Forest Shopping Center was deeded for what would soon become St. Irenaeus parish. Park Forest was a great success, although later it would become the subject of William Whyte's classic study of fifties conformity: *The Organization Man.*

Directly west of the city—another area of strong black growth—suburban white flight not only meant increases in existing suburban parishes as in Cicero and Oak Park, but also the creation of new parishes like Divine Infant and Divine Providence in suburban Westchester, St. John Chrysostom in Bellwood, and St. John the Evangelist in Streamwood.

Growth was so fast that the whole new diocese of Joliet was spun out of the westernmost counties of Chicago in 1949. Father Martin McNamara, a professor at Quigley Seminary, was selected as the first bishop and consecrated on March 7, 1949. The separation of Joliet resulted in the creation of several new parishes that had once been missions of churches now in the new jurisdiction, including St. Peter Damian in Bartlett and St. Raymond of Penafort in Mount Prospect.

Northwest of the city, parochial growth was initially slower but soon caught up to the rapid pace set in the city's burgeoning southwest. The first line of development was the well-to-do North Shore suburbs, which included Evanston, Kenilworth, Winnetka, Wilmette, Hubbard Woods, and Lake Forest.[19] Already by 1953, with the greatest expansion still ahead, Cardinal Stritch observed: "As things are going now we are building a new archdiocese on the perimeter of Chicago."[20]

The rapid growth of the parishes in the newly developing areas was amazing. Often these new parishes shared in the disorganization that generally plagued the development of these areas. Out of suburban mud and newly constructed streets and subdivisions, a Catholic community would be formed. It would take at least several months of holding services in temporary

quarters to collect enough funds to erect the first buildings of the new parish: a school with a large gymnasium. The gym would function as a church until a new structure, replete with rectory and convent, would be developed. In all, it is fair to say that despite initial worries about the tremendous costs involved, the Church kept pace with the development of the suburbs. Indeed, it was often among the first to raise an important social institution in the heart of a developing suburban community. Sometimes, within sixteen months of a parish's creation an entire complex was completed.

THE CHANGING CHARACTER OF THE CHICAGO CHURCH

Despite these positive developments, there were also troublesome issues. The main concern was for the plight of the urban parishes, which represented not only considerable financial investments but, even more important, strong loyalties and personal attachments. To deal with what was left behind, as the wealth and influence of Chicago Catholicism moved away from its traditional urban moorings, was no easy matter. But looming on the horizon was another question. As many of the Catholic flock moved rapidly into the comfortable middle-class status that had escaped them for years, what would suburban living do to the faith?[21] Andrew Greeley, a young curate in the flourishing Beverly Hills parish of Christ the King on the Southwest Side, was one of the first to systematically analyze the impact of suburban life on Catholics and sort out the meaning of these changes for the future of the church. Greeley was clearly cognizant of the fact that Catholic suburbanites were a new breed. Their affluence, their lack of concern for ethnic self-consciousness, and their inquisitive spirit convinced the young priest that he was not dealing with those of "the legendary simple faith of the Breton fisherman or the somewhat less simple faith of his immigrant grandmother."[22] Greeley had no doubt that readjustments and changes would have to be made.

But if his analysis of the new situation was on the mark, his suggestions for dealing with the new situation were more tacti-

cal than substantive. The notions of solidarity and the Mystical
Body ecclesiology embodied in the group dynamics of the
Christian Family Movement and Cana held for him the greatest
potential for reconstituting the Catholic community in suburbia.
He saw no need to alter the basic patterns of Catholic life and
institutional growth. Indeed, if the Church were truly to be an
effective spiritual force in the new environment, it would be
necessary to intensify its efforts to spread clear, rational, and traditional Catholic teaching. Greeley's solution to the problems
generated by an ethic of suburban affluence was simple: "Those
of us who believe in the timeless value of the fundamental principles of Catholic Social Action, would perhaps do well to dust
off our tattered copies of *Quadragesimo Anno* and see if it still has
something to say, even in an age of affluence."[23]

This same sentiment was echoed by Father Neil Hurley,
S.J., in an article in *America*. After carefully describing "the raw
material which Suburbia hands over to its Catholic priest,"
Hurley pointed out the tremendous potential for advance the
Church could make in this new and challenging mission field,
urging the formation of a true "spiritual community" that
would "activate the suburban Catholic's share in Christ's
priesthood." Hurley's prescriptions for this spiritual renewal
were drawn from the pages of the Specialized Catholic Action
groups: vernacular in the liturgy, lay leadership in non-sacra-
mental organizations, and adult study groups.[24]

In many ways, Greeley and Hurley were like the easterners
who had traveled to the vast expanses of the trans-Mississippi
West and attempted to apply the landholding patterns and
water laws they knew from their region of origin. The fit was
not quite right, to say the least, nor was there at this stage a clear
enough sense of the implications of suburban living on a faith
largely shaped by the urban environment.

There were voices that sounded a note of warning and did
not share the optimism and confidence bred by Catholic ideology. In his article "A Pox on Suburbia," written for the Chicago-
based Claretian magazine *Voice of St. Jude*, Paul Brindel expressed
some of the same fears for suburbanites that an earlier generation had expressed for European immigrants. The suburbs were
an unstable and risky financial venture for the government and

thus the support necessary for their development would probably be cut off. Even worse, Brindel commented, the suburbs
lacked the all-important Catholic institutions—schools, CYO,
Holy Name—in short, the support groups necessary to sustain
Catholic life. "Should you move to suburbia?" Brindel asked.
His response was an unequivocal thumbs-down. "Your decision
may well determine whether your children and their children
will be apostates." Lack of schools, anti-Catholic prejudice, and
the poor condition of suburban Catholic life would inevitably
result in the exodus of many hundred of previously safe
Catholics.[25] Protestant observers of the same phenomenon were
even less enthusiastic about the suburban flight of their commu-
nicants. Gibson Winter, in an insightful article in the *Christian
Century*, reflected on the effect of suburbanization on Church
life and concluded, in a passage that might have sent shivers
down Catholic spines:

> Suburbia has introduced its concept of success into the very cen-
> ter of church life. Advancement, monetary and numerical exten-
> sion of power—these are the criteria by which the suburbian
> measures all things.... The task of the churches as witnesses to
> Christ's lordship and to the power of the cross has been sub-
> merged.... Any remnant of corporate thinking which still existed
> in the Christianity of our century has been lost in this suburban
> encounter.... Suburbia is the prime representative of individualis-
> tic thinking. The church's captivity to it is the death blow to
> recovery of the biblical view of corporate life, corporate sin and
> corporate salvation.[26]

Certainly Catholic leaders recognized that something very
important was taking place. In 1962 the Archdiocesan
Conservation Council issued a fifty-two-page report officially
ratifying the fact that "Catholics now comprise a higher percentage of the suburban population than of the population of the
city of Chicago."[27] As co-director Michael Schiltz would tell the
New World: "It [the report] is the final historical evidence that
the American Church has passed through its immigrant phase
and now faces a new set of responsibilities and challenges."[28]

Despite Schiltz's announcement it is not known whether
the Catholic leadership stopped to consider the personality shift

Chicago Catholicism would undergo with the move to the suburbs. Initially this would not be easily detectable because, like the immigrants of former times, newly relocated urban Catholics would seek to replicate many of the features of Catholic life they knew from the city. Yet the fact that the majority of suburban Catholics did not dwell in multifamily units but rather in their own homes did not bode well for the maintenance of the community spirit characteristic of urban neighborhoods in Chicago. Suburban neighborliness was not the same. People may have shared the same socioeconomic status, but the yesteryear's ties that bound—ethnicity, common employment, common religion as well as sheer physical proximity—did not carry through in suburbia. Even though the first generation of suburban dwellers may have continued the spirit of the urban enclaves, there certainly was no guarantee the next generation would follow suit. It was less possible for the parish church to enjoy the status of a major social institution in the suburban community that it had been in the urban community.

THE EVANSTON CONGRESS: STRITCH'S RESPONSE

One of the by-products of the general blending of Catholics into the American mainstream was increasing interest in interdenominational activity. This concerned Stritch deeply and here his normal permissiveness gave way to uncharacteristic firmness. He was vigorously opposed to any interaction between Catholics and members of other denominations that might appear to weaken or dilute the truth of the Catholic faith. He regularly forbade his priests from participating in the National Conference of Christians and Jews (NCCJ), but did allow members of religious orders to do so. He cautioned them however: "Of course you must understand that we must not give any semblance of participating in interdenominational services.... It is difficult to find a formula for charity in the circumstances in which we find ourselves and at the same time avoid any sort of seeming approbation for heresy or infidelity."[29] He repeated this same advice to University of Chicago Catholic chaplain, Father Joseph Connerton who was also asked to participate in a course sponsored by

the NCCJ. "We must try very earnestly," Stritch wrote, "to avoid anything which would seem to minimize the truth."[30]

Anyone who knew Stritch would have been able to predict his reaction to the General Assembly of the World Council of Churches which met in Evanston in August 1954. Stritch first received notice of this in September 1953 and communicated it to Apostolic Delegate Amleto Cicognani.[31] Archbishop Cicognani informed Stritch of the Vatican's severe disapproval of Catholic participation in these events.[32] The issue of Catholic participation in the Evanston Congress lay dormant until formal invitations began to be issued to the Catholic press to cover the Evanston event. When *America's* Robert Hartnett, S.J., inquired of Stritch whether his magazine should accept the invitation, the Cardinal responded in the negative:

> The authoritative decision is that Catholics may not attend this Assembly in any capacity, even as observers. In the light of this decision, the question of Press representation has been considered and studied, and it has been decided that no organ or agency of the Catholic Press may send a reporter or staff member in a journalistic capacity to this assembly. This information I give you for your guidance and not for publication.[33]

At the end of June, Stritch issued a pastoral letter printed in handy pamphlet form for easy distribution among the faithful. He faithfully repeated the Vatican line (and no doubt his own) regarding such events:

> The Catholic Church does not take part in these organizations or in their assemblies or conferences. She does not enter into any organization in which the delegates of many sects sit down in council or conference as equals to discuss the nature of the Church of Christ or the nature of her unity, or to propose to discuss how to bring about the unity of Christendom, or to formulate a program of unified Christian action.

In unambiguous terms, Stritch formally forbade any kind of participation by Catholics in the Evanston meeting. "Accordingly, it is understood that the faithful of the Catholic Church may not in any capacity attend the assemblies or council of non-Catholics seeking to promote unity of the Church."[34]

Naturally, Catholic theologians like Father Francis Connell, C.Ss.R, dean of the School of Sacred Theology at the Catholic University of America, were quick to praise the pastoral.[35] However, from the Chicago-based *Christian Century* came an editorial entitled "The Gulf" with words of scorn:

> For those American Roman Catholics who have looked toward Evanston as an opportunity to increase understanding and good will between various branches of Christendom, Cardinal Stritch's letter will have almost as shattering an effect as Leo XIII's letter on the blight of "Americanism" had on liberal tendencies in American Catholic circles in the 1890s. Should "the faithful" observe the prohibitions laid down in the cardinal's letter ... dramatic emphasis will be given to the fact that there is a great gulf fixed between the papal church and all other churches. And the world will be told that this gulf yawns wide and deep because of the "infallible" teaching of the Roman communion.[36]

Protestant opposition notwithstanding, Stritch had no doubt that he had done the right thing and even prevented a group of nuns from taking a Gregg Shorthand seminar on the campus of Northwestern University (where the Assembly Sessions were held) during the month of August.[37] As he wrote Jesuit Father Charles Boyer, "On the whole the Meeting was a good piece of Apologetics for the Church, for it brought out in the clear the utter futility of Christian unity based on protestant [sic] assertions."[38] Yet, for the Catholic in the suburbs rubbing elbows with his Protestant neighbors, the Evanston declaration must have been unsettling. Even though the controversy died down, the plain fact that Stritch had to issue such a document was a sign that times had already changed.

For ecumenists and other progressives, Stritch's condemnations must have given pause. But the leadership of the Church during these hectic times did not allow a pause for quiet speculation and assessment. There were more pressing challenges to surmount, such as finding enough space to educate the growing number of Catholic children who were seeking admittance to Catholic schools.

CATHOLIC EDUCATION

Catholic education during these transitional years was a matter of supreme importance in Chicago and in the American Church at large. Not only was it linked with parochial expansion, but it was considered by Stritch and others a vital dimension to the Church's presence in the suburbs. A parish without a school was not really a parish. It is no wonder then that the Catholic school system reached the peak of its effectiveness and control over the Catholic school-age population in the period 1940 to 1965.

When he first came to Chicago, Stritch yearned to pour his efforts into teacher training, as he had in Toledo and Milwaukee. As with many other things in Chicago, however, he found that these areas were already attended to and jealously guarded as someone's private domain. He confided to McNicholas: "I wish I could do more in the field of teacher training. The setup here is most complicated. We have few Motherhouses. The two Universities and Mundelein College have Departments of Education."[39]

Stritch inherited an active system of Catholic schools welded together by the centralizing policies of Cardinal Mundelein. According to historian James Sanders, the elementary and high schools of the archdiocese prospered during the decade of the twenties. After a brief downturn in the early years of the depression, steady growth resumed and no schools closed or shortened their academic years. When the thirties ended, there was a higher percentage of children in Catholic schools than ever before.[40] Mundelein's last superintendent of schools, Monsignor Daniel "Diggy" Cunningham, proudly reported to Stritch in 1940 that there were 249 elementary schools in the city of Chicago and 121 outside its limits serving close to 150,000 pupils. In addition, 87 high schools and various academies served a total of 27,949 students.

In the postwar era, growth in Catholic elementary schools was phenomenal. By 1951 (after the separation of Joliet) there were 365 schools serving nearly 200,000 students. Stritch encouraged and even mandated this growth, insisting that

parishes spare no expense in providing for Catholic elementary education, even if it meant delaying the construction of a parish church. Over seventy-five new schools were built during his eighteen-year reign, at a staggering cost of $85 million. The greatest growth came in the newly founded suburban parishes in Cook, Lake, and DuPage counties, which, Sanders reported, added 92,000 new pupils between 1950 and 1965. In 1950 the suburban school numbers constituted 19 percent of the total school population, but by 1965 it was 41 percent.[41]

It was clear that during the period 1940 to 1965 a massive transfer of Catholic schools would take place from city to suburbs. Moreover, important developments in the field of high school education would take place as well.[42]

THE CATHOLIC HIGH SCHOOL:
STRITCH'S HOPES AND FISCAL REALITIES

It would not have possible to foresee that Catholic high schools would be an important priority when Stritch arrived in 1940. Mundelein had created a number of Catholic high schools in the prosperous twenties; but in the thirties, secondary-school expansion was largely confined to two-year commercial courses brought into empty classrooms in parish schools. High school education lagged in those last years of the Mundelein era primarily because the cardinal and his superintendent of schools were far more interested in establishing grade schools and colleges. Superintendent Cunningham, in particular, did not conceive his role as one of an initiator of school projects, and he tended to leave most decisions about the establishment of schools and their financing in the hands of local pastors. This would begin to change in the Stritch era and even more in the Meyer episcopate.

As a former superintendent of schools, Stritch brought a much more systematic and reasoned approach to Catholic education. In his previous assignments in Toledo and Milwaukee he had been the catalyst for the formation of a wider array of Catholic schools. Above all, he was an ardent proponent of high schools, which he felt were indispensable in properly forming

the Catholic mind. Stritch's concern for additional high-school facilities couldn't have come at a better time for the Archdiocese of Chicago, which was experiencing the need for this type of education as early as 1944. "We have not sufficient Catholic High School facilities to accommodate all our Catholic children," Stritch complained to Bishop Henry Althoff of Belleville.[43] Ten years later he wrote the same to a Jesuit educator at the seminary: "The Catholic high school problem is serious. We need more high school facilities."[44] But Stritch's hopes for a program of high-school expansion ran into the hard wall of reality. Existing schools were not located where Catholic population growth was the greatest and securing the capital to build in these areas was a nearly insurmountable task. The result was that Stritch made hesitant progress in high-school expansion until a new superintendent of schools, William McManus, broke the fiscal logjam.

Existing Catholic high schools did experience significant expansion, but more often than not these institutions were located in areas that were already beginning to experience the demographic changes described above. Stritch complained to one of his fellow bishops in Illinois: "In the archdiocese many families live at a distance from Catholic High Schools, and it would be unreasonable to expect them to send their children to school at such inconvenience."[45] If a Catholic high-school education was to be an option for Chicago Catholic teenagers, new high schools would have to be built close to their homes. But here the problem of financing such a venture entered in. The tremendous outlays required for their construction and equipment made cost-conscious and fiscally conservative archdiocesan planners think twice. Moreover, even if the schools could be built, equipped, and staffed, maintaining them required that they charge tuition, a practice uncommon for Catholic grade schools. Paying tuition was nearly impossible for parents of many Catholic teenagers, already strapped by mortgages and tapped by fund-raising appeals to build their newly founded parishes. Stritch sadly acknowledged this: "When I came to Chicago," he wrote to a fellow bishop, "we had a great many vacant desks in existing high schools. The difficulty was tuition."[46]

Raising the money for the building and staffing of a Catholic high school was enormously burdensome and often not possible without the sponsorship of prosperous parishes. No one parish or religious order could easily manage the construction of a Catholic high school on its own. Nor under Stritch's conservative fiscal policies could the archdiocese do much. As much as Stritch wanted Catholic high schools, he would not go into debt to finance them. Stritch wrote Father Robert Trisco in Rome: "Our people just want Catholic high schools for their children, and the building of high schools is a big work.... We don't want to go into debt in making this provision...."[47]

Lacking the finances, or the strong desire to raise money by episcopal fiat, makeshift solutions for providing high-school religious education were implemented by archdiocesan officials. One option was catechetical programs like that of the Confraternity of Christian Doctrine. In July 1941 the Confraternity of Christian Doctrine was introduced into the diocese under the leadership of Monsignor John R. Gleason. Taking advantage of released time programs enacted into law by the Illinois legislature in the late forties, student attendance in this popular program increased steadily until, by 1958, there were close to 50,000 children under instruction.[48] However, these programs were still considered less desirable than a full Catholic school education; and an impressive number of parents sent their children to a neighborhood Catholic school, or pressed for the establishment of such schools.

Released time and CCD were not adequate substitutes for Catholic education as far as Stritch was concerned, and he allowed local efforts to take the lead in establishing or enlarging high schools. But again because of the enormous financing involved, this was often a hit-or-miss proposition and Catholic high schools in communities that could have used them remained fond dreams or architectural drawings for many years. Even if there was seed money, sometimes the lack of coordinated leadership kept the planned high school from becoming a reality. A keen example of this was the effort to found a Catholic girls school on Chicago's North Shore. The progenitor of the idea was Monsignor T. V. Shannon, pastor of St. Mary's parish in Lake Forest. On his own initiative Shannon had writ-

ten Mother Evelyn Murphy, prioress general of the Sinsinawa Dominicans, urging the formation of a school and even offering a handsome donation of $150,000 to $200,000 to get the school rolling. Shannon repeatedly urged Mother Evelyn to lay the matter before Stritch. When she eventually did, Stritch wrote back and showed interest but let the matter drop for two years. The idea was resurrected by Monsignor Reynold Hillenbrand, who succeeded in arranging a meeting between Stritch and Mother Evelyn in early 1952. Again Stritch promised some action but nothing ever came of it and the school plan died.[49]

A similar circumstance occurred with the planning of a high school in the southwestern suburbs. Several parishes under the leadership of Monsignor Walter Croarkin, pastor of St. Agnes in Chicago Heights, organized to establish a central Catholic high school in the vicinity. Stritch again gave his blessing and fund-raising was begun.[50] But the school became a reality only when the Dominican Sisters of Springfield offered to assume a large share of the financing and staffing. Marian Catholic High School finally opened its doors in September 1958, nine years after Stritch had approved fund-raising for the endeavor.[51]

The best Stritch seemed able to do for a long time was approve the expansion projects that were occurring in nearly every existing high school in the archdiocese. Occasionally he made substantial grants to complete the projects, such as Notre Dame High School in suburban Niles, which received $200,000 to complete its new north wing. Given this pressing need, a new formula had to be worked out to establish Catholic high schools and provide for their funding and consistent leadership had to be provided. In 1952 Stritch made a step in this direction by inaugurating a five-year fund-raising plan to elicit voluntary contributions from local pastors for the construction of high schools.[52] With the funds he raised he was able to enter into agreements with religious communities for cooperative funding of high school enterprises.

But this voluntary arrangement was not nearly enough to supply the rising demand, especially in the suburbs. The flaw in the plan was that many of the suburban pastors who most needed the high schools were heavily burdened by fund-raising

and building projects for their parishes and had precious little to donate to the fund.[53] Moreover, the same areas were populated by Catholic families already burdened with mortgage and car payments plus the expense of raising families. Stritch did not have the heart to press for anything more than voluntary contributions from even the wealthier parishes. Clearly the archdiocese needed to play a more activist role than that involved in Stritch's voluntary program. This happened in 1957 when Cunningham stepped down from the superintendent's post and was replaced by William E. McManus.

THE McMANUS ERA

A native of Oak Park, McManus was ordained in 1939, one of a small group of diocesan priests sent to the Catholic University by Monsignor Reynold Hillenbrand for advanced studies.[54] McManus was slated to teach education at the diocesan seminary but discontinued his studies after attaining a master's degree in education. After a couple of years of parish life, spent teaching at St. Sebastian High School on the near North Side, McManus developed a deep love for secondary education. He wrote to Stritch: "I've paid particular attention to the high school because it seemed to need the special attention of a priest more than the grade school."[55] When NCWC Education chairman Dr. George Johnson died in 1945, his successor, Monsignor Frederick Hochwalt, suggested McManus for the number two slot in the Washington post. Stritch gladly gave his consent and when McManus returned to Washington to assume his new position, he was urged by Hochwalt and others also to resume his doctoral studies at the Catholic University. Laying this before Stritch for approval, McManus indicated that his area of concentration would be "the field of secondary education, for I believe that the greatest need for our schools is a Catholic curriculum for secondary education." As a general theme for a curriculum, McManus suggested a topic dear to Stritch's heart: "I have been fascinated by the possibilities of his [Dr. George Johnson's] 'Christian Social Living' as a core curriculum for high schools."[56] But plans for the doctorate failed because McManus's duties occupied more and more of his time.

Monsignor Hochwalt had very little interest in the internal workings of the Education Department and little regard for many bishops, spending most of his energies working with the National Catholic Education Association. This left McManus a relatively free hand to pursue his own agenda.[57] McManus was very much at the center of debates regarding federal aid to education which had begun with President Truman's proposals in the late forties. Not only did he testify before Congress on behalf of a Catholic share in whatever aid was proposed, he personally lobbied congressmen, took a hand in defeating the notorious Barden Bill, and filed *amicus curiae* briefs before the Supreme Court in the Everson, McCollom, and Zorach cases, which dealt respectively with busing transportation for parochial school students, the use of public school buildings for released-time programs, and the released-time concept itself.[58]

Years later, McManus reflected his personal excitement in being in the middle of these historic debates; yet the years 1945 to 1957 took their toll on him. He later complained that his duties "virtually laicized" him and he itched to get back to Chicago. He occasionally brought the topic up to Stritch during his vacations at the cardinal's winter resort at Hobe Sound, Florida. Finally in 1957, when Cardinal Mooney was pressing to have McManus appointed executive secretary of the NCWC, McManus pleaded with Stritch to allow him to come home and the cardinal agreed.[59]

McManus assumed the superintendency of Chicago's Catholic schools in the summer of 1957 and adopted a much higher profile and more active role than his predecessor. He inherited Cunningham's skeleton staff, consisting of Fathers Stanley Stoga and David Fulmer and some school visitators. Gradually he expanded the operation, enabling him to move aggressively on a number of fronts associated with the still burgeoning growth of Chicago's school system. By this time the issues were not merely where to put new schools or allocate the already insufficient numbers of sisters. More ticklish issues of school integration were also looming on the horizon.

McManus first threw his energies into the knotty high-school problem. Quickly appraising the situation, he observed that far too many Catholic young people were being turned

away from the schools. If this generation were to be saved for the Church, a greater number of high schools would have to be built. Stritch had wanted to do more but had been stymied by finances, and Superintendent Cunningham, already advanced in age, did not have the desire or the strength to push the high-school cause with the firmness it deserved. McManus would cut through the Gordian knot of finances and bring more energetic leadership to the high-school issue. Fortuitously for McManus, the restraining hand of Stritch's fiscal conservatism and his unwillingness to coerce money out of pastors would be replaced by the activist policies of Albert G. Meyer.

ENTER CARDINAL MEYER

Albert Gregory Meyer was born in Milwaukee on March 9, 1903, the youngest son of second-generation German-American parents Peter and Mathilda Thelen Meyer.[60] By 1917 he was admitted as a second-year student at St. Francis Seminary on Milwaukee's South Side. In 1921, at age eighteen, he was sent for advanced studies at the Urban College of the Propaganda, with residence at the North American College in Rome.

Meyer was ordained a priest on July 11, 1926, at the church of Santa Maria Sopra Minerva, by Cardinal Basilio Pompilj. His bishop, Sebastian Messmer, directed him to undertake advanced studies at the Pontifical Biblical Institute, and in 1930 he completed his licentiate in Scripture. Meyer returned to the United States in early August 1930 and was immediately assigned, for a one-year stint, to St. Joseph's parish in Waukesha, a small city west of Milwaukee. By the following June the newly appointed Archbishop Samuel Stritch assigned him to the faculty of St. Francis Seminary as professor of dogma and biblical archaeology. In 1937 he was appointed rector of the seminary. During the postwar flood of episcopal appointments in 1946 Meyer was named bishop of the Diocese of Superior in northern Wisconsin.

In July 1953 Meyer was appointed to succeed Moses E. Kiley as archbishop of Milwaukee. His five years there were spent coping with the tremendous growth of the Catholic popu-

lation of that archdiocese. In September 1958 the apostolic delegate announced Meyer as Stritch's successor.

With the accession of Meyer, McManus was given a green light to devise a bold fund-raising program to provide investment capital for new high schools. With Meyer's permission he called together pastors of areas that needed Catholic high schools and told them of plans to build. At the conclusion of the meeting, each pastor was handed an envelope by Vicar-General Casey indicating how much each parish would contribute from the funds they deposited in the archdiocesan central account. It was pure extortion, McManus later recollected, but it was far superior to the voluntary contributions of the Stritch era.[61] McManus raised nearly $50 million in this manner. With funds in hand he actively courted prospective religious orders with a tempting offer: if the orders would agree to staff and help build the new high schools, the archdiocese would contribute land and assist the building with a predetermined subsidy. Several religious communities jumped at these offers. Not only were their memberships expanding, thus providing a better cadre of well-trained teachers, but also the Catholic high school was far and away their best vocation recruiting device. Catholic high schools began to spring up around the archdiocese like so many weeds.

A perfect example of this archdiocesan/religious cooperation was the construction of Mother Theodore Guerin High School in River Grove. The need for a Catholic high school in this northwestern suburb had been determined by McManus's demographic projections and an offer of eight and one-half acres of prime property. When a one-million-dollar subsidy was made to the Indiana-based Sisters of Providence to build and staff a girls' school for 1,200 students, the offer was readily accepted. Mother Theodore Guerin High School was established and Sister Frances Alma McManus, (no relation) was the school's founding principal.

In addition to creating brand-new schools, McManus engineered the relocation of older central-city schools to newer growing areas and helped existing high schools with expansion projects. When all was said and done, over $45 million was expended for new high schools. When added to the $20 million

for new buildings and campuses of Chicagoland's six Catholic universities and colleges, plus $85 million for grade schools, expenditures for education totaled a staggering $150 million by the end of the Meyer years.

THE EDUCATION ACCOMPLISHMENT

A recapitulation of the building statistics brings home the almost epic dimensions of this building spree. From 1940 to 1958 Stritch had established seventy-five new grade schools and twelve high schools. Meyer's accession in 1958 saw a steady increase in the number of pupils in Catholic schools from 393,012 to nearly half a million. Confronted with this massive increase, Meyer continued to press for the establishment of new grade schools as new parishes were opened, giving only one new parish a temporary exemption from the traditional order of construction.[62] To meet the challenge of growth, Meyer founded two new high schools, approved the construction of twenty-seven new city elementary schools (to replace old or obsolescent structures), and okayed twenty-six additions to existing structures. But the real growth continued in the suburbs. Twenty-four new schools were created and fifty-six additions were made at the cost of $27 million. Even more significant, the number of high schools would increase in Meyer's short reign, with seven new ones built in the city, substantial additions to existing buildings, and eleven brand-new high schools established in the suburbs. The price tag for these schools: $54 million. The archbishops of Chicago ranked with the pharoahs of Egypt as the builders of brick and mortar monuments. The only difference was that the pharoahs built for the dead, the archbishops provided for the living.

What strikes the contemporary observer are the sheer numbers of children who attended Catholic grade school, high school, and even college. In many ways, the growth of schools, more than parish growth, was in the forefront of perpetuating Catholic culture. With improved facilities and instructors, Catholic schoolchildren in Chicago were exposed, in greater numbers than ever before, to a more in-depth experience of

Catholic teaching than were their parents. The number of college-bound Catholic youth increased dramatically, and thus the higher educational level of Catholic children was a contributing factor to the upward social mobility of the time.

TRAGEDY: OUR LADY OF THE ANGELS FIRE

Schools were one of the glories of these confident years. But a school also was the setting for one of the worst human tragedies of this era of Chicago Catholicism. On the afternoon of December 1, 1958, a pile of rubbish and old clothing caught fire in a stairwell at Our Lady of the Angels School on North Hamlin and Iowa Streets.[63] The blaze roared through the building, which held over a thousand pupils; before it was extinguished, eighty-seven children and three Sisters of Charity died and a number of children, leaping from the blazing building, had suffered fractured bones. Seventy-two children were severely burned. As this was in the days before area disaster planning allocated victims to numerous hospitals, all of the burned and injured were transported to the nearby St. Anne's Hospital. Ultimately the death toll reached ninety-two.

News of this tragedy was soon flashed all over the news media. McManus first heard of it when a *Chicago Sun-Times* reporter called his office requesting statistics of the school's enrollment. The superintendent hurriedly hailed a cab and arrived at the scene, where absolute pandemonium had broken loose. Meyer heard of the fire from his secretary, Monsignor James Hardiman, and also made his way to the scene of the tragedy, speaking briefly with the fire officials and priests who were consoling hysterical parents. He made a quick trip to St. Anne's Hospital, where screams of the children unnerved the usually calm archbishop. Later he returned to the school and then to the rectory, where he sat, impassive, almost in a daze. McManus broke his reverie by informing him that reporters were outside waiting for a statement. He spoke briefly with them:

> In this hour of supreme tragedy, my heart goes out in sympathy to all the bereaved families who lost children in this fire, as well

as to those who had loved ones among the children. Words cannot express the profound sense of grief which overwhelms us at a time like this. Our only recourse is to God in the spirit of faith and submission to His holy will.[64]

The funeral arrangements were long and taxing, with Requiem Masses for the sisters and a memorial service held in the Chicago Armory for the deceased children. Words of support came from all over the world, including a message and contribution to a growing relief fund from the recently crowned Pope John XXIII. A particularly thoughtful gesture was the presence of Francis Cardinal Spellman of New York at the doleful Mass at the Chicago Armory. Meyer was so moved when he saw the portly and benign Spellman in the vesting area that he burst into tears and sobbed on the shoulder of the older man.[65]

Once the obsequies were over, the difficult process of sorting out the causes of the fire and making restitution began. An investigative panel was commissioned by Mayor Richard J. Daley to explore the causes of the fire and to offer recommendations to the City Council. The panel's deliberations made regular copy for the city's dailies; the commission struggled for weeks to determine, with no success, what had caused the blaze. At times the forum became an opportunity to take swipes at the poor conditions in Catholic schools—the lack of safety doors, extinguishers, and sprinklers—and also to criticize the system of leadership which mandated that the superior of the school had to be consulted before a fire alarm could be pulled. Moreover, occasional letters to the editor also harshly criticized the poor conditions in Catholic schools. One even criticized Meyer's invocation of "God's holy will" at the fire scene as an evasion of his responsibility to provide safe schools for Catholic youngsters.

The results of the official inquest urged a sweeping revision of the city's fire code and mandated the installation of sprinklers and other safety devices in buildings of two stories or more to prevent a similar tragedy. At McManus's urging, Meyer retained the Schirmer Engineering Corporation to study the safety systems of schools and ordered a mass installation of sprinklers.[66] Anxious to go to every length to make restitution, Meyer directed archdiocesan attorneys to make generous settlements

in all the liability cases, paid for the hospitalization of the burned children, and had Catholic Charities provide free burial plots. For several years after the fire Meyer celebrated a memorial Requiem Mass to deflect charges that the archdiocese was seeking to sweep the whole matter under the rug. He even acceded, against McManus's advice, to demands that he tear down the relatively well-built Our Lady of the Angels school and built a new structure. The Our Lady of the Angels fire left many searing memories in the young priests who worked with the people during and after it.[67] The shock and trauma associated with the school fire were easily understood. For the new archbishop it was literally baptism by fire in the mass media of metropolitan Chicago.

EXPANDING THE SEMINARY SYSTEM

The schools were an important feeder system to Chicago's seminaries. Quigley and St. Mary of the Lake also participated in the rising tide of Catholic vitality that characterized the whole diocese. Again, overcrowding afflicted both institutions, especially the downtown Quigley facility at Rush and Chestnut Streets. Stritch had planned to build and formed a committee to study the issue, but he departed before the committee could initiate anything. Within a week of his installation, Meyer reconvened the committee and listened carefully as they urged a restructuring of the entire seminary program from its five-six program (five years of high school at Quigley and six years of philosophy and theology at St. Mary of the Lake) to a four-four-four system which would necessitate the creation of a freestanding college. Moreover, the committee members called for an additional minor seminary on the South Side to accommodate the growing numbers of area boys who wished to attend the seminary but found commuting to the downtown campus too difficult. Meyer approved plans for a new college department at the old St. Hedwig's Polish orphanage in Niles. Niles College, as it would be known, began as a two-year institution in 1962 and eventually expanded to a four-year curriculum in 1968. Later the school affiliated with Loyola University.

None of this expansion went on without some controversy. The acquisition of St. Hedwig's for the seminary college stirred up ill-will among some Poles who did not want to give up the facility. Others disagreed with the decision to build a second minor seminary. The argument was not that it was unnecessary but that it was too big. On the Board of Consultors the issue soon boiled down to the size of the chapel. Consultors Bishop Raymond Hillinger and former rector Monsignor J. Gerald Kealey wanted an enormous chapel as the focus of the new facility. McManus worried that this would drain funds for needed high-school expansion in the suburbs and fought the chapel vigorously.[68] Meyer listened carefully to all the arguments and deferred to the wishes of the older priests who favored the large chapel. Ground for the enormous chapel was broken on Seventy-seventh and Western Avenue in early 1960. On the site rose a magnificent new minor seminary that was simply known as "Quigley South." Classes began in the autumn of 1961 and would continue until Cardinal Joseph Bernardin ordered the closure of the seminary program at the end of the 1991 school year. The refurbishing of the seminary system stopped only at the restructuring of curriculum and the construction of new buildings. The major seminary was a particularly dismal place under Monsignor Malachy Foley, who would remain at the helm until Meyer's successor removed him in 1967.

CATHOLIC CHARITIES REORGANIZED

Changing conditions in the archdiocese were also reflected in the revised programs for the massive Catholic Charities. After parishes and schools, the programs of Catholic Charities touched more Catholics than any other single work of the Chicago Church. Thirty-nine agencies were attached to the central charitable bureau of the archdiocese when Stritch arrived in 1940. The original thirty-nine agencies had been geared to the needs of the depression, namely, orphanages and other institutions for dependent children; institutions for emergency and long-term care; and agencies for handling adoptions and foster care. Relief agencies also abounded, providing food, clothing, and household services to thousands of destitute families.

There were ten day-nurseries caring for children of working mothers and nine agencies engaged in settlement work. Only five archdiocesan homes for the aged existed in 1940. When postwar prosperity returned, Stritch urged new fields on the charitable bureau. By 1958 the number of agencies sponsored by Catholic Charities had expanded to eighty-seven, and the annual cost of the programs soared from less than $2 million to over $8.5 million.

The changing complexion and expansion of the agency had come about due to the work of Monsignor Vincent Cooke, who succeeded Monsignor William O'Connor. Cooke pushed the agency to consider the needs of the elderly and the retarded, as well as the growing number of juvenile delinquents in deteriorating Chicago neighborhoods. At the urging of Cooke and with the support of Stritch thirteen new homes for the aged were built. The deaf and the blind were also cared for under the expanding services of the bureau. Indeed, Catholic Charities became a kind of safety net for any needs that slipped through the cracks of educational or parochial apostolates. Cooke also swung the agency behind community organizing activities and adult education programs.

ORGANIZATIONAL REFORM

Under the umbrella of Catholic Charities was the Department of Cemeteries. This agency provides an excellent example for understanding some of the forces changing Chicago Catholicism. Cemeteries were and still are the most lucrative endeavors of Church life. The Chicago Catholic cemeteries had evaded the master-planning and centralization of the Mundelein years.[69] Even though Mundelein had created the post of director of archdiocesan cemeteries, ethnic groups with burial grounds refused to be amalgamated into the archdiocesan system. The first director, Father Samuel Lucey, was handicapped by the depression from setting up clear administrative policies. In 1934 Father William Casey was appointed to the post and made considerable efforts to organize and rationalize cemetery administration. Despite strikes by unionized cemetery workers in 1943, Casey was able to set down clear, workable

guidelines for the cemetery system. For the post of executive director of the cemeteries, Casey recruited George "Joe" Klupar, head of the Bureau of Public Welfare in Cook County. An administrative genius, Klupar made the Chicago cemetery system the envy of his professional colleagues in the business. Centralized planning of finances and management were the keys to Klupar's methods, and under his direction more was accomplished in less time with greater efficiency.[70] Klupar led the way in mechanizing the whole cemetery operation. Moreover, programs of cemetery marketing and perpetual care for graves reached out to the Catholic public.

Later Chicago's cemeteries pioneered the use of the community mausoleum, largely to satisfy a majority of Italian Catholics who preferred this form of burial. Chicago became the center of modern cemetery management and the headquarters of the National Catholic Cemetery Conference, which hosted an annual convention of cemetery directors. The strong direction of Casey, Klupar, and later Father Francis McElligott allowed the consolidation of the recalcitrant ethnic cemeteries, which could not fulfill covenants of perpetual care and provide the elaborate funeral arrangements afforded by larger cemeteries.[71] Suburban growth also threatened heretofore rural burial grounds. Though resistance to total consolidation with the archdiocesan system would continue, the reforms of cemetery administration provided the model of Archbishop Meyer's administrative reforms.

For all the growth and change that occurred in the Archdiocese of Chicago in the postwar period, archdiocesan administration remained a highly personal affair, mirroring the strength and weakness of its chief executive officer, the archbishop of Chicago. If Mundelein was able to effect a greater centralization, it was because his personality demanded it. By contrast, Archbishop Stritch was less interested in managerial details. His style of operation was more personal. Avoiding desk work, he traveled extensively inside and outside the diocese. Meetings and committee work for the NCWC took much time as did his voluminous correspondence. An important priority for him were the annual trips to Hobe Sound, Florida, the winter resort purchased by Mundelein.

More than any other archbishop before or since, Stritch relied on his subordinates to carry the day-to-day burdens of

running the Chicago archdiocese. To Stritch's credit, he seemed to trust most priests and religious, and was inclined to let them "have their heads" in plans or schemes that addressed an important area of concern. He insisted on knowing in general what was going on but rarely would make independent inquiries on his own—unless trouble developed. Because of this much of the social activism so closely associated with Chicago Catholicism was indirectly encouraged by Stritch. For decisions of moment, Stritch sought a great deal of advice before acting, often reaching back into his past for people he consulted. His early correspondence in Chicago was filled with letters to Milwaukee attorney Henry Kane, who continued to advise him on legal matters. His old friend Leo Dohn from Milwaukee gave him advice on Holy Name matters, and, above all, he maintained regular contact with his old secretary from Milwaukee, Auxiliary Bishop Roman Atkielski. Indeed, he had wanted to take "Romy" with him to Chicago, as he had taken the Josephite Father, Joseph Plunkett, with him to Toledo and Milwaukee; but Atkielski demurred.

In Chicago his chief advisors, apart from Monsignors Edward Burke and George Casey, seemed to have been Father John Clifford, S.J., the academic dean of St. Mary of the Lake Seminary, and his personal secretaries Monsignors John D. Fitzgerald and James Hardiman. In addition to Sheil, he enjoyed the services of Bishop William D. O'Brien (whom he playfully called "junior" or "junie," since Sheil designated himself the "senior" auxiliary) and Bishop Raymond Hillinger.[72] Hillinger had been consecrated a bishop by Stritch in the early fifties and was sent to take over the see of Rockford. While he was there, he suffered a serious nervous breakdown and Stritch graciously took him back into his own residence in Chicago. Neither of these men, nor Stritch's other auxiliary, Bishop William E. Cousins, exercised much clout in the diocese.

In addition to friends from Toledo and Milwaukee, Stritch had many close associates in the episcopate, including classmate James Griffin of Springfield and Stritch's successor in Toledo, Karl J. Alter. His closest relationships with fellow bishops were those with John T. McNicholas of Cincinnati and Edward Mooney of Detroit. Mooney was a contemporary of Stritch from seminary days and McNicholas had been Stritch's

metropolitan in Ohio. Stritch probably was closer personally to Mooney than either man was to the often irascible McNicholas, but the trio was, as we have seen, a powerful force in the affairs of the NCWC. Later Stritch and Mooney would be raised to the cardinalate together, while McNicholas, deprived of the see of New York by the death of Pius XI and the appointment of Spellman, looked on dejectedly.

Within the archdiocese, the administrative duo of Monsignors Edward Burke and George Casey virtually ruled Chicago. Both men were holdovers from the Mundelein regime. Casey, the older man, had been in the first class of St. Mary of the Lake Seminary and had been sent away by Mundelein for advanced studies in canon law. He returned to work in the chancery and made his way up the ecclesiastical ladder, eventually becoming the vicar-general, with broad authority over clerical appointments and finances. Casey was cautious and conservative, with a reputation for even-handedness. He worked indefatigably, so much so that in early 1946 he suffered a nervous breakdown and was compelled to leave Chicago for eight months of recuperation in Arizona. Accompanying him was his longtime friend Father Donald Masterson.

Casey's rival for power was the archdiocesan chancellor, Monsignor Edward Burke. He had also been selected by Mundelein for advanced work in canon law. He joined the chancery staff in 1935 and in 1943 Stritch appointed Burke chancellor. In contrast to the conservative and reserved Casey, Burke was a gregarious, glad-handing backslapper who enjoyed an active social life and could be the life of the party. Burke knew the pathways of power and used the patronage clout at his disposal to favor friends and causes that Casey might ignore. For example, although Burke was personally a conservative, he frequently served as frontman for many of the liberal social activists among the clergy, including John Egan and Daniel Cantwell. He also promoted the cause of Jewish layman Saul Alinsky.

The similarities between Burke and Casey were clear enough. Both were brilliant men, determined and ambitious. But the differences were obvious too. Because they were so temperamentally mismatched, their working relationship

involved very clear boundaries of jurisdiction and authority over which neither could transgress. Burke, a volatile man, needed much encouragement, and enjoyed socializing. Casey was steady, even-tempered, reserved (perhaps the cause of his breakdown), and led a more sedate life. Moreover, Burke desperately wanted to be a bishop and was nearly enticed into joining the staff of the military ordinariate by Cardinal Spellman as a means of realizing these hopes. Casey, on the other hand, reportedly turned down several offers of episcopal consecration.[73] Between Casey and Burke there was great and often ill-concealed animosity. During Stritch's tenure the two men carefully staked out their respective bailiwicks, but Casey's breakdown in 1946 permitted Burke to become more prominent in archdiocesan affairs. The feud between the two monsignori resumed when Casey returned, and priests of the diocese who cared about these matters defined themselves as either Burke men or Casey men—depending on whose patronage they enjoyed.[74]

Like his predecessor who had appointed the two diametrically opposed figures in the first place, Stritch was inclined to stay out of the quarrelling and avoid trouble wherever he could. He, too, observed the boundaries of their competence, calling on Casey for updates on archdiocesan finances and on Burke in matters relating to social issues or canonical affairs. The equilibrium continued until Meyer's arrival on the scene. By the late fifties serious problems developed stemming from their internecine feuding and Stritch's own lack of interest in hands-on administration. Mundelein's administrative structure began to crack. Calls for better management techniques arose from sources like the archdiocesan law firm, the bond house, and especially the cemeteries' executive director, George Klupar. These admonitions went unheeded until 1957, when a serious financial scandal rocked the Chicago chancery. A chancery accountant was found to have embezzled large amounts of archdiocesan funds from parochial assessments. Included in his "take" were even monies destined for the archbishop's residence. The theft, rumored to be in the neighborhood of $1 million, was discovered by a bright young chancery official, Monsignor Cletus F. O'Donnell.[75]

O'Donnell had been ordained in 1941 and served as an assistant to one of Casey's friends, Monsignor John Campbell. Casey grew to trust the young priest, who had also favorably impressed him by his splendid performance on the annual clergy examinations. Bright, handsome, and Irish (a winning combination in Chicago), O'Donnell was sent—at Casey's urging—to the Catholic University for studies in canon law. He received a doctorate and returned to Chicago where he served at the front desk of the chancery. Accommodating, hardworking, and blessed with the gift of clerical small talk, "Clete" endeared himself to virtually all the priests who came in on routine business. O'Donnell's discovery of the chancery scandal and his efforts to keep it quiet (the errant staffer was never prosecuted), greatly enhanced his reputation. Conversely, Burke, who had been a close friend and drinking buddy of the man accused of the theft, now labored under a cloud.

When Meyer arrived in 1958, he became immediately aware of the tense situation between Casey and Burke. Moreover, Meyer was far more devoted to administrative details than his predecessor. The showdown would be inevitable. Meyer was soon favorably impressed with young Monsignor O'Donnell and moved him into the episcopal residence, ejecting Bishop Raymond Hillinger, who had been living there with Stritch. Stritch's secretary/master of ceremonies, Monsignor James Hardiman, sensing that the old order had changed, requested a transfer to parochial duties. Burke, watching from the sidelines, eyed his rival's rise to power with suspicion. Burke had begun well with Meyer, but the chancellor's gregarious temperament did not resonate with the reserved and taciturn archbishop. Confronted with increasingly burdensome episcopal duties and the prospect of an ecumenical council in which he would be expected to play a significant role, Meyer needed new auxiliary bishops to carry more of the sacramental load that the older auxiliaries Sheil and O'Brien would not or could not manage. In 1960 Meyer consecrated O'Donnell and Aloysius Wycislo auxiliary bishops. This meant the end of the line for Burke, who was savvy enough to know that O'Donnell's rise meant his decline. The chancellor soon grew embittered with Meyer and wrote him in late December 1960:

In the light of the episcopal consecration last week, I find myself duty bound to ask you if my exit from the Chancery office would fit in better with your plans for the future of the Archdiocese. If so, I will gladly comply in as unobtrusive a manner as possible.[76]

Meyer turned down the offer, but by October of the following year Burke was out of the chancery and installed as pastor of St. Bartholomew's parish on the North Side.[77] Burke's replacement was the loyal and capable chancery bureaucrat Monsignor Francis Byrne. But Casey did not have long to savor the departure of his longtime rival. On July 5, 1963, while having cocktails in the Cathedral rectory, Casey suffered a massive stroke and died.

The passing of Casey, the elimination of Burke, and the death of real estate agent Robert Hoffman left the chancery with a number of administrative difficulties. Since these men had carried much archdiocesan business in their heads, their deaths meant a good deal of scurrying and guesswork and brought home the need for better record keeping. Casey's death opened up the way for the administrative talents of George J. Klupar, recently retired from the cemeteries staff. At O'Donnell's urging, Meyer commissioned Klupar to study the administration of the archdiocese and make recommendations for streamlining its management. Klupar's report emphasized the need for long-range planning for expansion, clear lines of accountability, job descriptions for archdiocesan personnel, centralized personnel procedures, centralized property procurement operations, as well as standing statistical bureaus to ascertain population shifts, and the direction of research. Moreover, Klupar urged the creation of a centralized self-insurance program to cover archdiocesan needs.[78]

Implementing these recommendations in the midst of the Vatican Council was difficult, but, acting under O'Donnell's advice, Meyer nonetheless approved their thrust and determined to professionalize central operations. He appointed layman William G. Simpson, Chicagoan and former deputy administrator of the Small Business Administration in Washington, D.C., to become the first lay administrator in the history of the diocese.[79] Simpson joined the chancery staff in

early 1964 and was handed an array of responsibilities related to building and construction programs, real estate and insurance activities, long- and short-term financial planning, budgetary analysis and control, personnel and salary administration, purchasing policies and procedures, and statistical research activities. But confusion soon arose over the scope of his authority in these matters. Simpson interpreted his authority in a broad manner but quickly ran into conflicts with various priests who complained to O'Donnell. The auxiliary bishop in particular, given broad delegated authority under the often absent Meyer, soon came to resent Simpson's intrusions in matters he considered spiritual. By late April, Simpson and O'Donnell were at loggerheads, and the auxiliary issued a "him or me" ultimatum to Meyer. Simpson was gone by the end of May 1964.[80]

Klupar was once again called from retirement to manage affairs; and reforms were resumed, including the retention of the auditing agency of Touche, Ross, and associates, and the placement of the $3-million archdiocesan portfolio with the prestigious Stein, Roe, and Farnham investment firm.[81] The inauguration of an archdiocesan program of self-insurance also occurred—a program emulated throughout the nation.[82] With these reforms Meyer brought the business and managerial policies of the archdiocese in line with the vast growth that had occurred in the postwar period. O'Donnell sang Klupar's praises to Meyer, "Klupar has been a great help and I only pray God will spare him at least until this work is better organized."[83]

Yet the brick and mortar, the new programs, administrative changes, and the population shifts tell only part of the story. An important characteristic of Chicago Catholicism was its yeasty social activism.

PARISH FAMILY ENROLLMENT IN ARCHDIOCESE OF CHICAGO

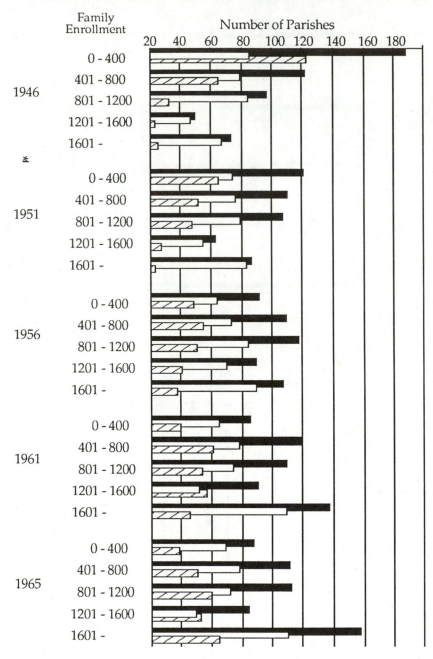

*In 1949 the counties of Will, Grundy, Kankakee, and DuPage were separated from Chicago to form the Diocese of Joliet.

Total　　　Urban　　　Suburban

NUMBER OF FAMILIES IN ARCHDIOCESE OF CHICAGO

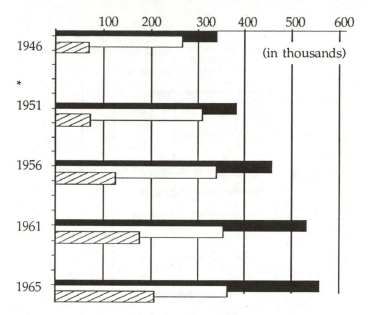

100 200 300 400 500 600

1946

(in thousands)

*

1951

1956

1961

1965

NUMBER OF MARRIAGES IN ARCHDIOCESE OF CHICAGO

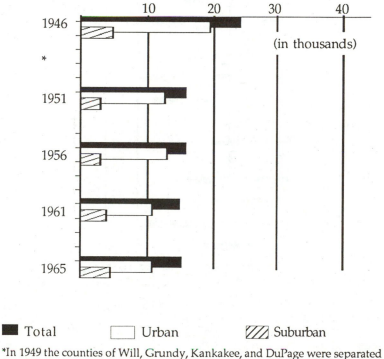

10 20 30 40

1946

(in thousands)

*

1951

1956

1961

1965

■ Total   ☐ Urban   ▨ Suburban

*In 1949 the counties of Will, Grundy, Kankakee, and DuPage were separated from Chicago to form the Diocese of Joliet.

URBAN/SUBURBAN PARISH COMPARISON OF MARRIAGES IN ARCHDIOCESE OF CHICAGO

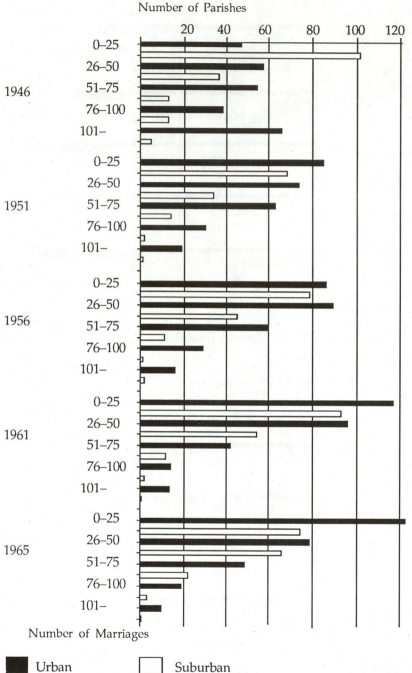

Number of Parishes

Number of Marriages

■ Urban   □ Suburban

NUMBER OF BAPTISMS
IN ARCHDIOCESE OF CHICAGO

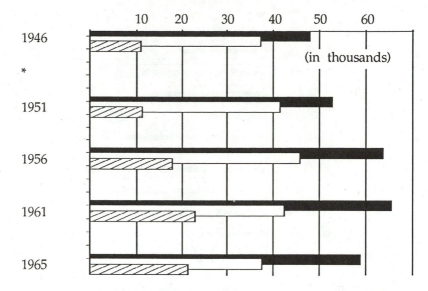

(in thousands)

SCHOOL ENROLLMENT IN ARCHDIOCESE OF CHICAGO

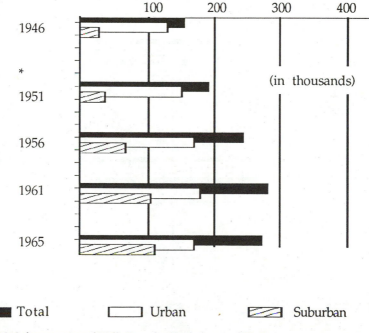

(in thousands)

■ Total ☐ Urban ▨ Suburban

*In 1949 the counties of Will, Grundy, Kankakee, and DuPage were separated from Chicago to form the Diocese of Joliet.

4

Bishop Sheil and Chicago Catholicism

On the morning of September 2, 1954, Monsignor Edward Burke received an anxious phone call from Stanley Pieza, religion editor for the *Chicago American*. Pieza had been contacted by the offices of Bishop Bernard J. Sheil informing him that the bishop had called a news conference for noon to announce his resignation from the Catholic Youth Organization. Burke was stunned and hurried to Stritch's office, where the cardinal was closeted with his consultors. Stritch too was shocked by the news and abruptly adjourned the meeting to huddle with Burke and Casey. Because Sheil's penchant for the unexpected was legendary, the trio worried that the well-known and articulate auxiliary bishop might say or do something that could be a public relations fiasco. Hoping to head Sheil off at the pass, Stritch, still in his house cassock, Casey, and Burke motored to the CYO offices to meet with Sheil and asked Monsignor Edward Kelly, archdiocesan director of the Holy Name Societies, to join them there. One can only surmise what was said and promised at the meeting with Sheil.

When the time came to meet the press, Stritch took command of the situation and defused it deftly by informing the reporters he had "reluctantly" accepted the resignation of Bishop Sheil and was appointing Monsignor Kelly as the bishop's successor at the CYO. Sheil himself stood awkwardly beside the cardinal and had nothing to add to the announcement. With that Sheil moved to the pastorate of St. Andrew's Church and into eventual oblivion. The man who had once

controlled what one historian called a "veritable social-work empire"[1] and who had been considered a candidate for every major diocese in the United States, watched from the sidelines as Kelly dismembered his once proud and energetic organization. Sheil lived another fourteen years, periodically reappearing to claim an honorary archiepiscopal title and a committee post at Vatican II; but, for all intents and purposes, his role at the center of events in Chicago ended on that September afternoon in 1954.

What had happened to Sheil? Only the year before he had been feted on the occasion of his twenty-fifth anniversary of episcopal consecration at a gala event at Chicago's swank Palmer House. In attendance were dignitaries from national, state, and local governments; labor union leaders, civil rights activists, and prominent businessmen, all of whom lionized Sheil in speeches that continued past midnight. There was much for which to praise him. The "Chicago" listing in the P. J. Kennedy *Catholic Directory* noted under Sheil's name and that of the CYO the directorate general of the Catholic Youth Organization, the pastorate of St. Andrew's Church, and positions as overseer of: the Mission of Our Lady of Mercy, the residence for women, Rita Clubs, vacation centers, the Catholic Salvage Bureau, the CYO Community Center, the Sheil House, the Chicago Interstudent Catholic Action (CISCA), and CISCA alumni association. Sheil had founded a new student campus ministry at Northwestern named the Sheil Center, an interracial residence known as Friendship House, the Lewis College of Science and Technology in Lockport, and the Sheil School of Social Studies.

Sheil's accomplishments were not limited to his work in the Archdiocese of Chicago. He was also well known as a friend of the Roosevelt and Truman administrations, as well as a strong supporter of the domestic and foreign policies of both presidents. His gifts for oratory had been effectively deployed in such causes as racial justice, the rights of labor, postwar reconstruction, and his favorite, the role of youth. Moreover, Sheil had been Mundelein's heir apparent. There were no two ways about it: Auxiliary Bishop Bernard J. Sheil was probably the best-known Catholic bishop in Chicago and possibly the nation. To

many, Sheil was the "labor bishop" or "the people's bishop," "the Bishop," or just "Benny." But by 1954 he was becoming a clerical nobody, tired and sick, beset by the worst kinds of financial problems and lacking the energy and drive to carry on the fights he had so vigorously waged against all kinds of opponents. On that September afternoon it became evident to him that he was moving into the oblivion he feared would be his fate when Samuel Stritch had become his superior nine years earlier.

WORKING WITH STRITCH

Initially, relations between Sheil and Stritch were cordial and gracious. Sheil orchestrated the enormous reception for Stritch at Union Station replete with hundreds of enthusiastic CYO members. Sheil conducted himself with dignity and charm during the days surrounding the installation. Stritch, for his part, went out of his way to be courteous and cooperative with his auxiliary. An example is the case of Cavalliero Umberto Nobile.

Nobile was a linguistic scholar from Italy who had been taken in by Cardinal Mundelein at the behest of Pope Pius XI. Not knowing what to do with the man, Mundelein pressed Sheil to find him a place at the Holy Name Technical School in Lockport, a position ill-fitted for a man of Nobile's training. The directors of the school soon grew weary of his complaining and wanted him removed. Nobile also did his share of complaining to Sheil, Stritch, and even the apostolic delegate, and insisted that they change the character of the technical school to accommodate his academic interests. Naturally, this was out of the question and Stritch wrote to the apostolic delegate, "It would not be prudent for me at this time to assume the responsibility for the conduct of this school which my demanding the continued active engagement of Prof. Nobile would impose on me." He reassured Cicognani, however, that he would "stand guarantor to this gentleman in the full measure which the agreement made by my predecessor clearly indicates."[2] However, getting rid of Nobile soon became a priority. Sheil came to the rescue and, using contacts in Washington, arranged to have the disgruntled professor sail back to Italy with the Italian diplomatic delegation

that sailed for Rome after the United States broke relations with the Fascist government in September 1940.

But their cooperation in the Nobile affair would be atypical of the relationship between Stritch and Sheil. Sheil was far too independent a character to confine himself to confirmations, altar consecrations, and religious professions—the usual agenda for an auxiliary bishop. While manifesting every intention of being a loyal and obedient auxiliary, Sheil knew enough to protect his turf and pushed ahead with a major reorganization of the CYO that more tightly centralized his control. The chief device for this was the creation of an archdiocesan youth senate under the auspices of the CYO, bringing about "a greater coordination of action" for the program.[3] In the reorganization Sheil turned over administration of the largely inert Holy Name Society to Stritch, who appointed Father Edward Kelly as its executive director. Stritch then set out to reorganize the society but found that many of the services they had performed so well in Milwaukee had already been subsumed by Sheil. As in the case of teacher training, Stritch found his options limited when it came to direct control over archdiocesan youth affairs. Stritch accepted the inevitable and meekly volunteered to his auxiliary, "If I can be of any assistance in furthering youth organizations in our parishes, you have only to call on me."[4]

Actual distrust began to develop between the two turf-conscious prelates even before fate threw them together in Chicago. Sheil and Stritch had earlier crossed swords over the auxiliary's attempt to nationalize his popular CYO program under the aegis of the NCWC Committee on Youth.[5] To Stritch, these efforts looked like nothing more than an attempt by Sheil and his chief supporter lieutenant, Father Robert Moore, at self-aggrandizement and grandstanding under the NCWC auspices. This scheme waxed and waned for several years, but collapsed finally in late 1939, when Stritch, as chairman of the Administrative Board, threw a monkey wrench into the plans. When Sheil and Moore sought the backing of the Administrative Board for a meeting in New Orleans to unite the CYO movement, Stritch refused to participate and directed Milwaukee priest Father Paul Tanner, an assistant director of the Youth Department of the NCWC, "to write [to Moore], in answer, that

I would have no part in arranging any Youth Meeting unless it had the approval of and was authorized by the Bishops' committee on youth." Referring to Sheil, he confided to NCWC Secretary Michael Ready, "Confidentially, I gathered some information which convinces me that a certain party is still determined to have his way, and his way is not for the best interests of Catholic Youth."[6] Sheil and Moore gave up their plans afterwards.

When he got to Chicago, Stritch apparently had not forgotten his misgivings about Sheil. And if he had forgotten, there is no doubt that his chancellor, Monsignor George Casey, who also disliked and distrusted Sheil, would have reminded him. In a very short time, Stritch sent a very clear signal of his opinion of Sheil when he refused to reappoint the auxiliary to the prestigious post of vicar-general. Instead he left the post embarassingly empty for two years (Stritch had done the same thing in Milwaukee) until it was finally filled by Chancellor George Casey. Other humiliations followed. Stritch let it be known, through his treatment of seminary rector Reynold Hillenbrand and others, that he did not favor clerical mixing in political or controversial issues: something that Sheil had done regularly under Mundelein. Nor was Sheil invited to be part of the inner circle of advisors who assisted Stritch in various matters. Moreover, Stritch also put some limits on Sheil's fund-raising by forbidding him to assess the parishes for blocks of tickets to CYO events. Although he did allow Sheil to send a letter eliciting voluntary contributions from priests for the CYO, the loss of revenue was considerable.

However, a broader perspective of the deterioration of the Stritch-Sheil relationship requires us to see more than personal animosity or grudges at work. The context of Sheil's marginalization in archdiocesan affairs was Stritch's desire quietly to move away from the policies and personnel of the Mundelein days. If the seminary was the apple of Mundelein's eye, Stritch paid off its existing debts and left it alone; if Mundelein scorned participation in the National Catholic Welfare Conference and petulantly refused to support the Catholic University, Stritch was chairman of the NCWC Administrative Board and sent many priests to the Catholic University; if Mundelein had looked

on Sheil as his heir apparent and alter ego, Stritch needed neither an understudy nor a rival in gregariousness. In the end
Samuel Stritch's suspicion of Sheil caused him to veto the auxiliary's possibilities for higher office.[7]

Yet Stritch did not have the temperament or personality to
forcibly rein in his auxiliary. He would occasionally fire off a letter to Sheil, inquiring about some activity or public position he
had taken that had embarassed him or contradicted archdiocesan policies. But Sheil knew that Stritch would never force a
confrontation and moved ahead without fear. Therefore, until
Sheil voluntarily resigned in 1954, he was a constant source of
concern for Stritch, who was compelled to explain to a steady
stream of complainants that he would "take care" of some offensive action of his auxiliary bishop. He never did anything more
than inform Sheil of his "concern."

A NEW DIRECTION

The disfavor of his Ordinary did not initially dim Sheil's
dream for a major diocese of his own and it probably sped up
the process of the transformation of the CYO, which had already
begun in the late thirties. Already by 1938 Sheil was plainly
bored with the athletic orientation of the CYO and wanted to
broaden its scope to meet a whole new set of changed circumstances and needs of Chicago's Catholic young people, many of
whom by now were adults. His public relations director, Italian
refugee Ralph C. Leo, would write in 1942 of this shift:

> The infant days of the CYO were at an end; the days that lay
> before would be days of adult achievement, of robust action, of
> major responsibilities, of democratic vistas.... For the first time ...
> the traditional notion that the CYO was a boxing organization
> began to give way before the rediscovery of the CYO as a symbol
> of youth work and youth achievement and as an expression of
> the democratic idealism that Bishop Sheil's generous humanitar-
> ianism and boundless social vision gave it.[8]

Sheil and others in his organization began to realize that his
efforts in behalf of youth, especially those who were most

deprived, had to include some concern for the kind of context in which they would mature. Although Sheil would grow remote from the hands-on work with boys that made him so popular in the first place, he was genuinely touched by the plight of people at the lower rungs of society. He encountered them everywhere: hanging around the CYO offices at 31 E. Congress; flocking to CYO athletic tournaments; derelicts and, later, parolees residing at the CYO hotels; blacks and all those others working long hours for low wages. Middle-class youth such as the alumni of the highly successful Chicago Interstudent Catholic Action organizations (CISCA) were appealing to Bishop Sheil for much-needed direction beyond the realm of sports and youth care.

In 1938 Bernard J. Sheil discovered the "social question." Between 1938 and 1954 he and his associates forthrightly discussed, and brought to public attention, every major problem confronting America in that period: race relations, labor organization, postwar reconstruction, liturgical reform, adult education, and the changing face of urban life.

THE EDUCATION DEPARTMENT

As a model for refurbishing the CYO operation with social education as its focus, Sheil took Franklin D. Roosevelt's New Deal. Like his friend Roosevelt, Sheil, too, wished to assemble a brain trust which would do research and write speeches on the issues that were uppermost in people's minds. Even before Mundelein's death, Sheil's reputation as a spokesman against anti-Semitism and racial injustice, in favor of labor unions, the poor and underprivileged was considerable. With the outbreak of the war, Sheil believed that he found the issue that would draw all his other concerns into one: democracy.[9] As the spokesman for democracy, he not only would appear as a patriotic, clear-thinking American Catholic, but he would also have an ideological basis to press for social reform. To assist him in this role, he created an Education Department in the CYO when he reorganized the organization in 1940.

The original aim of the new department was to be Sheil's brain trust and as such attracted scholars and writers who

would provide the fodder for the bishop's steadily increasing public speaking engagements. The first head of the Education Department was thirty-two-year-old Dr. Joseph Casey. Casey, a pupil of Fulton J. Sheen, had won a Ph.D. from the Catholic University with a dissertation entitled "The Primacy of Metaphysics." But Casey did not remain long in the post, for he enlisted in the Navy soon after Pearl Harbor.[10]

Casey's successor was the handsome and intelligent Father James V. Shannon, whom Sheil chose to head the Education Department and also gave the title director of social planning. Shannon was brought to Sheil's attention by a classmate, Father Joseph Ryan, who also happened to be an assistant of Sheil's at St. Andrew's. In addition to replacing Casey, Shannon served as the chief theoretician and speech writer during this new phase of Sheil's career. Shannon's had been one of the first doctorates in sacred theology to be awarded to a graduate of St. Mary of the Lake University. A nephew of former *New World* editor Monsignor T. V. Shannon, Father James had been first assigned as professor of English and religion at Quigley Seminary in 1931. A brilliant and sometimes erratic man, Shannon later admitted to his associate George Drury that he felt pushed into the priesthood by his family and that he suffered from alcoholism.[11] Shannon held liberal and even radical views on most social issues; his brilliant speech writing brought life to the bishop's new role as a spokesman for democracy.

But there were additional implications to the new program. In addition to speech writing, Sheil and Shannon agreed that more had to be done to amplify and build on what the bishop said. Earlier, Sheil's friend, the Baroness Catherine De Hueck, had called for the creation of "a school of social studies" and drew up a nineteen-page proposal that included two libraries (one open to the public, the other consisting of "condemned" books to be kept under lock and key and studied only by Shannon) and series of courses aimed at adults conducted by a stable of intellectuals who would also serve the bishop as a think tank.[12] Sheil and Shannon resurrected this proposal and it formed the nucleus of the Sheil School of Social Studies, one of the most successful and far-reaching educational programs ever conceived by the CYO Education Department.

Shannon had the brilliance to frame issues and to write for the bishop, but he did not have the requisite organizational skills to design the kind of educational program to amplify the meaning of Sheil's message. The formation of a program of adult education that more closely resembled a school than a lecture bureau was largely the work of Shannon's youthful assistant, philosopher George Drury. Drury, a native of Iowa, had lived on Chicago's West Side most of his life. He attended St. Mel's School and had gone to Quigley Seminary and St. Mary of the Lake. After Monsignor Reynold Hillenbrand had cashiered the young seminarian for writing a letter to a young woman using stationery he had pilfered from the rector, Drury drifted around Chicago's intellectual salons for about a year before Paul Kalinauskis, another former seminarian working for the CYO, suggested that he join Shannon. Drury eagerly accepted, remembering Shannon as one of his most brilliant teachers at Quigley and the two men set to the task of beginning the school. Drury recalled that after some floundering, the school began one November morning in 1942 when Shannon said to him, "Now let us begin our school."[13] Shannon and Drury had wide leeway in creating the school, since the bishop gave little direction other than insisting that the school was to concentrate on education for democracy and that no tuition be charged.

Shannon and Drury had plenty of examples of successful adult education programs in Chicago that provided worthy models. De Hueck's earlier outline for an education program was only one. In addition there was the Charles Carroll Forum, a series of lectures and forums organized in 1936 by Father James Magner "to make better known Christian principles and representative Catholic views on the leading topics of the day."[14] Other popular lecture series were sponsored by the Mercy Federation, composed of graduates of schools conducted by the Sisters of Mercy.[15] Chicago Catholics were also familiar with the labor schools created in the industrial neighborhoods of the archdiocese by Monsignor Hillenbrand and Father John Hayes. These courses extended over a series of weeks and acquainted laborers with Catholic social teaching, the history of labor movements, and parliamentary procedure.

When first getting off the ground, the school took the hodgepodge approach of other adult programs and public forums. While the program of the Sheil School incorporated the strengths of those formats (indeed, the first reports on the school referred to it as "Bishop Sheil's Labor Schools.")[16] The Sheil School of Social Studies announced its opening in a low-keyed way in February 1943 with a small article in the *New World*.[17] The first offerings were a miscellany of subjects, including "God, Liturgy, Survey of Science, Practical Writing, the Negro in America, Mathematics for Everyday Use, Panel Discussions on Women in Wartime."[18] The instructors included Shannon and Drury, who taught the theological courses, and other recruits from local colleges and universities. As per Sheil's request, no fees were charged, and all were welcome, regardless of color or creed. Sheil's name and the well-known location of CYO headquarters at 31 East Congress drew hundreds of Chicagoans to the evening sessions and weekend events. By July, the beginning of the third seven-week session, over two thousand adults had attended lectures or classes. Courses were offered in every imaginable field, including sociology, art, drama, current events, and foreign languages. One of the most popular instructors, Severino Sansolis Y Serra, a Filipino who taught courses in conversational Spanish, drew hundreds of students annually. Even the once scattered labor schools begun by Monsignor Hillenbrand and his associates soon came under the Sheil School umbrella. They were taught primarily by Edward Marciniak or Daniel Cantwell. In the basement of the building, Sheil made room for a library and, later, bookstore called St. Benet's Library, which had been in existence for several years under the supervision of septuagenarian Sara Benedicta O'Neill.[19] St. Benet's, which outlived even the Sheil empire, was eventually taken over by Nina Polcyn of Milwaukee and remained a favorite hangout for inquisitive Catholics. The CYO headquarters swarmed with Chicagoans availing themselves of the talented teachers who volunteered their services to the organization.

But Drury was not content with the odd-lot classes and one-shot lessons on how to conduct a union meeting that were the drawing cards of the school. He had originally been attracted to Sheil's service because it offered an opportunity to

do some serious work educating American Catholics in the correct principles of democracy. For the theoretical-minded Drury
that meant going deeper into the first principles of democracy
that were found in the natural law. Drury summed up the purpose of the Sheil School "to give to people, to all people, an ever
fuller knowledge of the truths of reason and revelation to enable
them to build a better world."[20] Knowing the truth about the
real origins of democracy would make better American citizens.

INTENSIVE EDUCATION FOR DEMOCRACY

As all of these developments were taking place, Sheil began
to take on more and more speaking engagements. He appeared
regularly at forums, conventions, and congresses around the
nation during the forties. He spoke frequently to the AFL and
was a regular fixture at the conventions of the CIO. He delivered
addresses and invocations at meetings of garment workers,
retail grocers, bartenders, foremen, building service employees,
stagehands, and motion picture operators. He lectured at conferences on welfare needs, recreation, industrial problems, and
juvenile delinquency. He testified before congressional committees on banking and currency, education, labor, jobs and security, housing and slums. He issued statements on minimum
wages, racial relations, fair employment practices, the Taft-
Hartley Act, and universal military training.[21]

But his speeches on democracy represent some of the
finest of Sheil's thinking and some of the ablest speech writing
by Shannon and Drury. Using their words Sheil hammered
away at the irony of fighting Nazis and Fascists to maintain
democracy while at the same time denying it to people here in
the United States. How, Sheil asked, could the United States
fight a war to abolish totalitarianism in the name of democracy
and still permit racial and religious discrimination? Sheil,
Shannon, and Drury were convinced that this disparity existed
largely because people did not understand the true meaning of
democracy. Those ideas were expressed in a speech, "Education
for Democracy," written by Drury and delivered in November
1943 to the Sheil School Forum. In this address the bishop elab-

orated the key ideas on democracy in concise terms. Sheil insisted that true democracy was a system that "rests upon definite intellectual convictions," namely, the natural law implanted in human nature by God. Democracy, he argued, was "based on a view of human nature that is profoundly philosophical—one may say even religious—in concept: that man is uniquely reasonable; that he is capable of making reasoned decisions; that he enjoys personal freedom with its concomitant responsibility; that he, precisely as man, possesses inherent and inalienable rights...."[22] Sheil decried "Kantian transcendentalism, the sociologism of Auguste Comte, and the naive materialism of the Marxian school," insisting that true democracy stems from "that Christian rationalism of which Saint Thomas Aquinas was so strenuous an advocate."

But as well-written as the speeches were and as eloquently and passionately as the bishop delivered them, they were not enough. Only intensive education in the first principles of democracy would help Americans live it in a much more consistent manner and make for more effective democratic participation. This was the keystone of Bishop Sheil's program and the guiding force behind Drury's activities at the school.

While working on speeches, Drury began to formulate a program of systematic study which would convey the all-important first principles of Christianity and democracy to a small core group, who would stimulate the kind of grass-roots transformation of society that would bring about a genuine and thoroughgoing renewal of American society according to democratic principles. In a manner similar to the Specialized Catholic Action movements, Drury proposed a program of intensive education with small groups of lay apostles who would be carefully formed in the first principles of sound social and democratic thinking and then be "turned loose" to reform society. If pondering these first principles of the natural law and its relationship to American democracy led an honest inquirer to seek further into the Catholic faith, so much the better. Catholicism was an authentic form of Americanism.

Shannon would eventually pass from the CYO scene, leaving Drury relatively free now to set the direction of the Sheil School as he thought best. In short order Drury drew up a core

curriculum that would embody the central precept of education for democracy and insist on firmly establishing democracy's first principles in the natural law. Drury's connections with academics all over the city, especially at the University of Chicago, helped him construct a program of intense study called, appropriately, the "Basic Course"—a layperson's equivalent of the first years of fundamental philosophy and theology given in the seminary curriculum. Drury's program was hammered out by his own seminary-trained mind and with help from George Schaeffer, a young scientist from the University of Chicago. In the school bulletin for the fall of 1943, Drury described the purpose of the two-year course:

> Before a man can plunge, for purposes of social action, into the welter of confused objectives, devious doctrines and strident bedlam of the modern world, he needs an accoutrement of truths.... Obviously for effective social action this intellectual equipment is of the utmost importance. It is to give people this panoply of ideas that [the] Sheil School introduces with this term its basic course.

Drury and Schaefer planned the course so that the matter could be "quartered into arts, sciences, philosophy and theology ... [moving] from the concrete to the abstract, reiterating on each level the fundamental truths expressed on the lower plane." But if the curriculum began simply with natural first principles, it was evident that it would end in supernatural life. Grace built on nature. Drury described the ultimate purpose of the Basic Course, "The whole resolves into the figure of Christ, the Man-God, Whose person is the summation, the epitome of all truth previously presented."[23] Good scholastic that he was, Drury's vision was truly synthetic: to encompass every aspect of human knowledge into one grand synthesis which found its complete expression in Christ. This even included course work in Christian Art. It made its debut during the summer of 1943 in the work of artist Ann Grill, an instructor in ecclesiastical design at the Chicago Art Institute.[24] With a solid theoretical basis, Christians could assume their roles in the Mystical Body of Christ and properly pursue the kind of radical social reconstruction that was the true goal of the Christian believer. Drury did

not abandon the popular lectures and general course work in languages or the like. But in his vision they were only "bait" to attract thoughtful Christians to the school, while it was hoped they would become acquainted with the larger purpose of education for democracy. Drury's approach made perfect sense to him and to the growing number of adherents of Specialized Catholic Action around the city who affiliated themselves with the school and enrolled in the Basic Course. With its first graduates in 1945, Drury bragged:

> It is a thrill ... to watch the implications of the tradition of truth and the Christian synthesis grow out through the person of the telephone operator, the department store clerk and the stenographer into the Natural Media of their lives. In our first band of graduates we have an example of the organism that is to come.[25]

Thanks to Drury and the wide array of offerings the school was able to present, the Sheil School was touted as an example of Chicago Catholic life at its finest. So active and prosperous was the school that James O'Gara, a veteran of the Chicago Catholic Worker House, wrote in *America* that the school was Chicago's "Catholic Time's Square, stay there long enough and you can meet almost anybody."[26]

Indeed, Sheil did attract an interesting medley of characters who inhabited nooks and crannies of the CYO building. Another important Sheil speech writer (after Shannon and Drury were bounced out) was Edward Joyce, another former seminarian. A multilingual and exceptionally astute young man, Joyce wrote a number of Sheil's important addresses in the late forties and even accompanied Sheil to postwar Germany in 1946 to survey the conditions of German youth and sit in at the Nuremberg trials.

Still another in this medley of characters was Harlem Renaissance poet Claude McKay. A native Jamaican, McKay had been deeply involved with the resurgence of black poetry and literature that emerged from Harlem in the twenties and thirties. His personal odyssey took him into Communism and sojourns abroad, including the Soviet Union. After growing disaffected with the left and the Soviet Union, McKay settled into an unproductive life in New York. Chronically ill, McKay recovered from

a serious illness in 1942 with the help of young Catholic volunteers from New York's Friendship House. He later became associated with Tom and Mary Keating, who were hired by Sheil for work in the CYO Vacation School program. At their urging, and that of Baroness Catherine De Hueck, Sheil "hired" McKay in 1944 to work as a "consultant" on black affairs. McKay offered a few courses in black literature, but his health faltered so badly he could do little more than occupy a desk. He eventually converted to Catholicism and was baptized by Sheil before his death in 1948.

The Friday Evening Sheil School Forums attracted some of the best spokespersons of the Catholic world to Chicago. Guest speakers including Jacques Maritain, Maisie Ward (who spoke to an overflow audience in the boxing arena of the CYO building), well-known journalists and politicians willingly came to the Sheil School to speak without fees or transportation costs. Added excitement came in 1944 when Sheil began to hand out an annual award named for Leo XIII. The first recipient of the award—which was a handsomely struck medallion designed by Pius XI's personal sculptor—was Sister Vincent Ferrer Bradford, O.P., a Sinsinawa Dominican who taught regularly in the field of social justice. Frances U. Sweeney, a librarian from Boston, won it posthumously in 1945. Subsequent recipients included Assistant Secretary of State G. Howland Shaw, Jacques Maritain, Frank Sheed, and Maisie Ward. In 1949 Sheil bestowed the award on Stritch, giving the cardinal the opportunity to tease the "senior" auxiliary about his erstwhile ways. With gentle humor, Stritch spoke to the awards banqueters at the Sheil School:

> There is one man who, having the sense of Christ's presence in the Church and the work of the Church, is doing so many things that even the Cardinal Archbishop has found it difficult to keep informed on all his activities.
>
> In Bishop Sheil, I would say there exist two outstanding qualities. The first I would call fecundity. For so prolific are his activities in behalf of the underprivileged that some of us cannot quite be sure what is coming next. His second outstanding quality is related to the virtue of fortitude. It is a quality of zeal, of

what I would call daring. Some of us possess prudence, others fortitude.... Many things would never be accomplished without daring. God wants certain things to be done which cannot wait on the virtue of prudence.[27]

VOICE FOR CIVIL RIGHTS

While the school went on, Sheil devoted a great deal of time giving speeches. As we have seen, his speeches on democracy contained a powerful, coherent, and confident message that Sheil, with his flair for the dramatic, was able to transfer to other issues, most notably to the issue of race. As he was able to demonstrate democracy's reliance on natural law so also Sheil was one of the first American Catholic bishops to actively apply the natural law to the thorny issue of race. For years, the CYO had encouraged interracial participation in its programs. Acting under the urging of Baroness De Hueck, Sheil began to make strong public statements regarding the race issue, and early in 1942 he welcomed the establishment of the Friendship House in Chicago. That same year, at the annual convention of the Conference of Catholic Charities in Kansas City, Sheil enlisted his oratorical skills in the cause of racial justice. Sheil informed the assembled delegates that delinquency among blacks was "a practical protest against a discrimination that is ethically indefensible, socially unjustifiable and radically unChristian." Voicing a complaint shared by many black groups throughout the country, Sheil declared, "It is the most dangerous kind of hypocrisy to wage a war for democracy and at the same time to deny the basic benefits of democracy to any group of citizens." He went on to bring the message home to Catholics "The church in this country at this moment is face to face with this problem. It must be met by a reaffirmation in action of the great Christian virtues of justice and charity. Jim Crowism in the Mystical Body of Christ is a disgraceful anomaly."[28]

In 1943, as racial tensions flared around the country, especially in Detroit, Sheil continued to hammer away at the theme that race discrimination was unworthy of America and made the crusade for democracy hypocritical. Moreover, Sheil urged black Americans to take pride in their heritage. In an article

titled "If I Were a Negro" in the popular *Negro Digest*, Sheil spoke out strongly for what in the sixties would be called "black pride," saying:

> If I were a Negro, I would be thankful for my heritage, for the traditions of my people, for a culture which presents such a hopeful contrast to the artificial and material elements now dominant in our modern civilization.... Above all, I would be grateful for that inherited spiritual strength fashioned in the crucible of persecution and suffering.[29]

The leading black newspaper in Chicago, the *Defender*, was quick to note Sheil's words, writing approvingly in 1942, "We welcome these words.... The bishop's words should supply material for a full page advertisement in some daily paper in every large center in the United States."[30] After Sheil's "If I Were a Negro" article, the newspaper once again hailed the fact that Sheil was "becoming ever more outspoken on questions which affect the Negro people." They were quick to point out as well, "the many Jim Crow Catholic schools that are maintained in Negro areas" and concluded, "The church is a power in the community. But not a power for unity, nor for equality and therefore not a power for winning the war or for creating the kind of America that will truly be the arsenal of democracy."[31]

Sheil did practice interracial inclusion in his hiring and personal practices. In addition to his sponsorship of the ailing Claude McKay, Sheil appointed a bright, young black Catholic woman, Dora Sommerville, to head the social service division of the CYO. Trained at the Catholic University to be a social worker, Sommerville would have a remarkable career in the field of social welfare.[32] Moreover, Sheil's efforts in the cause of civil rights was unflagging. In May 1946 at an address before the Chicago Council Against Racial Discrimination, Sheil thrust himself into the middle of one of the most hotly debated issues confronting Chicago in the postwar era: the question of restrictive covenants. These covenants amounted to a form of legalized segregation and were often the last bulwark of white neighborhoods seeking to ward off black expansion. Often the strongest opponents of black migration into white neighborhoods were local pastors who did not want to lose their white

parishioners. Sheil's speech blasted the "hideous question of restrictive covenants" and decried religious leaders who "under the plea of prudence have failed to appreciate or to teach fearlessly what the Brotherhood of Man means in terms of simple justice and charity for the poor, the underprivileged and the oppressed."[33] As a result of his interest in interracial justice Sheil was considered for a post on the Fair Employment Practices Commission when Roosevelt sought to reestablish it in 1943 after the resignation of its first set of members. (The post eventually went to the labor priest, Monsignor Francis Haas.)[34] Moreover, Sheil actively backed Truman's call for a civil rights bill in the late forties and urged the president, through Attorney General Francis Biddle, to press for such legislation forcefully.

Sheil was equally outspoken on the issue of anti-Semitism. His credentials in this area were firmly established in 1938 when he appeared as an opponent of the anti-Semitic oratory of Father Charles Coughlin. Jewish citizens in Chicago were so grateful that they took up a collection for Pope Pius XI in 1938–1939, and the money was given to Sheil, who responded with words of gratitude:

> My dear Jewish friends, I congratulate you on the magnificent and convincing demonstration you are now giving.... Your munificent gift makes all Catholics your grateful debtors. We sincerely hope that your kindly, beautiful and generous action will silence forever those few, very few, misguided, uncharitable Catholics who have so unjustly attacked your persecuted people. Be sure, dear friends, this noisy little clique are inspired neither by the doctrines nor the sentiments of the Catholic Church.[35]

From then on, Sheil became a fast friend to many important figures in the Jewish community and lent his prestige to important causes dear to the hearts of Jewish people. In 1942, speaking before a meeting of Temple Sholom, Sheil declared solidarity with suffering Jewry in Europe: "the ... quality of universality that makes the Jewish question not only a problem for Judaism, but also for Christianity—for our civilization.... The Hitlerian theory of Aryan superior of a master race, is not only directed at the Jewish people. By its implicit denial of the unity of mankind it strikes at the very core of our common Judaeo-Christian

civilization, the foundation of which is the belief that the God of Israel is also the God of mankind."[36]

In 1944 Sheil was appointed a member of the National Committee Against the Persecution and Extermination of the Jews, which had Supreme Court Justice Frank Murphy as its chairman. So closely linked to the Jewish community in Chicago did Sheil become that in 1948 the Decalogue Society, an organization of Jewish lawyers, voted him their award of merit for "waging incessantly that warfare which right and justice and truth must wage unceasingly against falsehood, hatred, ignorance and bigotry."[37] In 1951 he was the first non-Jewish recipient of the B'nai B'rith award.[38] So highly respected had Sheil become that he was singled out as one of the leading supporters of the State of Israel and a special friend of its government. In 1956 the Israeli ambassador to the United States, Abba Eban, visited Sheil for consultations and urged him to continue as a salesman for State of Israel bonds.

Sheil's friendliness with the Israeli government and his relationship with a number of Jordanian families made him a natural candidate as a goodwill ambassador to the troubled Middle East. Campbell promoted his friend in a memo to transportation magnate Jack Keeshin: "For many years in the United States, the Jewish population has regarded Bishop Sheil as one of the outstanding protectors of this minority. He has spoken publicly on many occasions and written numerous articles concerning Civil Liberties and equal rights for this segment of our population." Campbell went on to suggest: "In view of the foregoing circumstances it would seem that Bishop Sheil could be of great service to the Holy See either as a mediator between Arabs and Jews or as an official observer friendly to both sides in the present controversy."[39] Nothing ever came of it.

ORGANIZATIONAL EXPANSION AND DISARRAY

Sheil's warm relationship with the Jewish community had many important side effects, not the least of which were generous contributions to the financially troubled CYO. Not only did Sheil significantly expand the scope of CYO educational

programs but he also invested heavily in social welfare programs and recreation.[40] New programs included the opening of Nisei House on North LaSalle Street, a center for helping Nisei families with relocation problems and a haven for young Japanese Americans to discuss their problems. Sheil House on South Michigan Avenue was opened in a former Swift and Company clubhouse to provide recreational facilities for black youth in the area of St. Elizabeth's parish. Doddridge Farm in Libertyville was acquired from the Episcopal Diocese in 1940. It was first used for the Ladies of the Grail, a Dutch-founded women's organization, and later as a CYO boys camp.[41] A child guidance and speech clinic was established by Anna May Hawkeotte Smith, the wife of public relations chief Charles Carroll Smith, to help disabled youngsters.[42] These programs also included a Seeing Eye dog school, a community center on the West Side, and continued expansion of the popular Vacation Schools for Chicago youth in the city park system. Like a Chicago ward boss, whenever Sheil heard about needs, he tried to do something about them.[43] Personnel, organization, and especially finances were always secondary matters.

Although the Sheil School generated much enthusiasm and the Education Department provided the bishop with excellent speeches, there was internal dissension. Shannon was one of the first to go in the recurrent reorganizations of the enterprise. Shannon initially embraced Drury's notion of intensive education for democracy, but he soon grew tired of it and the whole Sheil operation. Shannon had done superior work for the bishop but, like so many others, he soon came to resent Sheil. As their personal relationship deteriorated even Shannon became increasingly caustic and disillusioned with Sheil. Sheil himself added to the dissatisfaction of the troubled priest. In one instance, Sheil claimed to have stayed up all night "writing" a speech that Shannon had already written for him. Another time, a GI from the Aleutians had written Sheil pointing out some flaw in one of Shannon's speeches, causing the bishop to twit the unhappy priest constantly about the matter. Shannon's unhappiness in the CYO resulted in a relapse of an earlier bout with alcoholism and caused a cabal of conspirators in the Public Relations Department, including Ralph Leo and Charles C.

Smith, to plot his expulsion. Shannon himself provided the fodder for his dismissal when on a trip to New York with Smith, he allegedly went on a binge and apparently made sexual overtures to a sailor. News of this went back to Sheil, who promptly dismissed Shannon and tapped Drury for the post.[44]

However, Drury would meet the same fate as Shannon when he antagonized the Public Relations Department. Growing dissatisfaction with Drury's Basic Program eventually undermined him. Smith and his associates grew tired of Drury's approach to adult education, which in their estimation was far too esoteric and therefore difficult to market. Drury personally considered the Public Relations Department out of step with the goals of intensive education for democracy, which he deemed central to Sheil's founding vision of the school. Open conflict between the Public Relations people and Drury erupted in 1945, when one of the PR staff scoffed at Drury's Basic Course as an attempt to replicate the *petite seminaire*. Drury superciliously corrected him by saying it was the *grande seminaire*.[45] Sheil was soon compelled to intervene.

Ironically, the issue that engaged Sheil in the direction of the school had nothing to do with the school's philosophy. It concerned the school's financing. Financial questions constantly clouded the future of the Sheil empire. CYO controller Scotty Haston, long accustomed to the erratic flow of money into the organization, frantically tried to decide which monthly bills he could let go and which he had to pay.[46] Drury's troubles began when one important source of funding, the Community Chest, began to ask some hard questions about the Sheil School, taking special exception to the highly Catholic nature of its program.[47] When this was brought to Sheil's attention, Drury's unwillingness to alter the "Basic Course" moved from being a minor irritant to a major threat to an already shaky financial picture. Moreover, Sheil was bored with the Education Department and this boded ill for Drury and his program.

Drury, for his part, had become increasingly disillusioned with Sheil, who seemed less the inspiring and popular bishop he had known as a seminarian, and more a shallow and insincere huckster of the ideas of others. The relationship between Drury and Sheil moved into open hostility when Drury

announced his intention in early 1946 to join a labor union, a course long advocated by Sheil for others but, ironically, not for his own employees. Sheil rightly feared that a strong union would reveal the pay inequities existing among workers in different categories and would publicly humiliate him. Moreover, Sheil would tolerate no rival to his authority over the CYO. When he heard of the incipient labor organizing going on in his own house, Sheil called Drury into his office and began dressing down the director with a series of "Listen guy" scoldings delivered through clenched teeth. Unshaken, Drury declared his intention to join the United Office and Professional Workers of America, to which Sheil retorted: "No Goldie Shapiro [the head of the Union] is going to tell me what to do."[48] Later, when CYO attorney William O. Burns heard of Drury's plans, he too called the philosopher aside and warned him to "watch it." Disregarding Burns's ominous words, Drury joined the union and sealed his doom. But, as Sheil feared, Drury's decision had its effect. Before long a movement for unionization of the sixty or more full-time workers at the CYO was underway, spearheaded by Nina Polcyn and Margaret Blaser, librarians at St. Benet's Library. After all, they reasoned in a circular to their fellow workers (in May 1946, the fifty-fifth anniversary of *Rerum Novarum* and the fifteenth anniversary of *Quadragesimo Anno*), "CYO is the first Catholic agency in Chicago to respond to the insistent and repeated call of the Church to organize.... The unquestioned leadership of our own Bishop Sheil in the field of labor gives added impetus to this drive to organize the CYO."[49]

The labor union decision was the only one of a bill of particulars that had already begun to be drawn up against Drury. Already in late 1945 a Policy Committee chaired by Attorney Burns was formed to suggest changes in the CYO. When the special problems in the Education Department were cited, Sheil appointed another committee composed of two Drury critics, Robert Burns (no relation to William), former member of the PR Department who was head of the South Bend chapter of the National Association of Christians and Jews, and Mary Elizabeth Carroll, professor of English at Barat College, and headed by Father Daniel Cantwell, professor of sociology at St. Mary of the Lake Seminary.[50] Cantwell was not directly connected with the inner workings of the Sheil School's administration but had

actively participated in the Labor School offering among Sheil School programs, via the Catholic Labor Alliance of which he was chaplain. Already a respected figure in the community, Cantwell probably had come to Sheil's attention on hearing him give the keynote address at an awards banquet at the Sheil School in March 1946.

The work of the committee was divided three ways: Carroll was to examine the problems of the school; Burns was to offer suggestions for its improvements; and Cantwell was to uphold the positive areas of the program. What Cantwell did not know was that prior to the deliberations of the committee Sheil had already decided to dismiss Drury. Cantwell recognized the antipathy for Drury on the part of the other two committee members; he nonetheless worked tenaciously at a report only mildly critical of some of the current operations, believing that great things could happen in the future. The report was delivered to Sheil in June 1946. Cantwell focused on the difficulties at the school in a letter to Sheil: "The staff of the School and the committee are certainly in agreement about the work to be done by the Church in contemporary society. What disagreement exists concerns the selection of means to that goal. In judgments concerning the selection of means no one should attempt to be apodictic." Cantwell further suggested "discussions between the staff and the committee," which in his estimation "would be the best way to resolve these disagreements."[51]

Despite Cantwell's recommendations, the report offered Sheil a pretext for firing Drury, and this is exactly what he did in July 1946. Indeed, after this decision was announced to a shocked Cantwell, Executive Director Charles Carroll Smith admitted:

> The decision to re-organize the Sheil School was made prior to Bishop Sheil's trip to Europe in December 1945. It was abundantly clear, even then, that George Drury did not fit into that re-organization. The desire for a re-organization grew out of dissatisfaction with the over-all operation of the school; a dissatisfaction with which George Drury was and is, thoroughly familiar.[52]

Cantwell, who had known Drury since grade-school days at St. Mel's, was heartsick and enraged by the decision. In a desperate attempt to save Drury, Cantwell sent a salvo of telegrams

to a number of priests, sisters, and distinguished participants in the Sheil School programs, eliciting letters of support for Drury. The telegrams were of no avail because Drury was already gone.[53] Sheil refused to return Cantwell's telephone calls, prompting the priest to write one of the strongest letters extant in his papers.

> Why should I have spent several days of nervous anxiety over George Drury's dismissal? Why should I have bothered and worried about it? Why should I not have let it pass as an internal matter within the Sheil School ... simply because I knew that its worst effect would be to injure a man whom I regarded filially and loving—namely yourself. I believe that a great injustice has been done to George Drury. But I believe that a much graver injustice has been done to you, to your great name, to the inner respect that simple people have in their hearts for you....just a few days after I had begun the committee work, I became aware that the committee was biased against George Drury and that at best I could only temper its report and that at worst I was simply being used.[54]

As with the phone calls, Sheil did not bother to respond to Cantwell's letter. The decision to fire George Drury was Sheil's. He ungraciously allowed Smith, Carroll, and Burns to take the rebukes for his own petulant act.

Even before Drury was gone, Sheil had prevailed on Father Edward Cardinal, C.S.V., former president of St. Viator's College, to head the school. Mary Elizabeth Carroll was hired as Cardinal's day-to-day operations chief. The school did continue to prosper and attracted many people to the well-known Sheil School Forums on Friday nights. By 1948 Drury's "Basic Course" disappeared from the curriculum and the Sheil School became a think tank for Sheil and a highly popular forum for lectures by prominent figures, as well as a hodgepodge of popular courses in language, art, and politics. Drury's vision of a school that would produce lay apostles educated in the first principles of democracy would shift to the rapidly growing Specialized Catholic Action groups around the diocese. Sheil's treatment of Drury and his humiliation of Cantwell account, in large part, for the mistrust and even disdain many Jocists felt for Sheil and his

operations. Father Cardinal eventually drifted away from the work when he was made pastor of St. Viator's parish, and Mary Elizabeth Carroll found herself left out after another of Sheil's periodic shake-ups of the Sheil School organization.

Ironically, the group that had engineered the overthrow of Shannon and Drury found themselves on the outs by the end of the decade, when Irene Lundgren Wiltgen rose to prominence in Sheil's firmament. Irene Lundgren was married to a young serviceman named Wiltgen who perished in the war. Mrs. Wiltgen had first known Sheil through the work of another Sheil enterprise in the forties: a campus center for Catholics at Northwestern University known as Sheil House. The prime driving force behind the Catholic presence at Northwestern had been Father Cornelius McGillicuddy. Sheil had taken an interest in the work of the campus priest and, even when he was transferred to a parish outside of Evanston, Sheil cajoled Stritch into allowing him to continue his work.[55] Eventually Sheil got a wealthy Jewish stockbroker, Barnet Rosset, to contribute $50,000 for the purchase of a three-story house on Sheridan Road which became a Catholic center in 1940.[56] While still in mourning, Wiltgen went to work for Sheil and soon became his personal secretary, effectively shielding the increasingly beleaguered, busy bishop from anyone she did not want him to see.

Wiltgen apparently convinced Sheil in late 1948 that he needed new blood in all the departments of the CYO. Accordingly he dispatched artist Jerry Keefe to New York to hire all new people for the main departments of the organization. The arrival of the "Wise Men from the East," as the displaced CYO department heads called them, was supposed to bring a new era to the CYO, but Sheil's heart was no longer in it.[57]

Nina Polcyn, one of the few survivors of the periodic staff shake-ups, reported occasionally to Drury about the inner politics of the school. On a trip to France she wrote to Drury: "I called Cogley before taking the plane on Wednesday to find that Beth Carroll is meeting the same fate as you. Her successor, one Gargan-guy from Boston College is en route to Chicago. She has not heard the news! All this on the eve of your anniversary. How ironic."[58] The "Gargan-guy" Polcyn referred to was historian Edward Gargan, who directed the program from 1952 to 1953—

one of the last full-time directors of the Sheil School. Gargan lasted only one year in Bishop Sheil's employ, resigning as soon as he could find full-time academic work.[59] The Sheil School closed in 1954 and was succeeded by the Centers for Adult Education, which were advanced by Daniel Cantwell and directed by Russell Barta.

FINANCES: THE BÊTE NOIRE

The beginning of the end for Sheil came in 1948 when his competent and long-suffering controller, Scotty Haston, resigned. Haston, a longtime associate of Sheil from the thirties, had kept the financial picture of the CYO together "with Scotch tape and staples," according to one worker.[60] Finances were the bête noire of Sheil's career and the cause of his deteriorating relationship with his Ordinary and his fellow priests in Chicago. Even those who admired him often shook their heads in sorrow when they discussed his financial affairs. From the onset of his career Sheil's two greatest problems were a lack of consistent attention to assigned duties and a tendency to be unconcerned with fiscal matters. His obvious lack of talent to manage money and his impulsive decisions to create programs and hire people was an unstable combination. If a petitioner convinced Sheil that something "ought" to be done, Sheil would jump in with both feet and somehow secure the money for the enterprise. After his fall in 1954, a former staffer recollected, "He was the single indispensable man in this operation." Another manager said, "It wasn't our privilege to think about finances; that was the bishop's job. Why, he used to explode like a firecracker if I'd even suggest we couldn't afford something. He used to say to me, I'll decide whether we can afford something. You just tell me if it ought to be done."[61]

Sheil's difficulties with money were rooted in his earliest days with the CYO. Mundelein probably recognized that. One suggestion has been that the reason Sheil was appointed to St. Andrew's was to relieve a financial crisis in the CYO. As early as 1935 the CYO had run up debts in excess of $50,000. Monsignor Griffin, former pastor of St. Andrew's, had accumulated that

exact amount in parish accounts and Catholic Bishop of Chicago bonds during his years of stewardship. Sheil's successor at St. Andrew's has suggested Mundelein installed his senior auxiliary in the parish so that Sheil could help himself to this tidy sum—a minor fortune in depression days—and end the CYO's fiscal crisis.[62] If this were true, Mundelein probably intended the transaction to be only a short-term loan that the CYO would repay with interest. But either Sheil found it too difficult to keep the accounts of the CYO and St. Andrew's separate, or he simply considered the parish an extension of the CYO. At any rate, the intermingling of parochial and CYO funds continued and would create a bookkeeping nightmare for his successors in the CYO and in the parish. Perhaps this misuse of money created some sparks between Sheil and Mundelein before the latter's death. Some unpleasant rumors also arose during the interregnum that he used archdiocesan funds at his disposal as administrator of Chicago to pay off his CYO debts.[63]

Stritch was even less inclined to cater to Sheil, because he was far more fiscally conservative than his predecessor and was saddled with Mundelein's considerable debt. Even if Sheil had been a model of fiscal responsibility, Stritch's conservative financial philosophy alone would have depleted Sheil's access to archdiocesan funds. Stritch shut off the archdiocesan spigot (although he did pay for the milk for the Holy Spirit Vacation schoolchildren and did fund Sheil's programs for the Japanese and Puerto Ricans) and, as we have seen, refused to allow Sheil to assess parishes for blocks of tickets to CYO events. Instead he allowed the bishop to send out a voluntary appeal for funds to the pastors. Many of them, glad to be free of Sheil's "extortion," simply threw the requests in the wastebasket and blasted hapless CYO workers who phoned seeking donations. This undoubtedly netted him less than the enforced ticket sales and a goodly number of the tickets ended up in garbage cans. Losing the parish revenue was a blow, but Sheil was able to tap public sources of support, such as National Youth Administration funds as well as the Chicago Community Chest for his broad-based programs of social welfare. But even these steady transfusions were unable to overcome the shortfalls in revenue that became worse each year.

To make up for the deficit, Sheil was forced to turn to other resources and become a full-time fund-raiser. A favorite fund-raising scheme was the sponsoring of dinners at which prominent Catholic entertainers were featured. Every May, Sheil's friends would host a party at the Palmer House or some other expensive hotel to commemorate the bishop's anniversaries of episcopal consecration or priestly ordination. An annual corned beef and cabbage dinner, hosted by Arch Ward of the *Chicago Tribune* and the sportswriters, brought in a handsome sum. Among the more elaborate fund-raisers was a barbecue dinner hosted by the Knights of Columbus at the Chicago Stadium. Frank Sinatra, Jimmy Durante, and singer Lena Horne were among the leading supporters of this event. Sheil's relationship with entertainers like Sinatra involved occasional personal counseling and friendly advice for the often hot-tempered singer.[64] Durante was introduced to the bishop by mutual friend Judge Abraham Lincoln Marovitz. One memorable evening Sheil gave the comedian a rosary that had belonged to his mother. Years later as Durante lay dying, Marovitz observed that he tightly clutched Sheil's rosary.[65]

With William Campbell's help, Sheil also tapped into the larger financial community of Chicago. Jack Keeshin, a transportation and trucking mogul, was especially generous to Sheil, as was the head of the Public Service Company of Northern Illinois, Britton I. Budd. The owner of Sportsman's Park, Charles Bidwell, contributed funds for a time. Later, Leo Lerner, the owner of a chain of neighborhood newspapers with extensive contacts in Chicago's Jewish community, became a close friend of the bishop and opened for him the doors to Jewish wealth in the city. Sheil's outspoken attacks on anti-Semitism had endeared him to the Jewish populace of Chicago. In one of his few projects as pastor of St. Andrew's, Sheil assembled an interdenominational group of clergy into what was called the Lake View Citizens Council, out of which grew an annual Thanksgiving service and an Interfaith Brotherhood Dinner, which often coincided with Sheil's February 18 birthday. Lerner's community papers promoted the bishop and his projects with gusto and fervor.

On the Catholic side, Sheil's leading benefactors were Frank J. Lewis and his wife. Lewis supported Sheil in the formation of

the Lockport, Illinois, aeronautical school which bore Lewis's name. It was eventually transformed into a liberal arts college and university by the Christian Brothers who assumed its management. One of Sheil's more grandiose schemes that was assisted with Lewis money was the establishment of an FM radio station in 1949. Always receptive to new ideas, Sheil had first been introduced to the potential of FM broadcasting in 1942 or 1943 by E. F. McDonald, Jr., president of the up-and-coming Zenith Radio Corporation. Sheil had grown so enthused at the possibilities of Catholic broadcasting, especially through his own speeches and radio talks, that he had sent a lengthy memorandum to Stritch urging a Catholic radio station. But wartime restrictions and other difficulties forestalled Sheil's plans. By early 1949, with a sizable grant from the ever-generous Lewis, he bought equipment and secured a broadcast license for station WFJL and put the whole operation under the leadership of artist Jerry Keefe.

WFJL, its transmitting tower perched atop the Lincoln Towers downtown, began broadcasting May 22, 1949. Besides a staff of thirty-one, it had an accredited overseas correspondent in Brussels and broadcast a combination of religious programming, music, and news commentary provided by Dr. Karol Ripa, former consul general from Poland and postwar refugee from the Communist regime. Sheil's station was an independent operation that sent reporters to Korea to interview GIs and broadcast a wide array of speeches by prominent public officials. Although the broadcast day was only fifteen and a half hours, Sheil accepted no advertising and the expenses began to mount precipitously. Moreover, FM programming receivers were still in their infancy. Few "average" Catholics could afford an FM radio, and although it broadcast to 270,000 listeners, it was a tiny share of the large Chicago market. When PR chief Robert Burns offhandedly joked that the station could reach more people by opening the studio window and shouting, Sheil was not amused. As in all other Sheil operations, the bills mounted and the complaints poured in.[66]

Sheil's problems with money soured his relations with Stritch, who was clearly nervous with his spendthrift senior auxiliary. Only reluctantly he brought himself to challenge his

financial dealing. Sheil knew that Stritch would not really do much to rein him in and reacted with indifference when Stritch offered mild criticism about the establishment of WFJL: "I am not familiar with the plans for financing the radio station. You asked me at one time to assist in this financing, but at that time there was no definite decision given in this matter."[67]

Stritch was not completely intimidated by his auxiliary and, in matters that directly involved archdiocesan credit and permissions, did attempt to be more stringent but with little success. The occasion of a serious financial problem was a huge bill run up by the auxiliary for extensive repairs to St. Andrew's. Sheil added an upper floor to the rectory which included a sauna in the bathroom, a personal chapel, a huge formal banquet room with a marble fireplace and an elevator that went directly from the heated garage to his personal quarters. (The assistants of the parish were never permitted on the upper floor.) In his sun-filled, knotty-pine-paneled office, Sheil did most of his desk work, gazing at walls decorated with letters and photographs from numerous dignitaries and well-placed friends. In late 1948 it became evident that these improvements on the rectory, plus repairs on the school and gymnasium, cost far in excess of what the archdiocese had approved. Sheil did attempt to seek approval for more money from the archdiocese, but when he refused to give a specific figure, Stritch reacted cautiously, wanting to know just how much was needed. From his vacation in Florida, Stritch lectured Sheil:

> You certainly agree with me in my wanting to know your contractor's careful estimate of the cost of the balance of the work in question. I must arrange loans and without knowledge of the approximate cost of the balance of this work I cannot make any such arrangements. It is not a question of the usefulness of the provision for the parish but of the extent of the indebtedness of the Catholic Bishop of Chicago. There are many things I would like to do but cannot afford to do in the Archdiocese.[68]

Stritch did not approve the increase, but Sheil went ahead and contracted the work on the parish and told the contractor to bill the archdiocese. Eventually the unpaid contractor complained to Stritch, revealing that Sheil had authorized over $600,000

more than the sum for which he had permission. Stritch was furious and curtailed his Florida vacation to meet with his consultors to decide what to do in the matter. But Sheil again presented him with a *fait accompli* and the archdiocese had to hand over the money. When Sheil was forcibly retired from St. Andrew's in 1967, the parish was over $1.4 million in debt.[69] Moreover, the rectory and gymnasium (often used for CYO events) were the only buildings to receive much attention. The rest of the plant, even the rectory and the church building itself, was in a sorry state when Sheil's successor, Monsignor John S. Quinn, took over in 1967. Stritch was kind enough to allow his auxiliary free rein in building his empire and even more gracious in picking up the pieces when it all fell apart in 1954.

ISOLATION AND DECLINE

Sheil was isolated from his fellow bishops, whose company he generally scorned and whose organization he openly disdained (especially after the rejection of his youth organization plans). He once commented to Drury on the pleasure he took being photographed coming out of the White House when he was supposed to be at a bishop's meeting. He bragged to Drury: "I said nerts to them and their discussions and went over to the White House."[70]

One of his chief antagonists among the bishops was James Francis McIntyre, auxiliary to Cardinal Spellman and later archbishop of Los Angeles. Sheil's first clash with McIntyre occurred in October 1945, when the New York-based Committee of Catholics for Human Rights bestowed an honorary award on Sheil. McIntyre heard of this and wrote disapprovingly to Sheil about the organization, adding: "My comment is to ask if you are acquainted with Emanuel Chapman, the inspiration behind this movement and the character of the movement. It tends very much to anti-clericalism."[71] Sheil dismissed McIntyre's concern and attended the dinner: "I am astonished, to put it mildly, to hear that the Committee of Catholics for Human Rights tends to anti-clericalism. My astonishment only increases in re-reading the list of honorary board

members, including Archbishop Lucey, Hon. Frank Murphy, Philip Murray and George Meany."[72] Trouble erupted again with McIntyre when Sheil received an invitation to another affair in New York, this time a dinner sponsored by the National Religion and Labor Foundation. What irked the New York auxiliary was that the honoree for the event was none other than Bishop Francis J. McConnell, a local Methodist Episcopal leader known as "America's Red Bishop" because of his strong support for organized labor. This time McIntyre decided not to confront Sheil directly and complained instead to Stritch: "May I venture to say that the appearance of Bishop Sheil on this program would be seriously injurious to the cause of the Church in the country, and it would be difficult for us to explain the many inquiries that will certainly arise from the recognition of Bishop McConnell by a Catholic bishop."[73] Stritch responded sympathetically and promised to restrain Sheil. But Sheil went anyway.

Stymied again, Bishop McIntyre tried a third time to trip up Sheil. This time the issue was the making of Jesse L. Lasky's movie *The Miracle of the Bells*. McIntyre went ballistic when he learned that the role of a priest was to be played by Frank Sinatra, then a teen idol. He was even more incensed when he learned that Sinatra, a regular contributor to the CYO, had intended to donate the proceeds of the film role to the organization. McIntyre dashed off a hand-written letter to Stritch: "Sinatra" he wrote, "has been promoted professionally as the idol of the 'bobby-socks' youngsters and in a way that would seem to disqualify him for the proposed role."[74] In his letter to Stritch, McIntyre enclosed a copy of a letter from an official of the Motion Picture Association referring to a telegram Sheil had sent to the producer of the movie congratulating him on the selection of Sinatra.[75] Stritch wrote to his auxiliary a few days later recounting McIntyre's complaints, closing with words that must have been on his lips many times: "We must get together so as not to have any unfortunate conflict or seeming division in this matter.... I know you understand how much I want to avoid any difficulties in this matter."[76] In this, as in so many other instances, Sheil did not respond to Stritch.

McIntyre was certainly more intransigent and socially conservative than most bishops of the time, but these conflicts simply illustrated Sheil's poor reputation with his brother bishops.
The effects of this reckless jousting with Cardinal Spellman's
chief aide probably closed the doors to higher appointments in
the Church. Antagonizing Spellman in those days was like teas-
ing a cobra: you knew it would strike back. Spellman's influence
with the Holy See neutralized any possible good impression
Sheil or his work would have had with Roman officials. His go-
it-alone approach, coupled with his aggressive social commentary and the rumors of his notorious financial profligacy made
many shun him as a kind of rogue elephant.

By 1953 he knew he was through. Recurrent bouts with res-
piratory ailments plagued him throughout the fifties. He
seemed susceptible to colds and the flu, and in 1951 he was
stricken with such a severe case of pneumonia that his life
seemed in danger.[77] Sheil regularly slipped away from his office
affairs for vacations to the Caribbean or to the mountains, sending Stritch hurried notes as he left the city. Sheil's deteriorating
health and his isolation may well have been aggravated by his
being bypassed for episcopal promotion. Rome's inattention to
him had become obvious as early as 1946, when Sheil failed to
receive a promotion to a diocese of his own in the first rash of
appointments that came from the Holy See after World War II.
Even though his friend Agnes Meyer of the *Washington Post*
supposedly angled for his appointment to Washington and
Newsweek magazine announced in July 1946, "authoritatively,"
that Sheil had been summoned to Rome so that the pope could
"proclaim the Chicago prelate the new Archbishop of St. Louis,"
it never happened.[78]

Perhaps the most vexatious issue in the Stritch-Sheil relationship was the auxiliary's tendency to speak as the official
voice of the archdiocese of Chicago—a prerogative jealously
guarded by Stritch. Sheil's high public profile often gave his
words a weight that other auxiliary bishops did not enjoy, as one
disgruntled packinghouse owner, whom Sheil had publicly
attacked, complained: "Considering the fact that many people
are prone to think a man as high in the Church as Bishop Sheil

speaks ex cathedra, his quotations are given weight wholly undeserved by his knowledge on the subject."[79] Stritch was basically powerless to stop Sheil, but from time to time he did try to take action. When Bishop William O'Connor of Springfield informed Stritch that University of Chicago sociologist Frank Flynn, speaking on behalf of Sheil, had lobbied for a welfare bill before the Illinois legislature and had taken a position opposite that of the Illinois Catholic Conference, Stritch tried again to harness his auxiliary. He wrote O'Connor:

> I am definitely writing to Bishop Sheil and telling him that leg-islative matters, as far as people in this diocese are concerned must be cleared with me and that when they are cleared with me I shall refer them, according to our custom, to our organization. It is bad for us to have the confusion which obtains, and I shall do my utmost to remove it.[80]

As with previous complaints, Sheil made no reply to Stritch. But already in 1953, Sheil was running out of steam. Before his exit from public life, Sheil stirred up one last controversy, this time over the issue of anticommunism—an issue that would also be related to his swift departure from public life.

Sheil had long been preoccupied with communism and railed against it in speeches to labor unions and others. His approach to combating communism, however, avoided the red-baiting that was becoming increasingly popular among American Catholics, especially after the war. Sheil expressed his own approach in a letter to Bishop John Noll of Fort Wayne. Noll, a strong anti-Communist, had expressed concern about Sheil's support for certain labor unions in Gary that were sus-pected of communist influence. Sheil replied:

> I am somewhat perturbed over what I can only consider your over-emphasis of the Communist danger. Undoubtedly, Communism is a danger; I am well aware of that. Undoubtedly it is a potent threat to everything we of the Catholic Church hold dear. Yet, I believe that your great concern over this danger and threat is out of all proportion to the strength and influence of Communism.... I have always believed that Communism is no danger in a society where justice and charity prevail.

> Communism, I believe, is no threat in a decent and human economic structure.

Sheil drove his point home,

> It seems to me, then, that we Americans, and especially we American Catholics, should work indefatigably to bring about a Christian economy in accordance with the magnificent teachings of our Popes. If we do this, we shall strike the greatest possible single blow to Communism.... We Catholics possess the most far-reaching and radical (in the best sense of the word) plan for social reconstruction; we *must*, we are bound to put it into effect.[81]

Sheil publicly challenged assaults on his loyalty. When radio commentator Upton Close accused Sheil of being one of the "liberals whose logic lays down the red carpet in the United States for smirking Communists to stride to power upon," Sheil blasted Close in a radio broadcast, defying him to prove his statement. In a 1947 speech before the national convention of American Veterans in Milwaukee, Sheil decried the "regrettable tendency to find communistic influence in almost every proposal for legitimate social and economic improvement....even now if anyone points to the evils of modern industrial society, the smear brigade goes into immediate action."[82]

Sheil's sentiments on the Communist threat seemed to change a bit when the Cold War shifted into high gear during the Korean War. In a speech in September 1950 before the Polish American Journalists Guild, Sheil maintained that "Poland was turned over to Stalin at Yalta and Teheran through the influence of leftist liberals." Moreover, "the shocking effect of 'liberal influence' upon the State Department had been revealed only within the past year. It was the liberal influence which placed Alger Hiss in vital and strategic foreign office work at Dumbarton Oaks, Yalta, and in the Far Eastern Division of the State Department."[83]

But this flirtation with red-baiting never included the unqualified support of the leading American Catholic politician of the time, Joseph McCarthy. McCarthy's wild accusations reawakened the old social reformer in Sheil, and the fact that McCarthy was supported by Sheil's old nemesis, Cardinal

Spellman, did not help either. McCarthy, a Republican, had boldly marched into Democratic Chicago on St. Patrick's Day, 1954, to speak before an Irish-American gathering at the Palmer House. Although a number of important Irish-Catholic civic leaders were present, neither Stritch nor Sheil came. McCarthy was warmly received by the partisan Irish, but his effect on the Catholic community was negligible. Less than a month later, Cardinal Spellman had signaled his support for McCarthy by appearing with him at a breakfast meeting of Irish-Catholic policemen in New York. Sheil grew incensed over "McCarty" and contacted *Commonweal* editor John Cogley to make up a speech to blast the junior senator. Sheil had already been the principal narrator of a film produced by the New York-based Freedom House, an ecumenical organization designed to oppose totalitarianism wherever it reared its head. In the film he had decried the McCarthy tactics as totalitarianism in disguise.[84]

Even before the film was released Sheil made national headlines with an attack on McCarthy. At the annual CIO convention in Chicago's Opera House, a crowd to which Sheil had spoken on numerous occasions heard him open fire on McCarthy using Cogley's words:

> Are we any safer ... because General [George] Marshall was branded a traitor? No we aren't. But we are a little less honorable.... Are we any safer because nonconformity has been practically identified with treason? I think not.... Are we any more to be feared by the Communists because of all the hundreds of headlines the Senator from Wisconsin has piled up? I don't believe so. This kind of ridiculous goings-on is seriously described as anti-Communism. If you will pardon a very lowbrow comment, I say 'Phooey!'[85]

The attack on McCarthy by the bishop won loud praise from some quarters, scorn from others. Sheil later went on to underscore his opposition to McCarthy by appearing on Edward R. Murrow's television show, repeating his criticisms of the senator.[86]

Anyone who knew Sheil's feelings about McCarthy and McCarthyism would not have been surprised at his assault on the already faltering junior senator from Wisconsin. However, because of its proximity to Sheil's resignation, many thought

there was a connection between the two events. Typical was a letter to Stritch from one angry Sheil-supporter from Missouri:

> I was very much disturbed about Bishop Sheil's resignation from the CYO. Many of my non-Catholic friends gave him 'a month' when he spoke his mind about Senator McCarthy. I can't but help believe myself that his 'stand' hurt him with many of our high-ranking clergy.... Cardinal, I'm not asking you to think my way.... But please let's not take the stand that just because a Senator is Catholic he can do no wrong.... Forget McCarthy is Catholic and consider the things he stands for ... and then decide.[87]

Other letter writers and commentators drew the same conclusion: Sheil was punished for his bold denunciation of McCarthy. Indeed, this has been repeated as recently as 1989 in Sanford Horwitt's book, *Let Them Call Me Rebel*.[88]

The truth is less dramatic. Anyone who knew Stritch knew that the cardinal was a life-long democrat and deplored McCarthy and McCarthyism. Although the proximity of the events (denunciation-resignation) may lead some to make a connection, the real cause of Sheil's abrupt resignation was the collapse of his finances. The final straw was Sheil's suspicion that the chancery was beginning to dip into his reserved list of contributors by making overtures to long-time CYO contributor Fred Morelli, president of the Century Music Company, a purveyor of jukeboxes and owner of the Blackstone Hotel. However Sheil's growing isolation caused him to lose touch with reality. The truth of the matter was just the opposite. The archdiocese did not wish close ties with Morelli and indeed Stritch had such serious doubts about Morelli's character that he blocked Morelli's nomination for papal honors in the early fifties. Nonetheless, Sheil believed Stritch was now poaching on his fund-raising preserve. Isolated and perhaps prone to paranoia, Sheil figured the game was over. For this reason the famous press conference announcing his resignation was called.[89] The mountainous debt Sheil and the CYO had accumulated, which by one wild rumor stood at nearly fifteen million dollars, finally compelled Sheil to accept "charity" from the very people he had attempted to bypass for over fourteen years.

DISMANTLING THE EMPIRE AND EXILE

Sheil retired to his palatial suite at St. Andrew's and watched from the sidelines as Monsignor Edward Kelly of the Mission of Our Lady of Mercy set about the task of deciphering the total indebtedness of the CYO as well as proposing plans for its reorganization. Kelly set to work, immediately requesting reports and financial records from each of the six departments of the organization. Two weeks after Sheil's resignation, Kelly made a preliminary report to Stritch, cataloging all the programs of the Sheil empire and their financial status. "The total debt, insofar as I know is approximately $429,000." Kelly concluded, "The Mission of Our Lady of Mercy is part of the CYO Corporation and I believe that we have at the Chancery Office enough to cover these debts in Catholic Bishop of Chicago notes. I should be very happy with your permission to give these to the organization to straighten out the financial difficulties."[90] But taking care of the debt was only half of Kelly's problem. By his calculation the CYO, as it was then constituted, would need $600,000 per year to maintain operations. Moreover, Kelly was critical of the whole "liberal philosophy" of the CYO program, which, he felt, did not sufficiently emphasize religious motives but seemed more dedicated "on character training than on promoting a religious philosophy of life."[91]

Pressed by the financial needs of the organization and the desire to make it more self-consciously religious, Kelly proposed outright elimination of programs such as the Sheil School, Sheil Institute, the CYO Band, WFJL, and the Arlington Polo Farm. He further suggested that some programs be absorbed by existing archdiocesan agencies. For example, Catholic Charities would take over the Sheil Guidance Service and the Sheil Reading Service, Sheil House, the West Side Community Center, and the Puerto Rican Program. The Confraternity of Christian Doctrine would undertake the Vacation Schools, and the Lewis School of Aeronautics would be transferred to the Diocese of Joliet. What remained was the original athletic program. That, Kelly suggested, ought to be operated in a decentralized fashion "to secure greater participation." With Stritch's blessing Kelly impaneled a new board of directors for the CYO and spent the

next year effecting the reforms proposed in his report of September 1954. In general, the reorganization was a success. St. Benet's Bookstore, one of the most popular hangouts for Catholic liberals, was transferred to the ownership of long-time Sheil worker Nina Polcyn. The Sheil School was reorganized as the center of Adult Education, overseen by Monsignor Daniel Cantwell and executive director, Russell Barta. Even before the dust had settled on Kelly's reorganization, George Higgins wrote Cantwell: "The dissolution of the CYO empire may turn out to be a blessing in disguise if it results in bigger and better programs under the auspices of the CLA [Catholic Labor Alliance.]"[92]

For the remainder of Stritch's tenure Sheil had little to do with diocesan affairs, even omitting the administration of Confirmation. When Albert Meyer succeeded Stritch in 1958, he made gestures of friendship and respect to the aging prelate, but no efforts were made to bring him into the loop of archdiocesan life. In 1959 Sheil received a small consolation prize when he was created a titular archbishop. He also wangled himself a spot on the pre-conciliar commission to draft a decree on communications; but he rarely attended meetings, nor did he go to any of the sessions of the Council, pleading illness. Meyer generally humored Sheil and offered no opposition to his honorary titles. He did restrain the hand of the bishop when Sheil sought to tap wealthy concessionaire Andy Frain for a fund-raising project at the same time Frain had committed himself to raise funds for the college seminary. Meyer also insisted that Polish refugee and Sheil associate Dr. Karol Ripa cease using the name and prestige of the archbishop of Chicago on the letterheads of his news release service. But Meyer was far too busy to do what his successor, Archbishop John P. Cody, did: compel Sheil's retirement. By his death in 1968 Sheil was a sad, pathetic figure. He lived in exile in Tucson, Arizona, with his secretary, Irene Wiltgen, thoroughly embittered with the diocese and the Church he had so faithfully served.

Mary Elizabeth Carroll's biting article in *Harper's* in 1955 had called Sheil a prophet without honor.[93] With an honesty and candor unusual in treating ecclesiastical subjects of those times, she took the Church to task for not recognizing Sheil's accom-

plishments. But she was equally hard on Sheil for his fiscal irre-
sponsibility and flare for the dramatic. Carroll's insights rang
true for anyone who knew or worked with the bishop. Even
more perceptive were the insights of the man Sheil fired in 1946,
George Drury. Drury, who had observed Sheil from the time of
the 1926 Eucharistic Congress through the experience of the
Sheil School, was struck early on by the importance of Sheil's
athletic past.[94] Drury remarked on the similarity of Sheil's personality with those of athletes or actors. This, Drury insisted,
made for a certain restlessness, which allowed him to generate
so many programs and bring so many good ideas to practical
expression. It also meant he easily tired of people and projects.
He was capable of intensive engagement with people and projects, as are athletes who would give their all to a specific game
or team. But when the game ended and the teams changed, it
was time to move on to newer challenges. Drury's insights are
best taken with other features of Sheil's life. Sheil's limited
attention span, the weighty financial problems of his organization, his health problems, and his conflict with the redoubtable
Spellman brought him down with a crash.

Drury also accentuated Sheil's flair for the dramatic.
Edward Gargan described his first meeting with Sheil: "I sat
completely in the dark and the bishop sat on an elevated dais
with soft lights playing off him."[95] Sheil loved displays of power.
The smell of the crowd, the dramatic moment, at the Chicago
Coliseum with John L. Lewis at his side, or at the scene of an accident where he would throw his coat over a victim—these were
moments he savored. They were also the moments that made his
career and won him the adulation of people everywhere. When
he was "on," the resonant voice, the famous flashing smile, the
engaging personality that could even melt the heart of a hard-bit-
ten Saul Alinsky, all came into play. But a vast gap existed
between the public persona and the real Sheil. Between engagements, he was like an athlete between games, low and nonde-
script, almost a nobody. He was an engaging man, but he seemed
to lack the substance one would have expected for a person in his
position—tragically incapable of doing anything more than
hawking the thoughts and ideas of others as his own. This fatal
flaw made the last years of his life a tragedy.

Yet for all his failings, he attracted people of depth and quality to his various organizations and the programs he approved and erratically funded attempted to respond to critical human needs and drew unashamedly on Catholic ideology as the raison d'être for social amelioration. The infusion of holiness in the marketplace was the theme of Sheil at his best. Reynold Hillenbrand would move this message even more deeply to the core of the Chicago Catholic experience.

5

Hillenbrand and His Disciples

While Sheil's juggernaut rolled on, winning the attention of the news media and prominent politicians, the work of social reconstruction was taking place in other ways less flamboyant and more intense. Social reconstruction was on the agenda of every committed and thoughtful Catholic in the thirties, forties, and fifties. But, as Sheil's conflict with George Drury revealed, there were vast differences over how best to attain these goals. Drury's advocacy of intensive Christian formation clashed with Sheil's egocentric vision of himself as the single catalyst for social reform as well as with that of the CYO's fretful Public Relations Department, which feared Drury's overtly Catholic program "would not sell." When Sheil exiled Drury and humiliated Cantwell in 1946 he indirectly rejected the father of much of the intensive Christianization movement in Chicago, in the person of Monsignor Reynold Hillenbrand. This seems truly unfortunate, especially when one speculates about the possibilities of an alliance between the charismatic bishop and the dynamic seminary rector. Among the many parallel movements for social reform, Hillenbrand's efforts penetrated the minds of a Chicago Catholic elite far more deeply than Sheil's multifarious projects.

LITURGICAL ISSUES

Hillenbrand's work at the seminary had progressed relatively unimpeded during the Mundelein era. With Stritch, however,

he had to proceed more cautiously, especially in liturgical matters since the archbishop was highly conservative in that regard. Given this, it is significant that Stritch gave his blessing to the first meeting of the National Liturgical Conference, which met at Holy Name Cathedral in the fall of 1940. Hillenbrand took an active role in this gathering modeled on the Belgian Semaine Liturgique, which had been held since 1910 at the Abbey of Mont César. The conferences offered opportunities for priests and religious around the nation to share the latest research on liturgical studies. In the United States, Fathers Virgil Michel, O.S.B. and Gerard Ellard, S.J promoted "Liturgical Days," but it was not until two years after Michel's death that plans for a full week of liturgical study were made by Father Michael Ducey, a Benedictine of St. Anselm's Abbey in Washington, D.C., and head of the newly founded Benedictine Liturgical Conference.[1] From October 21 to 25, 1940, interested persons from around the nation gathered in the Cathedral basement to discuss "The Living Parish," a theme selected by Hillenbrand himself. Each day was marked by a special Mass that stressed communal participation.[2] Hillenbrand gave the keynote address, summarizing the history of the liturgical movement, and lamenting the fact that the liturgical week had not come to reality sooner.[3]

As a result of this meeting, plans were set in motion to organize the National Liturgical Conference and Hillenbrand served as an officer in the organization for many years. Hillenbrand also kept alive the interest stirred in liturgical matters by organizing a Summer School of Liturgy at Mundelein, Illinois, in July 1941. In 1943 a special three-day meeting (a concession to wartime restrictions) was held to discuss the newly issued encyclical *Mystici Corporis*.[4] An offshoot of the the 1946 Week in Denver was the formation of the American Vernacular Society by Hillenbrand and Morrison, a group dedicated to the promotion of an English liturgy. This group's small quarterly, *AMEN*, was begun in 1951 and continued until 1961, when Apostolic Delegate Egidio Vagnozzi insisted on its suppression.[5] Hillenbrand's other services to the liturgical movement, included organizing conferences, writing for *Orate Fratres* (later renamed *Worship*) and later using his parish in Hubbard Woods as a showplace of liturgical reform.

How much effect did Hillenbrand's ideas have on the liturgical life of an average parish in Chicago? It is difficult to answer this question, since most parish histories fail to account for any changes in liturgical practice until Vatican II and not all liturgical innovations were attributable to him. For example, the *Missa recitata* (dialogue Mass) was in use among the Servites of Our Lady of Sorrows Basilica on Jackson Boulevard. Father Hugh Calkins, O.S.M., encouraged subscribers to the popular *Novena Notes* to "Pray the Mass," and in 1940 a movie explaining the Mass was made at the popular basilica. Other groups of Chicago Catholics helped to disseminate Father Stedman's Sunday missal, a pocket-sized handbook which had all the chants and readings for the Sunday liturgy, along with brief explanations and pictures of various rituals of the Eucharistic sacrifice. Father Bernard Laukemper, pastor of St. Aloysius Parish on LeMoyne and Claremont, made his parish a showplace of liturgical reform. A native of Germany, Laukemper hosted a local liturgical week in 1936, replaced his ornate high altar with a simpler one, and introduced such "innovations" as an offertory procession and the dialogue Mass in his regular Sunday schedule.[6] As more and more priests came out of St. Mary of the Lake Seminary under Hillenbrand's liturgical influence, the tempo of reform increased. By 1939, Gerard Ellard reported in an article in the November issue of Orate Fratres, that sixty-five of the two hundred fifty city parishes in the city of Chicago had the dialogue Mass.[7] Moreover, institutions of higher education such as DePaul University and Rosary College reported regular use of the *Missa recitata*, as did seventeen of sixty-six Catholic high schools.

SPECIALIZED CATHOLIC ACTION

In tandem with the liturgical movement Hillenbrand strongly pushed the cause of Specialized Catholic Action. As with the liturgy, Stritch had misgivings about these movements as well, stemming from official concerns for any project that bore the name "Catholic Action." When he came to Chicago in 1940, Stritch intended to coordinate and centralize official Catholic Action as he had in Milwaukee by reinvigorating the

Holy Name Societies. Independent specialized Catholic Action groups were a cause of concern to him and supporting them was not high on his list of priorities.

Hillenbrand cautiously sought permission from Stritch for the activity of the Catholic Action cells, which were growing in popularity around Chicago. Already in September of 1940, Hillenbrand held a meeting for the priests associated with cell work in Chicago and formed an informal federation of Catholic Action cells, directed by a board of seven priests chaired by Father Martin Farrell of St. Malachy's parish. Chaplains were appointed to oversee high school girls, high school boys, normal-school girls, college boys, working men, working women, and professional men. Stritch gave some direction to these priests in the cell movement in a meeting with them on September 18, 1941, encouraging the movement but cautioning against competition with official Catholic Action, like the Holy Name Society. Above all, he insisted that the work of the groups receive no publicity. "That would spoil it. It is a quiet work, even unknown to the general Catholic public."[8]

Hillenbrand did not allow Stritch's lukewarm endorsement to deter him and indeed seemed to go directly against the prelate's wishes by working harder to insist on clear distinctions between his Catholic Action cells and other Catholic Action and Catholic activities, especially the study group technique. Typical of this was a letter to one young apostle:

> Let me make it clear to you that the Catholic Action cell technique is not to be used in any Sodality....the cell should not be part of the Sodality. These are two distinct organizations. The movement is a specialized one, which means that you must have the same kind of people in the cell so that they can remedy the defects in their particular environment.[9]

Hillenbrand left no doubt in anyone's mind which brand of Catholic Action was superior (i.e., closer to what the popes had intended)—Specialized Catholic Action. Hillenbrand also began writing and distributing a newsletter for priest chaplains. In June 1941 one of the first Summer Schools of Specialized Catholic Action was held at Holy Name Cathedral. This study week was the first of many conducted by the individual federations and

provided structured opportunities for deepening the ideas and methodology of Jocism. Eventually the big-hearted Monsignor Morrison provided a central meeting place for the movements at an old school building owned by the Cathedral at 3 East Chicago. Jocist groups also began drawing up their own inquiry programs as part of their ongoing formation in Christianity. Timely topics, such as movies, gossip, dating, and theological topics, such as the Mystical Body and the liturgical movement, were covered in these inquiries. The end product was always some action. Even though the war took away many of the members of the male cells, Hillenbrand and the federation priests continued to meet to define and structure the cell movements.

In 1944 the general Catholic Action cells were further broken down into more specialized groups of students and workers. young women's groups even began to publish a small periodical called *Impact*, which reported cell activity and efforts to reconstruct the social order on the part of young apostles. Once the war was over, two young women, Mary Irene Caplice and Edwina Hearn, visited Europe to observe the movements in their native environment. They came home aware of the fact that the American environment would have a distinct impact on the nature of the groups here. After their return the name "Jocism" became more regularly used among the cell groups. In 1947, after Hillenbrand attended an international meeting of the Young Christian Workers in Montreal, the breakdown of the cell groups into Young Christian Students and Young Christian Workers was made.

Stritch's attitude toward the Catholic Action movements continued to be ambivalent throughout his years in Chicago, but he was more kindly disposed to them than he was to liturgical reformers. Indeed, even after he had dismissed Hillenbrand from the seminary, he wrote some encouraging words to the Jocists at a luncheon meeting for priests at the Stevens Hotel in April 1945. Although he did not personally attend, Stritch sent a letter that was read to nearly a hundred gathered priests which said:

> In Catholic Action there is a distinct place for quiet constant work of small groups of devoted Catholics. This is not a secret work or a wholly hidden work. It is a quiet, unobtrusive work. Little

bands form and work on the basis of a well-thought-out program. They undertake no large public programs and confine themselves to effective quiet activity. Living deeply in the Life of the Church, these workers seek to lodge Christian principles in the individual and social life of those with whom they come in contact.... I have followed the work of the Catholic Action Cells and I approve it wholly and hope from it, ever increasing good. It is my wish that it continue and expand and that the Directors under your guidance meet often to study programs of action and exchange experiences.[10]

Stritch also used an opportunity to support the cell work when he was dragged into a dispute over the participation of faculty members from Quigley Seminary. The rector of Quigley, John M. Schmid, had reiterated strict rules in 1945 that priest instructors were to have no outside activities. Since the professors did not live under Schmid's watchful eye (Quigley priest faculty lived in parishes, not in a common seminary residence), they ignored the rector's ruling and actively participated in novenas, open forum work, and even teaching in other schools. Early in the 1946-1947 school year, Schmid decided to crack down and reprimanded two priests, James Voss and Charles (Jules) Marhoefer, who had been active with Cana work and Catholic Action Cells. Voss and Marhoefer promptly complained to Cardinal Stritch, who wrote Schmid:

> They tell me that they will be able to take care of all their needs at Quigley and keep up their interest in the Cell work by devoting to it a single evening period each week. In this it seems to me that with this understanding we cannot really interpret the interest in this work as being an outside activity in any way conflicting with their duties at Quigley. It simply means they will do all their work at Quigley and in their spare time interest themselves in this other work.[11]

Schmid wrote back to Stritch painting a dire picture of how the work of Voss and Marhoefer required "numerous telephone calls" which "have frequently embarrassed us in the official business of the Seminary and have caused the pastor of one of these young men to complain bitterly that the same confusion exists in the parish house." Schmid also complained, "They

started with one group and added others as they progressed in this work.... most of their evenings every week were spent in this work."[12] Stritch replied to Schmid with an understanding letter and promised to "call these young men and have a very definite understanding with them. They will be told that the regulation stands and that they must limit their activities in Catholic Action Cell work...." But Stritch indicated, "There is a difficulty of course in that we don't want to forbid reasonable legitimate leisure time activities. I see the good that is to be done in proper [sic] directed Catholic Action Cell work. In fact I am quite in favor of this work."[13] Stritch did write to Hillenbrand repeating some of the complaints of Schmid and restating the regulation prohibiting outside work by Quigley professors. He also called in Marhoefer and Voss and gave them a "talking to."[14]

STRITCH AND SEMINARY REFORM

While Hillenbrand was diligently tending these movements in the forties, his work at the seminary also kept him busy. Mundelein's insistence on five years of study at Quigley and six at St. Mary of the Lake had always been an awkward arrangement for the forces that wanted to see better organization of the courses. Interestingly, Stritch (and St. Francis Seminary Rector, Albert Meyer) had been part of an official visitation team to come to the Mundelein seminary in the late thirties and recommend some expansion of the collegiate years of the seminary program. Soon after Stritch's arrival as archbishop, Hillenbrand was permitted to add an another year of study to the curriculum, a year that would include additional course work in the liberal arts and education. Stritch initially seemed favorable to making a change that Hillenbrand had wanted for a long time—adding diocesan clergy to the major seminary staff.

It was Stritch's original intention to have most of these priests take advanced course work in education in order to prepare them to be school visitators.[15] Hillenbrand managed to expand their role and had them trained in economics, sociology, religion, and other fields of endeavor. The teachers for these new classes would be taken from the diocesan clergy; the rector selected a number of bright young priests to complete higher

studies at the Catholic University of America—a place off-limits during the Mundelein era. Hillenbrand was delighted with this decision and wrote to Dean Roy J. Deferrari: "I am very happy with the fact that at long last Chicago is sending priests to the Catholic University."[16]

This corps of men included some of Chicago's brightest priests and was known collectively as "Hilly's Men." They included George Higgins, William Rooney, William McManus, Martin Howard, John Kelly, Henry Wachowski, Aloysius Wycislo, and Daniel Cantwell. Other archdiocesan priests like James Killgallon, John Fahey, and William Boyd were recruited to substitute for the priests at school. But the effects of these policies, plus the introduction of loyal retainers to the seminary staff, exacerbated tensions with the Jesuit teachers of the seminary.

TENSIONS AND DISMISSAL

Tensions developed in 1942 when seminary students began to seek out the more popular diocesan priests for spiritual directors. The anger of the Jesuit faculty at this development prompted Stritch to command the seminarians to choose the Jesuits.[17] Hillenbrand's chief antagonist through these years was long-time faculty member, Father John Clifford, S.J., who became academic dean in the fall of 1941. Clifford was a moral theologian who became very close to Stritch and served as his unofficial theological advisor until the Jesuit's death in 1953. Hillenbrand also had critics among the diocesan clergy as well, in particular the two prefects of discipline for the philosophy and theology departments, Fathers Frederick Stenger (a contemporary of Hillenbrand's who had been a class prefect when they were classmates) and Daniel Culhane. Stenger and Culhane were constant critics of the rector, especially of his long absences from the seminary while on speaking tours.

In 1943 Culhane had written a complaining letter to Stritch at the end of the summer session requesting policies regarding lectures, movies, and entertainments, and asking "whether there ought to be *Missa Recitata* in the main chapel every day

and whether prime or compline should be substituted for morning or night prayer." Culhane also questioned the wisdom of allowing extracurricular activities, such as the seminarians' weekly liturgical bulletin.[18] Stritch, as we have seen, strongly disapproved of liturgical "innovations" at the seminary and hinted at his displeasure in a talk to the seminarians in the fall of 1943. This encouraged Stenger, who later wrote: "If it is not out of order, may I say that I was very much pleased with your Excellency's opening talk at the seminary this year. There seems to be a rather strong tendency to exaggerated views in certain phases *de re liturgica.*"[19]

Liturgical innovation was not something Stritch encouraged anywhere in his archdiocese, least of all in the seminary. It was one thing to host the National Liturgical Conference at his cathedral, it was another thing to have priests, especially young priests, do some of the things the liturgists advocated. Indeed. Stritch was genuinely wary of liturgists and at one point sought to dilute their impact on the national scene by diverting their activities to the control of the NCWC Department of Education.[20] When he heard of liturgical innovations going on in the archdiocese, he regularly took steps to stop them. One such incident involved the Ladies of the Grail, a women's movement at Doddridge Farm in Libertyville. At one of their summer schools, a Mass was held where liturgical activists introduced an offertory procession. Upon hearing of this, Stritch "forbade [the procession]...as being contrary to the Liturgy."[21] When the participants argued that the practice "went back to history," Stritch refused to alter his decision, stating, "I had simply to stand on the grounds of my authority.... Things which are local customs in monasteries and cloisters and approved or tolerated for these places may not be made general practice."[22] The Ladies of the Grail ultimately packed their bags and left the Chicago archdiocese.

But reports came to Stritch from pastors around the archdiocese that the Grail "innovations" were only the tip of the iceberg. Indeed, liturgical reform seemed to be spreading around the diocese like an infection, promoted by the newly ordained priests from St. Mary of the Lake Seminary. Hillenbrand's young levites, it was reported, would insist on such liturgical

novelties as the *Missa recitata* or an end to daily Requiem Mass in favor of the Mass of the day. When pastors protested they often invoked the name of the rector as justification for their "insubordination."

To make matters worse, Stritch and Hillenbrand were not personally compatible. Apparently Stritch had been nettled by something Hillenbrand had said at a National Social Action Conference in Milwaukee in 1938 and had told him so. In 1941 the two of them had a bitter exchange over the exclusion of representatives from the Illinois Manufacturers Association from the Catholic Conference on Industrial Problems meeting in Chicago in June that year. Edward Kerwin, a vice-president of the Brach Candy Company had written Stritch in early May, protesting that "only one representative of industry is on the program, and he is not even a Christian." Kerwin went on to single out a mimeographed labor bulletin that quoted Hillenbrand "in what amounted to a vigorous attack on business." He ended his letter:

> I have a boy in his first year at Quigley. Of his own choosing, thank God, he has decided to be a Priest and our prayers are that his vocation will be completed. But I look forward with some regret to the possibility of his coming out of Mundelein (built, I understand, largely through gifts from businessmen) with his mind warped on this point, as apparently are the minds of many of the newly-ordained young men in the last few years.[23]

Stritch wrote back to Kerwin, assuring him that "Business is a right function in the society body and businessmen have work to do for the welfare of the whole. To say or intimate that all businessmen are practicing injustice or even that business is not animated by high social ideals would be wrong."[24] Kerwin, along with Illinois Manufacturers' Association officials James L. Donnelly and Homer Buckley responded to Hillenbrand's bias by proposing a series of luncheons and discussions between industrial leaders and Church representatives to deal with such issues as labor-management relations and the relations of government and industry.

Stritch responded favorably: "I think the time has come when we must discuss very freely and frankly our whole

economic problem and recognize the great difficulties which presently beset private business."[25] When Stritch requested that Hillenbrand and his associates participate in the IMA-sponsored program, the rector sent Stritch a copy of a "very anti-labor" report issued by the association and informed the archbishop: "I think that the record and influence of the Association are definitely not for the good. They are inheritors of an evil tradition."[26] Stritch replied with a stinging letter to the rector, upbraiding him for so "confining the expounding of Catholic principles to one social group as to make the other group hopelessly damned enemies of all good. This is not the Catholic ideal." He blasted the rector:

> I think that your mental attitude towards this group will hinder your going among them trying to understand their problems and expounding to them Catholic principles.... So as not to embarrass you, I withdraw my request that you and some of the young priests associated with you attend as Catholic priests the meetings which will follow the luncheon.... I am not interested in any Catholic labor activities which contribute to the building up of a class society or assumes as hopeless the conversion of management and ownership in industry to Catholic principles.[27]

The aftermath of this incident was nowhere near as tense as Stritch's letter suggested. When Hillenbrand met with Stritch to smooth over the situation, he recalled eight years later to Daniel Cantwell:

> I went in to see him. He shrugged it off and said to forget it—as if it were just another letter. He didn't even enlarge on it or want to talk about it—and wasn't at all offended as I thought he was from the letter.[28]

But Stritch was not at all amused by the rector's social activism which bordered on political activity. Shortly after the IMA incident he complained in a letter to McNicholas about the strong social emphasis of Hillenbrand and others:

> I am very fearful at the tendency to over emphasize the social phase even of the virtues. It is alright but it must not be over-done....while of course we must keep in mind the social man we

must not forget individual sanctification. How easy it would be to slip into social welfare and even controversial policies.[29]

Hillenbrand continued his service to organized labor throughout the forties. Interestingly, despite his strong pro-labor stands, he served as a labor mediator in a couple of cases involving the Ornamental Plasterers Union. But it was his service in behalf of the organization of retail workers for the Montgomery Ward Company that brought him into his final conflict with Stritch.[30]

Hillenbrand's involvement in the Montgomery Ward strike is an example of the kind of actions Stritch feared. Hillenbrand had been instrumental in the organization of the United Retail, Wholesale and Department Store Employees of America—a CIO union—at Montgomery Ward in 1941. Ward's management had refused to deal with the union until compelled by an order of the War Labor Board and personal pressure from President Franklin Roosevelt. Then the company's president, Sewell Avery, entered into a one-year contract with the union, but bided his time and in 1944 refused to sign a new contract. This prompted the union to walk out (a practice foresworn during the wartime emergency) and forced Roosevelt to seize the company and administer it under the auspices of the Commerce Department. Widespread publicity attended the strike and the government takeover in April, 1944, including a now famous incident—immortalized in picture—of federal guardsmen carrying Sewell Avery out of the Ward's building.

Hillenbrand was outraged with Avery's high-handed tactics and decided to publicly show his support for the strike. In early May, on the eve of the National Labor Relations Board election, Hillenbrand issued this message to the company's workers, which was reprinted on the pages of the Catholic Labor Alliance's periodical, *Work*, and picked up by the local dailies:

> This is the time for the Ward workers to put the Union [Local No. 20] over, to prove that three years fight and the strike were not wasted. Everybody should VOTE—and vote for the union. A vote for the union means that the union is in Ward's to stay.[31]

Hillenbrand later shored up his message of support by marching with the picketing employees. The attendant publicity added to Hillenbrand's already shaky reputation among city business leaders and was more than Stritch could take. The archbishop loathed public controversies, especially those involving his priests. The Montgomery Ward's case had already caused him problems when he first came to Chicago because of some ineptitude by Father Bernard Burns and the Association of Catholic Trade Unionists [ACTU].[32] Now, Hillenbrand was immersing the Church in these matters again.

The Ward's situation was probably the straw that broke the camel's back. Sometime in late July, Stritch called the rector in and demanded his resignation. Hillenbrand dutifully accepted Stritch's decision and bade farewell to the students at Mundelein in a touching Mass on August 5, telling them: "Every day of my life there shall be a *memento* at Mass for you and succeeding seminarians. We may be separated, but at Mass we are all together doing the same thing—you in my Mass, I in yours."[33]

While Hillenbrand kept a dignified silence about the reasons for his dismissal, people around him reacted with shock. Father John Hayes wrote from Texas, where he was recovering from tuberculosis, "In time, perhaps a long time, we shall no doubt discover some supernatural advantages in this change. You see, I still have faith, if no good works. As for your position [Cantwell's], I feel fortunate by comparison, t.b. and all."[34] Many, like George Higgins, speculated as to the reasons for this abrupt dismissal:

> How much of a hand did Stenger and Culhane have in undermining Hilly at the Chancery? I have my own suspicions. Was Hilly's participation in the M.W. strike the straw that broke the camel's back? These are questions which Hilly's friends in Washington are asking.[35]

In reality the dismissal was probably an act of rashness on Stritch's part. Hillenbrand himself hinted at this later in a letter to Daniel Cantwell when he wrote: "These outbursts are to be expected, because he hears things from people and acts on them impulsively. We have to put up with it and understand it."[36]

Hillenbrand's next assignment was to the prosperous Sacred Heart parish in Hubbard Woods. To Hillenbrand's votaries, Stritch added insult to injury by appointing Quigley Seminary rector Malachy Foley to the major seminary post. A benign but thoroughly unimaginative mathematics instructor, Foley dismantled virtually every initiative of the Hillenbrand era, including the eventual dismissal of all the diocesan priests specially trained by Hillenbrand. Andrew Greeley wrote bitterly of Foley's administration: "It was ... a caricature of paradise, a sick institution, presided over by sick men and training priests many of whom would fit badly into the post-World War II society and even worse into the post-Vatican II world."[37]

But all was not darkness. As in many of his "hard" decisions, Stritch relented somewhat and gave Hillenbrand enough assistant priests to allow him to continue, unhindered, his work with Specialized Catholic Action and liturgical projects. Hillenbrand's productive career continued for many years, but his effectiveness was somewhat curtailed by the loss of the rectorate and a nearly fatal auto accident in 1949. Hillenbrand had been traveling through Oklahoma with a group of Young Christian Students when a truck driver who suffered a heart-attack struck his car head-on. Hillenbrand's right leg was shattered and his hip broken, and he suffered serious internal injuries when a suitcase hit him in the stomach during the collision. His injuries left him hospitalized in Oklahoma for over a year and slightly disabled afterward. During his long months of recuperation his priest friends dutifully visited him and collected money to pay his mounting medical expenses.[38]

When he returned to Chicago, Hillenbrand was able to resume most of his duties. Through the fifties he kept busy with the parochial work combined with his participation in the national organization of the Christian Family Movement and the Liturgical Conference. According to Father Gerard Weber, a close friend of Hillenbrand, most of his time was taken up by the Young Christian Workers, a group he believed to be more malleable to the kind of intensive formation necessary for effectively Christianizing the world. Sacred Heart parish became a center for liturgical life and the site of liturgical celebrations which made the parish well known nationwide. In 1952 Stritch

gave Hillenbrand and others permission to experiment with proposed revisions in the ritual of Holy Week. Hillenbrand was positively elated at performing the restored Easter Vigil ceremonies at their appropriate hour, and he even rounded up five children from one family for baptism. He wrote glowingly to Stritch of the evening:

> I should say the people gathered in a way not hitherto possible, three profound impressions: the transition from darkness to light, from death to life; the tremendous meaning of Baptism; the joyful impact of the first Easter Mass.[39]

In 1957, Hillenbrand launched a major renovation of the church, turning the altar to face the people and commissioning sculptor Ivan Mestrovic to produce new statuary and holy water fonts. When the changes of Vatican II began, Hillenbrand was chosen to serve on the first Archdiocesan Liturgical Commission created by Cardinal Meyer under the chairmanship of Auxiliary Bishop Aloysius Wycislo.

But after the accident he was a changed man. Always something of an autocrat, he became even more dictatorial and irritable as time went on. Sometimes his manners were downright rude. In one episode, after Christian Family Movement leaders Patrick and Patty Crowley and others had arranged an ordination anniversary party for him and presented him with a statue, Hillenbrand wrote a nasty letter to Crowley: "The giving of the statue ... was in poor taste and embarrassed me.... I shall give [it] away. It brings up an annoying remembrance."[40] This act of ingratitude even ruffled the normally placid Cantwell, who upbraided his former mentor.[41] That he could irritate the Crowleys and Cantwell who revered him deeply, is a testimony to the depth of his irascibility. In 1958 he even fell out with Monsignor Jack Egan over Egan's decision to take on the University of Chicago in the Hyde Park-Kenwood Project.

Part of his difficulty was physical. He freqently suffered from migraine headaches and often took it out on the younger priests assigned to him and with whom he had once been so popular. Ironically, after working so hard for liturgical reform all his life, he became highly critical of the actual course of liturgical change after Vatican II. And older ideas about the liturgy, which

seemed fine in classrooms or symposiums but awkward in actual practice, he held to with tenacity. For example, he clung to the notion that the liturgy was the chief teacher of Christian social life and insisted that the children in his school attend the Eucharist daily at the inconvenient hour of 10:10 A.M. When teachers complained about this or disputed his contention that the liturgy could teach children, he retorted with contempt and insisted by his authority as pastor that the practice would continue. He was especially scornful of some of the new liturgical music that he felt lacked the depth and dignity befitting worship. The irony of a man who had once suffered persecution for his liturgical ideas now persecuting others was not lost on many.

Perhaps what troubled him most was the apparent lack of a sound theological basis for liturgical renewal: a theological basis grounded in the corporative view of society that was the heart of his own social and liturgical vision. He clung to the repetition of papal documents as the final authority, even after Vatican II had nuanced the interpretation of these texts by its emphasis on episcopal collegiality. After the uproar over *Humanae Vitae* in 1968 and 1969, Hillenbrand's stubborn insistence on the papal encyclicals seemed outdated and rigid. He was especially incensed that his two close friends in the Christian Family Movement [CFM], Patrick and Patty Crowley, had been among those who recommended a change in papal teaching. Eventually he had fallen out with most of his old clerical companions and had practically to be forced out of the chaplaincy of the CFM in 1971. In 1973 conditions at Sacred Heart were so bad that Cardinal John Cody sent Father Thomas Raftery to become administrator of the parish. A year later, just a few months shy of his seventieth birthday, Cody forcibly retired the aging pastor.

Hillenbrand retired from the active ministry in 1974 and lived in obscurity as pastor emeritus of his parish in Hubbard Woods. Although he eventually reconciled with many of his former antagonists, he felt lonely and abandoned as death approached. He tearfully confessed to his former confidant Monsignor Jack Egan that he felt he had wasted his time working to organize small groups of Catholics and that his work was unknown and unappreciated.[42] Egan went to great lengths to assure him that he had not lived in vain. Hillenbrand died in

1979 with few Chicago priests knowing him or his considerable influence on the life of the Church in Chicago,[43] despite the fact that over five hundred Chicago priests had passed through the Mundelein Seminary for at least a portion of the time Hillenbrand was there. Father Dennis Geaney, O.S.A., longtime friend and confidant, summed up the once popular cleric's career:

> How do I explain the waning of Reiny's charisma a decade before he died in 1979? ... He never saw human freedom as central to Christian life. His papal blueprints for reordering society and the church became dysfunctional as we entered the era of Vatican II, which sponsored a pilgrim church, people going with the flow, trusting the Spirit to pull together our brokenness. Vatican II theology pulled the rug from under his hierarchical theology of the laity, social action and liturgy.... Reiny's genius lay in his insight that lay formation, social action and liturgy were integrative elements of a new church, but the intuition could not flourish under his authoritarian thumb in an American church that had a new awareness of the democratic spirit.[44]

Geaney's words about Hillenbrand were sadly true. For a man who had devoted his life to building up community, he had virtually no community when he died because of his autocratic tendencies.

HILLY'S MEN CARRY ON

Although Hillenbrand's direct personal influence had begun to wane after his dismissal from the seminary and long before his death in 1979, he continued to cast a long shadow over Chicago Catholicism. This influence was felt through the movements he fostered which were lead by men and women he had trained. This was especially true of Specialized Catholic Action movements and the marriage and family life programs that had begun independently of diocesan authority in the forties. Indeed, after World War II these programs grew so rapidly that archdiocesan officials recognized the need to given them some order and direction. It was chancellor Edward Burke who pointed out to Stritch:

Both the Catholic Action Work of the Archdiocese of Chicago and the Cana Conference have progressed so rapidly that it seems propitious to take two men and devote their services exclusively to these two projects.[45]

Consequently, after consulting Hillenbrand, Stritch appointed Father William Quinn, ordained about eight years, to be the head of the Catholic Action federations around the archdiocese.[46] Quinn was formerly an assistant to Father James D. Hishen at St. Gall's parish on the South Side. Hishen was the most tolerant of pastors and had allowed Quinn leeway to organize a successful parish Jocist group, which had actually drawn some young men into the organization (a rarity during the war years). Quinn set up offices in the same Cathedral-owned property, at 3 East Chicago Avenue, that had originally housed the Jocists. There he worked assiduously with the various groups developing around the city.

At the same time that he appointed Quinn, Stritch appointed Father John Egan, a curate at St. Justin's parish on the South Side, to head the flourishing Cana Conference.[47] Egan was born in New York and educated at DePaul University and Quigley Seminary. He had been a protege of Hillenbrand, whom he served as a typist for the 1938 Summer School of Catholic Action. Ordained in 1943, Egan had much experience with Jocist organizations, including participation in a Michigan Study Week in 1944 and the chaplaincy of a students' group at the Chicago Teacher's College. His appointment as director of the fledgling Cana Conference in Chicago was the launching pad for his distinguished career.

CANA AND EGAN

Though the pre-Cana and Cana conference work became virtually synonymous with Chicago Catholicism, their real origin was in New York and the work of Jesuit John Delaney. In 1943 Delaney adapted from Europe a series of exercises, known as "Family Renewal Days," which discussed the challenges and struggles of marriage in the context of a day-long retreat or day of recollection.[48] Eventually these days of recollection became

very popular, not only for their content, but also as an occasion to meet new people and forge new friendships—something that would become increasingly difficult in the diffused neighborhoods of suburbia.

In 1944 the men's and women's Catholic Action cells sponsored Family Renewal Days in Chicago. That same year the name of the program was changed to Cana Conference. By early 1946 Cana retreats had become so widespread throughout the diocese that the adult cells approached Cardinal Stritch for formal approval and archdiocesan sponsorship of the program. Stritch referred the matter to his chancellor, Monsignor Edward Burke, who had expressed deep concern over some of the marriage cases that had come to his desk during the war years. Often lonely GIs had entered into quick marriages that ended in divorce. In trying to "straighten out" these tangled marriage cases so that the parties could marry in the Church, Burke realized the need for better Catholic instruction and support to keep existing marriages alive as well as to adequately prepare engaged couples for their new vocation. Consequently, Stritch approved the Pre-Cana and Cana programs and elevated them to the status of the official family retreat movement in the archdiocese. With Burke's support and Egan's superb organizational skills the Chicago Cana operation thrived. Setting up shop in the rectory of St. Carthage Church at 7315 South Yale, Egan worked tirelessly at the promotion and expansion of the Cana movement in Chicago and around the nation.[49] He unified the various Cana programs throughout the archdiocese and opened up a network of friendships and contacts with those involved in the work around the country. By the end of the forties Chicago was acknowledged as the unofficial Cana capital of the American Catholic Church.

Cana was for those already married. For those preparing for matrimony, a similar program was established called Pre-Cana. Originally devised by Father James Voss and layman Clem Lane in 1946, the structure of a Pre-Cana program was similar to Cana, consisting of a day-long Sunday conference beginning with Mass and breakfast, followed by conferences, discussions, Benediction of the Blessed Sacrament, and a preview of the wedding vows. Pre-Cana and Cana were highly

successful in the Chicago archdiocese, attracting thousands of young couples. Egan used many occasions to trumpet the statistics. In the year 1946–47 650 couples attended Pre-Cana. Cana figures were even more impressive. In his 1950 annual report to Cardinal Stritch, Egan recapitulated all the figures of attendance and parochial participation. In 1946, three institutions hosted four conferences consisting of ninety-three couples. The very next year, under Egan's direction, the number of host parishes jumped to twenty, the number of conferences to twenty-four, and the number of couples to 826. By mid-1950, when the report was turned in, thirty-one parishes had sponsored thirty-one conferences for 2,346 couples.[50] A small newsletter, *Couplet* edited by John and Eileen Farrell, appeared in the late forties and was sent to Cana programs around the country. Egan solidified Chicago's hegemony in the Pre-Cana and Cana movement by publishing a series of talks from a national meeting of Cana priests, at the Dominican Priory in Chicago in the summer of 1949.[51] This volume became known as the Cana Manual. A companion to it was developed the following year when a second meeting was held in Chicago under Egan's direction.[52] In 1957 the manual was again revised and reissued by Father Walter Imbiorski, Egan's successor.

The dynamics of the day, the refined quality of the presentations, and the appeal to Catholic families all combined to make the Pre-Cana and Cana programs a success. Even more important was the effect they had on people's thinking. When Egan asked one of the newly engaged if any of her ideas had been changed, she told him: "I never could see why birth control was so terrible, but now I know."[53]

The success was not confined to Chicago. Even though Stritch had insisted that Cana not become a national movement, this is exactly what happened.[54] Cana and Pre-Cana became nationwide programs by the early 1950s, assisted by Egan, who went on the road at the request of Monsignor Loras Lane, chancellor of the Archdiocese of Dubuque. Egan and a team of chaplains, doctors, and lay couples conducted a series of workshops for interested parties in Dubuque. After the Dubuque meeting requests for information flowed into Egan's office and into the chancery, and the "road show" became an important feature of

the pre-Cana and Cana movement.[55] Chicago's influence in the Cana movement reached a peak when it took over operation of The Grail magazine, published by the Benedictines of St. Meinrad's Abbey. Later the magazine was titled *Marriage* and featured many articles by Chicago-based writers.

In 1957 Egan's interests turned to urban affairs and he handed over the reins of the pre-Cana/Cana operation to Father Walter Imbiorski. The Cana movement eventually peaked in the late fifties and began to ebb in the early sixties, but the pre-Cana program was adapted into successful pre-marital preparation programs in place even today in Chicago and in many dioceses across the country. The ferment of the post-conciliar period, confusion surrounding family issues, and internal disputes over birth control sapped the strength of the local organizations. However, Cana served Egan well. His association with the powerful Monsignor Burke won him a good friend in the chancery office and Burke served as a "front man" for many of Egan's later endeavors. Egan's association with Cana brought him into contact with a large number of religiously active lay Catholics and also acquainted him with many of the problems associated with urban life in the postwar period. Highly popular as a speaker, carefully deferential to his ecclesiastical superiors, and at times combative and aggressive with those who challenged his authority or questioned his views, Egan used the Cana experience as an important springboard for other kinds of activism.

THE CHRISTIAN FAMILY MOVEMENT

Although not formally linked with pre-Cana and Cana, a highly successful Hillenbrand-inspired organization dealing with marriage and family issues developed in the postwar era— the Christian Family Movement (CFM). The roots of CFM were in the Specialized Catholic Action movements of the early forties. Hillenbrand's insistence on ideological purity had separated the various cell groups according to vocation and gender. When large numbers of these young activists began marrying, it became increasingly difficult to maintain separate meetings. Moreover, the need for a Christian support group for young

married couples and their growing families became increasingly pressing. Developed simultaneously in Chicago and in nearby South Bend, Indiana, the Christian Family Movement employed the observe-judge-act methodology of the Specialized Movements and attempted to form families according to principles of Christian social teaching. Catholic lawyer Patrick Crowley and his wife Patty became the leading couple in Chicago, while Burnett Bauer and Father Louis Putz, C.S.C., led the movement in South Bend.[56] The union of these groups, under the general chaplaincy of Reynold Hillenbrand, resulted in one of the most popular family-oriented movements in American Catholic history.

Thousands of couples joined CFM groups and hundreds of Chicago priests volunteered their services as chaplains to these families. A popular manual, *For Happier Families*, drawn up in 1949, directed families to seek not only their own sanctification but the larger goal of rechristianizing the world. Indeed CFM, like Cana, also provided a point of human contact for Catholics moving more and more into their suburban enclaves and away from the enforced closeness of urban housing and neighborhoods. The popularity of CFM and Cana in Chicago was further evidence of the increasingly middle class character of Chicago Catholicism.[57] In its heyday, thousands of CFMers would meet annually at Notre Dame or other Catholic campuses to hear talks by Hillenbrand and others.

With his ambivalent feelings about Specialized Catholic Action, Stritch was characteristically detached from CFM. Although he appeared occasionally at CFM events and offered courteous, if not always effusive, praise for their activities he never could feel comfortable with these movements. Indeed, his discomfort was actually suspicion and he demonstrated this when he turned thumbs-down on a proposal to award the Crowleys Notre Dame University's prestigious Laetare award. He wrote to Father Edmund Joyce, C.S.C., of Notre Dame, who asked Stritch for his opinion of the Crowleys:

> Personally, I would not recommend the Crowleys. They are good people, doing good work. Both of them have fine enthusiasm. However, I think it is a little bit too early to give this sort of recognition to the work in which they are engaged. It is going along

fine and I think that we are showing in it more and more necessary maturity. However, I don't think that this work has reached
the stage yet where we can say that it deserves the recognition
which the giving of the Laetare Medal would bring not only to
these individuals but to the work.[58]

The couple did receive the award after Stritch's death.
Archbishop Meyer also regarded CFM with caution, because he
had had problems with the movement in Milwaukee.[59]
However, by the end of his years, he had vigorously embraced
the movement, referring to it as his "strong right arm" in one
public statement. Unlike Cana, which found a new incarnation
in the marriage policies of the post-Vatican II era, CFM did not
survive long after the council. A major division erupted in the
movement between those who wanted to focus on internal family issues and those (led chiefly by Hillenbrand) who wanted to
continue the social reconstructionist thrust of the founding
vision. Racked by internal difficulties and increasing tension
between Hillenbrand and the CFM leadership, the movement
lost steam and shrank during the seventies.[60]

What were the effects of these movements on the quality of
Catholic life in Chicago? The analogy of "leaven in the dough,"
of which the Jocists were so fond, was certainly appropriate in
describing the effects of these movements on the character of
Chicago Catholic life. CFM, like Cana, also had a profound
impact on the Catholic values of its adherents. In particular, its
strong emphasis on Catholic social teaching led many to a deep
commitment to Catholic viewpoints on social issues. The impact
of these highly motivated men and women would be felt in the
larger community of the Chicago scene as they became public
officials, educators, and were well represented in professions
like law and medicine. Clearly, the intensity of the movements
and the charisma of men like Hillenbrand, Egan, and Quinn
deeply affected a number of young Chicagoans. According to
Mary Irene Zotti, the historian of the Young Christian Workers,
roughly 40 percent of the total membership of all the specialized
movements were residents of Chicago. Chicago was the national
headquarters for these movements and the source of much of
the intellectual impetus behind them. In a later survey of the
Young Christian Workers, Zotti received an abnormally high

response to a lengthy questionnaire sent to all the former members she could track down (600 out of 1,000). Of these six hundred, she found only a few who had either abandoned the Church altogether or were deeply disillusioned with it. The vast majority, around 80 percent, described themselves as practicing Catholics; and a significant number indicated that their involvement in the Church was more than regular Mass attendance. A large number indicated that they served as lay ministers in various ways (Communion distributors, lectors, on parish councils). Moreover, a high proportion of the active Catholics indicated a sense of social consciousness regarding current issues in their local communities.[61]

Since people grew older and moved on, the Young Christian Workers, like the Young Christian Students, assumed only a temporary commitment, the CFM held the allegiance of its members for a much longer time than the YCS or YCW, and exercised an even greater impact on their members' becoming strongly attached to the Church in their participation in its liturgical and communal life. Moreover, the effects of the social action inquiries on the formation of their political, ethical, and moral systems of belief were, in all likelihood, quite significant. Some former members of the specialized movements, like Michael Schiltz, went to work with Catholic organizations in order to better the community. Father Vincent Giese, who began a Specialized Catholic Action group for young blacks in his inner city parish, reported that a number of them attained high stature in city, state, and federal government. Priests like Martin Farrell and lay Catholics like George Drury and Russell Barta all traced their concern for social issues to the impact of the Cardijn methodology on their lives.[62] Others, as we have seen, would be put off by the movement's insistence on racial justice and leave the organization.

DANIEL CANTWELL

Quinn and Egan were two priests who rivaled Hillenbrand in single-mindedness and zeal, but one other who would have a significant impact on the shape of Chicago Catholic life was Father Daniel Cantwell.

Cantwell was perhaps the priest most formed in Hillenbrand's image and likeness.[63] Born in 1914, the son of a union truck driver, he grew up in St. Mel's parish on the West Side of the city. He had entered the archdiocesan seminary system and was ordained in April 1939, the last class raised to the priesthood by Cardinal Mundelein. His first assignment was to Christ the King parish in the prosperous Beverly Hills neighborhood. In 1940, at Hillenbrand's urging, he was sent to the Catholic University of America for studies in sociology in preparation for a place on the faculty of the major seminary. At Catholic University he came into contact with John A. Ryan, Francis Haas, and public housing advocate John Ihlder, all of whom reinforced his determination to "go back and [try] to do something in his own community."[64] After completing a master's thesis entitled "Facts in Negro Segregation," he returned to Chicago and began his work at the seminary. With the example and encouragement of Hillenbrand and his practical knowledge of sociology, he becamemade him a popular faculty member who branched out into a number of areas, including public housing, race relations, and labor organizing.

Cantwell's graduate work gave him a solid grasp of the mechanics of housing and racial issues, as well as a strong ethical framework to guide his positions on these issues. He was a member and later chairman of the Chicago Public Housing Conference, chaplain for Friendship House and the Catholic Interracial Council (which he helped form), and chaplain of the Catholic Labor Alliance. All of these groups were lay organizations with their own respective boards of directors, executive secretaries, and internal concerns and workings. None of them were directly sponsored by the Archdiocese of Chicago. Each had constantly to scramble for funds to survive, and all of them turned to Daniel Cantwell for guidance. Cantwell, in turn, served as their liaison with archdiocesan and public officials.

The Catholic Labor Alliance was a clear reflection of the deep influence Hillenbrand had on Cantwell. It was born of a general Catholic concern for the rights of labor. This concern was spearheaded by Bishop Sheil in his association with the CIO and with the work of Reynold Hillenbrand, John Hayes, and William Boyd in establishing and staffing Church-operated

labor schools. The labor schools not only assisted the incipient unions in winning some scuffles with management, but also served to keep out the Communist organizers who were seeking to capitalize on the social unrest bred by the depression.[65]

Another organization which tried to curtail communist influence was the Association of Catholic Trade Unionists [ACTU]. In 1939 a Chicago branch was formed, and Mundelein appointed Father Bernard Burns as its chaplain.[66] The ACTU, a popular movement in New York and Detroit, had rough sledding in industrialized Chicago. Its president, reporter Harry Cyril Read, was actively involved in the CIO efforts to organize the Newspaper Guild in the two Hearst papers of Chicago, the *Sun* and the *American*. He also wrote a popular manual of parliamentary procedures for labor union meetings. Read's wife Lucy was equally immersed in the struggle, even to getting herself arrested in a demonstration against the Hearst papers.[67] Read's interest and the natural inclination of many Catholic labor people toward the CIO unions provoked the ire of AFL workers, who resented the Catholic blessing on this strike. So bitter were the rivalries that Catholic laborers split along AFL and CIO lines and held two separate Labor Day Masses—the CIO in Holy Name Cathedral and the AFL in St. Peter's Church on Madison Street.

In 1940 an action of Burns brought the ACTU under archdiocesan scrutiny. Burns had been active in gaining recognition for CIO workers in the Montgomery Ward situation and, just when it looked like his efforts to win approval of the union were succeeding, Ward's backed away. This snafu was one of the first things on Stritch's agenda when he came to office; it embarrassed him greatly and tipped him off that the ACTU meant trouble.[68] Things got worse in 1941. The monthly periodical *Catholic Labor Leader* came under suspicion by the FBI in 1941 as "subversive," and agents contacted the new archbishop about the matter. Stritch was able to reassure federal agents about ACTU loyalty, but called in Chaplain Burns and admonished him to keep the organization in line.[69] The FBI investigation was only one of the organization's troubles. Earlier that year, Harry Read had left for Detroit, and Burns was unable to handle the recurrent crises within the organization. He chose to enter the

military service with the onset of World War II and left the organization dangling. Eventually, the Chicago chapter of the ACTU became a casualty of division and of the wartime work orders which quelled much labor unrest. Mayor Kelly made industrial peace in Chicago a point of pride.[70]

The loose reins of leadership in Catholic labor circles were picked up during the war by three men: Edward Marciniak, a veteran of the Catholic Worker house on Blue Island Avenue and an employee of the typesetters union; Frank Delaney, a regional attorney for the wage and hour division of the United States Department of Labor; and Monsignor Hillenbrand. In long discussions, Hillenbrand, Marciniak, and Delaney addressed the need for an ongoing Catholic labor organization that would educate Catholic workers, keep alive salient issues, and serve as a force for the Catholic voice in local and national labor affairs. In order to avoid the mistakes of the ACTU, they envisioned an organization that would tread a careful line between AFL and CIO rivalries, would embrace Catholics and non-Catholics, and assume concerns beyond the bread-and-butter unionism of the AFL. This would be a Catholic Labor Alliance, a voice for workers and an agency of social reform embracing issues such as racial relations, housing, and social justice. The organization even enrolled businessmen, seeking to find a way to overcome the traditional antipathy between labor and management. In substance, the Catholic Labor Alliance was a vehicle for social reconstruction according to the lines of the social encyclicals.

In early 1943 Delaney, Marciniak, and Hillenbrand approached Archbishop Stritch with plans for the new organization. The prelate approved and suggested that it take as its official foundation day the feast of St. Joseph, March 19, 1943. Their goals were stated clearly: "Our aim is to labor 'energetically and effectively'—in the words of Pius XI—that this world, this country, this city may advance in the spirit of justice and charity as the proper preparation for that Home where only the Just and the Charitable shall enter."[71] The means to accomplish this goal were twofold: by action—doing something about the economic and social problems as individuals and as a group—and by education—influencing the attitudes of men and women to encourage them to join in the work of the new social order.[72]

Immediately, the three leaders set to work to finance the new venture and to secure a broader base of support and publicity. They wrote letters of appeal to the clergy and solicited contributions from lay people. After they had secured about $3,000, Monsignor Morrison gave them office space at 3 East Chicago Avenue, the building which housed the Specialized Catholic Action groups. New members were recruited to the Alliance, including Edwin R. Hackett of the Commercial Telephone Workers Union, James J. Szalkowski of the United Auto Workers, John L. Yancey of the United Transport Service Employees, CIO, Frank Gillespie, International Brotherhood of Teamsters. Even Harry Read and Andrew Taft, former ACTU officials, signed on as honorary members.

By July of 1943 a successor to the *Labor Leader* rolled off the press. Edward Marciniak became the guiding force behind the monthly tabloid entitled *Work,* the official organ of the Catholic Labor Alliance. Marciniak boldly led a group of seminarians to the gate of a large Chicago factory and distributed 2,000 copies of the first issue. *Work's* hard-hitting editorials and labor reporting made the tabloid a hit with working men and women throughout the city. By the late forties it had a circulation of around ten thousand, six thousand of which were paid subscriptions at a dollar a year. The Alliance later recruited journalist Robert Senser, a free-lance writer who also had some experience as a newspaper man on the *Hammond Times.* Senser and Marciniak continued to write for *Work* into the fifties, long after Catholic concern for labor issues had evaporated.

The Alliance's first chaplain was, Father John Quinn, who held the post until 1947 when he was sent to Rome for advanced studies in canon law. He was replaced by Cantwell, who had been part of the planning and early days of the Alliance and who faithfully shuttled back and forth on the North Shore Railway to meetings of the Alliance in the Loop. After Hillenbrand's dismissal in 1944, conditions at the seminary grew progressively more uncomfortable for Cantwell and for the whole coterie of diocesan priests Hillenbrand had recruited. Finally, in 1947, Cantwell too was removed from the faculty at the request of Monsignor Foley and sent to St. Philomena's parish on the Northwest Side of Chicago. After one year at St. Philomena's,

Cantwell wrote to Stritch, asking permission to serve as chaplain to the Labor Alliance, Friendship House, and the Catholic Interracial Council. He explained the reasons to his Ordinary:

> We have not been able to revive the Labor Schools that flourished before the war. We have not been able to give this vast industrial city the kind of carefully planned study and apostolate that is necessary among the workers. We have not been able to come to know as many of the leaders of workers as we should have. Meantime, the efforts of the Communists have not slackened.[73]

Although Cantwell offered to subsidize his own salary, Stritch not only gave him the requested permission to work full-time with these groups but also paid his salary and benefits for the duration of his chaplaincy, while allowing him to live at St. Finbarr's parish at Fourteenth and Harding.

A quiet and genuinely unassuming man, Cantwell hovered behind the scenes of the organizations he mentored, offering advice when asked and allowing a great deal of latitude to his lay associates. But his gentle voice, premature baldness, and gray fringe, belied a vigorous mind and an iron will. Like Hillenbrand, Cantwell held tenaciously to his reading of Catholic social teaching and was capable of explaining and defending it when the occasion required. Cantwell's approach was firm and unyielding on many topics, but he was generally low-key, always courteous, and deliberately nonconfrontational. Like his mentor Hillenbrand, Cantwell was able to handle a large volume of work in a kind of balancing act. By dint of this hard work and his obvious commitment to causes not always popular or well understood, Cantwell built a reservoir of tremendous moral authority which persisted even into the nineties.[74]

Cantwell was shrewd enough to avoid some of the mistakes of Hillenbrand, particularly with regard to ecclesiastical authority. He realized his presence in these labor groups might create controversy and set up the same wave of ill-feeling that eventually toppled Hillenbrand. Cantwell was generally very deferential to Stritch and faithfully reported in writing and in person on his activities. This diplomatic attitude won the Catholic Labor Alliance critical recognition in the *Official Catholic Directory* as an agency of the Catholic Church. This

meant they could speak with some legitimacy for the Church (subject to careful chancery monitoring) and, even more important, do fund-raising as a legitimate Catholic organization.

Working quietly and with deference to the lay character of the Alliance, Cantwell set to work acquainting public officials with official Catholic positions on matters of general and local concern on labor, housing, and racial issues. CLA officers and Cantwell himself wrote letters to legislators, cooperated with local and national organizations including the Office of Price Administration, the Chicago CIO Industrial Union Council, the Chicago Federation of Labor, and the Mayor's Committee on Human Relations. The Alliance also hosted an annual Labor Day Mass at Holy Name Cathedral which drew huge crowds and featured a prominent cleric who spoke on some facet of labor relations.

Cantwell was equally committed to the CLA's educational programs. He, like Hillenbrand, believed social change occurred when one changed hearts, not institutions. Cantwell's strong belief in the power of education led him to launch one of the most popular labor education series, the John A. Ryan Forums. The idea originated in the fall of 1948 when the finance committee of the Alliance suggested a series of four lectures as fund-raisers for the chronically strapped organization. The lectures were named for the recently deceased moral theologian Monsignor John A. Ryan, and the lead-off speaker was Ryan's colleague Bishop Francis A. Haas of Grand Rapids, Michigan. Haas's talk, given to a packed audience in the grand ballroom of the Hamilton Hotel, was a smashing success. After Haas, Cantwell arranged for a galaxy of important labor speakers, including big names such as Walter Reuther of the United Auto Workers, Philip Murray of the CIO, Joseph Keenan, national director of the AFL League for Political Action, James Carey, secretary-treasurer of the national CIO, and Meyer Kestenbaum of the Chicago clothing firm Hart, Schaffner, and Marx. The forums provided some of the necessary funds for ongoing lectures and generated publicity for further programs.

The educational outreach also included a link with the Sheil School of Social Studies which enabled the CLA to offer Neighborhood Labor Forums. These labor classes were derived from the old labor school curriculums and offered in the fall and

spring for a period of six weeks. Most classes were held in the CYO building at 31 East Congress; but under the Sheil School auspices the Labor Forum could also hold sessions at Corpus Christi High School, Back-of-the-Yards, and Bridgeport. Offerings included "You and Your Job," "Christian Social Principles," "Why Labor Unions?" "Parliamentary Law and Public Speaking," and "Current Problems Forum." Instructors included clergy, members of trade and industrial unions, university professors, and members of the social service branches of government.[75]

When the Sheil empire collapsed in 1954 the labor schools were already dying, but interest was growing in the whole concept of adult education. Stritch encouraged Cantwell to find a way to continue the adult education program of the Sheil School. In 1955 Cantwell proposed a new adult education program that would offer advanced courses in religious and theological topics. Stritch approved the concept and generously funded the operation with monies from Catholic Charities. Cantwell headed a committee composed, among others, of Sheil's old nemesis, George Drury, and chose former seminarian and sociology professor, Russ Barta, to head the new agency. Barta had long been affiliated with Specialized Catholic Action and the Catholic Labor Alliance. Under his careful leadership and with Cantwell's support the Adult Education program sponsored any number of important speakers, events, and workshops on a host of topics.[76]

Under the auspices of the Adult Education program, Cantwell introduced priests to some of the newest scholarship emerging in the fields of Scripture and theology. In 1959 he organized the first of many successful summer schools in Scripture for the priests of the archdiocese. The idea of summer sessions went back to the days of the Summer Schools of Catholic Action so popular and effective in the thirties and forties. Monsignor Malachy Foley refused to allow the use of the seminary campus for the event, but Cantwell was able to secure the Maryknoll seminary in nearby Glen Ellyn. At these sessions many Chicago priests received their first exposure to the historical-critical scholarship that had been developing in Catholic scriptural circles since the forties. It was at one of these gatherings that Cardinal Meyer was first acquainted with this scholarship and

where he met the man who would be his chief *peritus* at Vatican II, Passionist Father Barnabas Mary Ahern. Eventually the Adult Education Centers and the Catholic Interracial Council all shared common headquarters in a building at 21 East Superior.[77] The building had been taken over in 1951 by the two Cantwell-directed organizations. The address alone became synonymous with the confident enthusiasm of Chicago Catholics.

Eventually all these organizations underwent some degree of transformation, given the changing conditions of Chicago Catholic life. This was especially true of the Catholic Labor Alliance. Although there had been considerable labor unrest after World War II, labor issues gradually diminished as "hot topics" for Americans in general and Catholics in particular. The organizing days of the thirties and forties were over, and this was reflected in the declining appeal of Alliance programs. In a 1947 report to the governing board of the Alliance, Marciniak complained that the labor classes held at the Sheil School were not attracting significant numbers.[78] In subsequent years attendance continued to drop. In 1955 the union of the AFL and the CIO put an end to their internal rivalry, and this too had implications for strong pro-labor organizations like the CLA. In short, the new mood compelled a reorganization of the Catholic Labor Alliance. This brought forward issues that had only been dealt with in a lateral fashion, such as housing, racial relations, and urban affairs, and made them the center of a new agenda. To symbolize the shift in emphasis, the Alliance was the Catholic Council on Working Life (CCWL). Explaining this to a Jesuit priest at Mundelein, Cantwell stated:

> We are of the opinion that in the Church's Social Action movement in this country we have over the years succeeded in making the Church's position on the right to organize so clear that no reasonable person would any longer question that. This having been accomplished, we judged that a change was advisable in order to move forward and to strike out towards new goals.[79]

The CLA's traditional interest in organized labor was still present and resurfaced in the early sixties, when the plight of migratory workers became a hot topic. However, the reorganization was only a holding action before the organization's eventual decline

and extinction. The social composition of Chicago Catholicism reflected less and less the blue collar constituency that had been the object of the CLA's efforts. Eventually however, old stalwarts of the movement, like Sensor and later Marciniak departed for other fields of endeavor. *Work* went out of publication even though it was briefly succeeded by a slick magazine called *New City*[80] and Cantwell was transferred to parochial duties. The CCWL and *New City* folded quietly in the late sixties.

HILLY'S OTHER MEN

Because the Hillenbrand groups were united by a common formation and a common social vision, there was a great deal of cross-fertilization among these various organizations and interests. Meetings or conventions of Cana or CFM, talks at the John A. Ryan Forums or the forums of the Catholic Interracial Council, and rallies of Specialized Catholic Action groups often brought many of the same people together. Cantwell, Egan, Quinn, Killgallon, Weber, Hillenbrand, seemed to represent the vital core of the movement. Many priests, especially those who had been seminarians during the Hillenbrand years and their immediate aftermath, were strong supporters of these movements and served as speakers, chaplains, and guides on the local level. Naturally there were opponents (although they kept their voices muted after Quinn's and Egan's appointments by Cardinal Stritch in 1946), and there was always the larger group who were wholly indifferent or too caught up in other duties to pay attention in any consistent way.

It is true that these movements were popular and highly profiled and won a great deal of attention in the post-conciliar era, especially because they seemed to anticipate changes that occurred in the areas of lay leadership in the Church, social activism, and liturgical reform. But the relative handful of priests who were deeply involved in them probably felt somewhat beleaguered and turned to one another for support. To reassure each other, and perhaps to plot strategy, many of these priests gathered on Sunday evenings in the rectory of Annunciation parish, where Father Jake Killgallon, a Hillenbrand ally, was an assistant pastor.[81]

These meetings were sociable and informal but also stimulated discussion and, occasionally, some real action. For example, at one of these gatherings a general dissatisfaction was raised with the popular "Cogan Catechism," an instructional text drawn up for those in black conversion work by Father William Cogan. Father Leo Mahon challenged Killgallon and Father Gerald Weber to devise a new catechism to supplant what they considered the other's deadening pedagogy.[82] Taking up the challenge, Weber and Killgallon turned out the tremendously popular *Life in Christ* or "Chicago Catechism," which was highlighted in the Jesuit weekly, *America*, and went through numerous copies and editions.[83] Although following the question-and-answer method, each item of Christian doctrine in the Chicago Catechism was introduced by a passage from the Scriptures and concluded by suggestions for action. In short, the inquiry methodology used in Specialized Catholic Action meetings was now crystalized in catechetical form. The catechism was printed by a small firm in Ohio and was so tremendously successful that Weber and Killgallon devoted the remainder of their careers to writing catechetical texts that were readable, theologically sound, and pedagogically appealing.[84]

The Sunday night group also welcomed occasional newcomers such as Father Andrew Greeley. Ordained in 1954, Greeley was assigned to the prosperous Beverly Hills parish of Christ the King. Greeley was one of the first to observe the impact of suburbanization on the Catholic community from his catbird seat at Christ the King, and he made his findings known to the Sunday night group who "adopted" him and promoted his career as a sociologist.

Another gathering spot for the social action minded priests and lay persons for many years was a retreat center northwest of the city called Childerly.[85] This was a five-acre farm which had been owned by Dr. and Mrs. Francis Lillie. Dr. Lillie, the dean of the Division of Biological Sciences at the University of Chicago, had taken an interest in the Calvert Club, an association of Catholic students at the university. Mrs. Lillie, a social activist and a friend of prominent social workers Ellen Gates Starr and Jane Addams, administered the Crane Fund for Widows and Children. A former Episcopalian, Mrs. Lillie established a

chapel on the property after she converted to Catholicism in 1928. Members of the Calvert Club and Catholics at the University of Chicago were often guests on the farm. In 1940 Mrs. Lillie deeded the property to the Calvert Club.

What evolved during the thirties was a gathering spot for Catholic intellectuals. Priests of various religious orders would visit the place, and conduct interesting discussions on secular and religious topics. But since the University of Chicago had been on Cardinal Mundelein's hate list, he studiously ignored the community. When Stritch arrived Jerome Kerwin pleaded with him to appoint a chaplain to the group who met there regularly. This he did in the person of Father Joseph Connerton. Connerton built on Kerwin's initiatives and Childerly became a mecca for Catholic intellectuals. Many conversions to Catholicism were made because of Childerly conferences, and Hillenbrand used the facilities for his Catholic Action activities. Indeed, at one point he referred to Childerly as "his guest house."[86] Childerly was a gathering place for Catholic social actionists to recharge their batteries, deepen their spiritual lives, and plan new initiatives that would keep the visions of social reconstruction alive. Unlike Mundelein, Stritch encouraged the development of a Catholic presence at the University of Chicago.

Nearly all of the Hillenbrand priests had a kind of suspicion of Cardinal Stritch. Since he had fired their mentor in 1944 and undid all Hillenbrand's reforms at St. Mary of the Lake, they worried about his conservative instincts and their own fates. How would they fare if their activities demanded as controversial a stand as Hilly had been willing to take in the Montgomery Ward episode? Moreover, Stritch's southern attitudes on the race issue worried and, at times, discouraged them. When Stritch departed in 1958 and Meyer's appointment was announced in the late summer, Cantwell and his forces were ready. In a memo to the heads of the organizations he served as chaplain he wrote: "When the new archbishop gets to Chicago, we must help interpret Chicago to him. We ought to be thinking about how to do it." [87]

Few in Chicago knew what to make of "that Dutchman" Meyer, and this was especially true of Cantwell's social action crowd. Ostensibly Meyer was a much more conservative man

than Stritch. But years of episcopal ministry, especially in Superior, Wisconsin had taught him the virtue of patient listening. Chicago's urban problems were a source of worry and consternation to many, and Meyer had no illusions about the tasks ahead of him. He quickly realized that Cantwell and his associates represented a precious fund of expertise and knowledge on urban issues and relied heavily on Cantwell and the organizations he had nurtured. For example, two memorable clergy gatherings, one on race and another on the role of the lay person, were largely crafted by Cantwell and his coworkers. Cantwell also provided the ideas and backing for the 1963 Conference on Race and Religion. Cantwell himself felt much more comfortable under Meyer's administration and remarked to a friend: "Happily we have in Archbishop Meyer the most aggressive leadership we have ever enjoyed."[88]

Hillenbrand's vision of social reconstruction according to the principles of the social encyclicals of the thirties and forties clearly prepared the way for the activities in the fifties. Major challenges awaited those who remained in the demographically and racially changing city. Urban affairs and race relations would occupy a prominent place in the efforts of men like Egan and Cantwell.

6

Chicago Catholicism and Urban Issues

The Great Depression and the Second World War were like glaciers freezing the urban landscape of Chicago. The economic desperation of the depression had ground to a halt the natural expansion of the metropolis. Even though World War II rekindled the city's economy, wartime shortages limited the growth of housing and simultaneously flooded the city with servicemen and defense workers. Two decades of pent-up growth demanded attention in the postwar era and summoned the energies of all those concerned with the welfare of the city. This included the Chicago Catholic leadership.

In terms of sheer numbers the Catholic Church had a large stake in the city of Chicago. In 1940 there were 262 urban churches, representing about 80 percent of the 1.4 million Catholics in the whole archdiocese. The total insured valuation of all archdiocesan property was around two billion dollars. But even more important than its considerable material assets was the extent to which Catholicism in Chicago was identified with its urban setting. From the affluent North Shore to the industrial South Side, a symbiotic relationship existed between the church and the neighborhood. Chicagoans more so than other urban dwellers associated themselves with their neighborhoods as a kind of "social skin" and often identified their home turf by responding to the question: what parish do you belong to? The shifting demography of their urban neighborhoods after World War II would alter this relationship and the character of Catholic life in the Archdiocese of Chicago.

187

The largely non-Catholic, poor black population pushed into previously all-white neighborhoods, provoking bitter resistance and conflict. In response, a large number of Chicago Catholics emigrated to the suburbs, where they could enjoy single-family dwellings, better schools and social services, and freedom from urban crime and blighted housing. Those who stayed, either by their own choice or because they could not afford to move, grew increasingly sensitive to urban issues. The reworking of the urban landscape through the placement of controversial public housing and the location of freeways caused issues of serious concern to pastors, parishioners, and church leaders.

HOUSING

Housing was the premier urban issue. The depression had stalled home building in the metropolitan areas, causing a severe housing shortage. Government efforts to deal with this housing crisis in Chicago began during the New Deal when the Public Works Administration (PWA) constructed three low-rent housing developments in the city.[1] In 1934 the Illinois Legislature passed a state housing act calling for the establishment of housing authorities to regulate and control the federal housing projects. After the enactment of the Wagner Housing Act of 1937, the Chicago Housing Authority (CHA) was established and undertook the management of three PWA projects, the Jane Addams Houses, the Julia C. Lathrop Homes, and the Trumbull Park Homes, and soon began to plan and construct housing on its own. In 1939 the Ida B. Wells Homes, with 1,662 units, were built on the near South Side. Plans were drawn up for the Frances Cabrini Homes on the near North Side along with the Robert H. Brooks Homes.

The urgent need for housing during the war pushed public housing construction high on the government's war priority lists. Projects like the 128-unit Lawndale Gardens and the Brooks and Bridgeport Homes were rapidly constructed. In 1943 the federal government planned construction of 1,500 temporary family dwellings in the Calumet area to accommodate workers in the steel mills. Altgeld Gardens on the far South Side

was created to meet this need.[2] By the end of that year, Chicago's public housing was supplying homes for 5,765 families.

Whatever affected neighborhoods affected the Catholic Church and so it is no surprise that Catholic priests like Father Luigi Giambastiani played small roles in the selection of these public housing sites. Stritch, too, had been an early supporter of government-subsidized housing in Milwaukee, where he had spoken approvingly of two proposed federal housing projects.[3] On coming to Chicago he took an early interest in the work of the CHA and encouraged Father Giambastiani in his work with the Frances Cabrini Homes. Stritch also had an interest in housing issues and indicated it in a letter to CHA executive secretary, Elizabeth Wood,[4] and even more directly to a young mother who appealed to him for help in securing housing:

> There is no social problem which gives me greater concern than the housing problem.... Despite much that has been done by the government in helping families to build homes and in providing public housing projects the solution of this problem in the main must come from a change of conscience in private owners. I want you to know that I have not once but many times spoken and written of the urgent need of finding a solution for this problem.[5]

But the name most closely associated with Catholic concern for housing in Chicago was that of Father Daniel Cantwell. Cantwell's interest stemmed from his graduate school days at the Catholic University, where he had become involved with the Alley Authority, a public housing agency for the District of Columbia. Having seen some of the problems of homelessness and squalid living that existed among that city's black population, his own master's thesis[6] analyzed housing conditions in Chicago and found similar and sometimes worse circumstances. Cantwell laid the blame for these horrendous conditions at the doorstep of restrictive covenants, clauses written into housing agreements wherein owners pledged not to sell their homes to blacks or Jews. The result was to confine black Chicagoans to an increasingly cramped ghetto, even if they had the money to move out to better housing.[7]

If existing conditions were bad when Cantwell studied them in the early forties, they were destined to get worse

because the city's black population was growing. Between 1940 and 1950, 214,534 blacks took up residence in Chicago, an increase of 77.2 percent over the migration of the previous decade. Between 1950 and 1960, 350,372 more blacks moved to Chicago, bringing the total number to over 800,000 or 22.9 percent of the population of the city.[8] Housing conditions for these newcomers were simply unbelievable. Men, women, and children lived in basements, garages, coal bins, and other scarcely habitable spots simply because they could not find any decent or affordable place to live. In 1942 a private group, the Metropolitan Housing Council, reported:

> Approximately 25,000 Negroes have moved here since 1940, and constitute in themselves a tremendous problem ... sixty percent of the units occupied by the colored people are substandard. When you have more than 300,000 people bottled up and forced to live in indesirably [sic] horrible, hazardous and unhealthy quarters, piled up on top of one another, you have all the ingredients for an explosion.[9]

A good idea of the crowding is given by historian Arnold Hirsch, who reports that 375,000 blacks lived within areas only equipped to deal with 110,000.[10]

When Cantwell returned from graduate studies in 1943, he set to work bringing his own expertise and the social teaching of the Church to bear on Chicago's housing problems, becoming a leading Catholic spokesman for justice in housing policies. The depth of Cantwell's commitment to justice and his desire to cast these long standing problems in moral rather than political terms was evident early on as reflected in an incident related to restrictive covenants.

In 1944 Cantwell became part of a steering committee of interested citizens who formed a Chicago chapter of the National Public Housing Conference (NPHC).[11] This nationwide organization had begun during the war and included among its members Monsignor John O'Grady of the National Conference of Catholic Charities.[12] The first work of the NPHC was a crusade against the practice of restrictive covenants. The Catholic Labor Alliance's periodical *Work*, at Cantwell's urging, had already begun the attack with a forceful editorial against them:

Restrictive covenants against Negroes are a racket. They have made it possible for real estate agents and property holders in slum districts to reap gold mines on dwellings which they don't have to bother keeping in repair. They have cut off the supply of available housing on the bulging southside where the population has increased by 33,000 persons since the 1940 census.[13]

The Mayor's Conference on Race Relations underscored this in a report issued in February 1944:

At present Negroes are confined to restricted areas with bad houses and exorbitant rents. They are confined to these districts by an atmosphere of prejudice, and specifically by conspiracies known as restrictive covenants. This Committee has by formal vote declared itself opposed categorically to restrictions of race, creed, or color on the place where any of Chicago's citizens may live. We propose to continue to work earnestly with other effective agencies to rid the city of arbitrary restrictions on the living space of any group.[14]

A spirited public debate on the issue took place between the NPHC and representatives of the real estate industry. Real estate operator Newton C. Farr launched the discussion when he appeared before the prestigious City Club in early 1945 to defend the practice of restrictive covenants as a means of guaranteeing property values. In response, NPHC president George Quilici spoke to the same group and urged the "quick eradication" of the covenants, arguing that they "do not protect property values but actually destroy property values by causing overcrowding and overuse of property."[15]

Cantwell was glad that the battle had been joined and wanted to inject a moral tone to it from the outset. To this end, even before Quilici's appearance before the City Club, Cantwell had proposed a strong resolution to a statement being prepared by the NPHC, denouncing restrictive covenants as not only an economic curse but a moral cancer on the city of Chicago. Cantwell's strong words created a ripple of unease in the organization not only from Chicago Housing Authority chairman Robert Taylor, who served on the board, but also Robert Weaver, a black who would later be the first secretary of housing and

urban development under President Lyndon B. Johnson. Weaver expressed discomfort with Cantwell's moral indictment of restrictive covenants and urged Taylor:

> While it is true that there are moral questions incident to the operation of race restrictive covenants, I doubt that the NPHC of Chicago is primarily in the area of moral evaluations. I should like to see the first section concentrate upon the economic aspects of race restrictive covenants and minimize, if not exclude, reference to the moral problems involved.

Weaver also objected to Cantwell's insertion of a pledge of cooperation with the Chicago Council Against Racial and Religious Discrimination (an organization Cantwell had also helped found) "in its efforts to abolish restrictive covenants." He noted: "It would be extremely unfortunate to limit our cooperation or to imply we are limiting it to this one organization." He went on, "other organizations such as the NAACP, the Urban League, and the Mayor's Committee have all taken steps to fight restrictive covenants before the Chicago Council Against Racial and Religious Discrimination announced its program."[16] Cantwell however was not deterred by Weaver's attempt to short-circuit the moral dimensions of the issue. He wrote to Taylor:

> I was not aware that the N.P.H.C. of C. was organized to 'concentrate upon the economic aspects' of housing or of any of its allied problems. I was under the impression that we were concerned primarily with the people who needed housing, with human persons who have, through their spiritual nature, feelings, worth, dignity, and rights that find their recognition and partial guarantee in moral principles. If I have been wrong in that impression, I was also wrong in joining the organization.[17]

Cantwell's forcefulness pushed Taylor off the fence. "Restrictive covenants are an assault upon the dignity and spiritual value of the human being," he wrote to the priest. "The primary and compelling basis for opposition to restrictive covenants should be predicated upon these principles."[18] The moment was typical of Cantwell's approach to social issues. They were all moral. Although he could be consumately political in dealing with his

ecclesiatical superiors, Cantwell rarely flinched on a matter of moral significance. He drew strength from the certitudes of Catholic social teaching and hewed to his principles regardless of the cost. And often this adherence to principle paid off. Under the assaults of the Housing Conference and other like-minded groups, restrictive covenants began to melt away as judges increasingly refused to honor them. By the time the Supreme Court declared them unconstitutional in 1948, historian Arnold Hirsch attests, "restrictive covenants in Chicago served as little more than a fairly coarse sieve, unable to stop the flow of black population when put to the test."[19] The breakdown of restrictive covenants meant the complete collapse of any successful efforts to repel black immigration into white Chicago neighborhoods.

Cantwell continued to serve on the board of the Housing Conference until 1948 when the political orientation of the group caused him to resign and distance himself from them for a time. However, Cantwell's work with the NPHC provided an important liasion between the Catholic Church and local activists. Cantwell was elected to the board and immediately commissioned to recruit new members and help raise the sum of $4,000 to attract matching funds from Chicago businessman, Marshall Field III. Cantwell wrote to Catholic dignitaries including auxiliary bishops of Chicago—O'Brien and Sheil—as well as to Stritch. Sheil donated handsomely. Stritch called Cantwell in for a discussion, after which he donated a small sum of money. Despite its paucity the organizers were elated with Stritch's token response. Milton Shufro, the information officer of the CHA, wrote to thank Cantwell: "The fact that the Archbishop himself contributed, as a result of your discussion with him, is, of course, of considerable importance—much more than the actual donation."[20]

Cantwell also touched base with virtually every official who had some connection with housing issues. This included not only Shufro of the information office, but Robert Taylor, the chairman of the CHA Board, and the executive secretary, Elizabeth Wood. They in turn were glad to have Cantwell "on-board." When Cantwell voiced support for the Altgeld Gardens project at 130th Street and Langley, Shufro wrote a note of thanks saying: "You may know by this time how appreciative all

of us are for your interest and help in our program."[21] The Catholic Labor Alliance became an important springboard for Cantwell's concern for housing; it soon formed a housing committee and the pages of *Work* were often dedicated to discussion of housing issues.[22]

His high visibility on housing matters also won the attention of state and local officials such as Mayor Edward Kelly, who in 1946 invited Cantwell to become a member of the Veteran's Emergency Housing Committee.[23] Likewise, Governor Dwight Green asked him to serve on a state committee to study the housing shortage and propose measures to the Illinois State Assembly. However, when Green made derogatory comments about "New Deal type solutions" to housing issues during a radio broadcast, the utter integrity of Cantwell shone through and he rejected the Governor's invitation:

> It seems to me, that there can be no solution to the housing problem without the help of the type of governmental program presented to Congress by Senator Taft along with Senators Wagner and Ellender. Whether or not that program can be labeled "New Deal" interests me little. It seems to me that your statement which accompanied your letter is so obviously partisan that a committee launched with that as its guidepost is hopelessly limited in its scope and effectiveness.[24]

Cantwell's voice was heard also in the thickening controversy that surrounded the placement of public housing in the city. At the outset public housing was based on an "up and out" premise: Once people got on their feet they would move out of public housing and into single family dwellings.[25] However, after the war public housing became the permanent refuge of the poor, many of whom were black. This made the placement of public housing problematic, especially in neighborhoods seeking to protect their property values. Underlying the issue was the racial composition of the housing developments. Originally there had been racial and income restrictions on the people who could reside in the public facilities. But the income restrictions had dropped away when salaries rose sharply during the war. Rather than evict war workers who exceeded the income limit, a graduated rent policy was adopted by the housing authority. Strict racial composition rules, mandated originally by Interior

Secretary Harold Ickes, required that the racial balance of a neighborhood should not be disturbed by public housing. Hence, if there were no blacks in the area of a project, the project could only take whites. If it was 80 percent white and 20 black, the same had to obtain in the unit. This policy held firm during the war.

In 1946, however, at the instigation of Elizabeth Wood and Robert Taylor, the CHA changed its integration policy and set aside the neighborhood composition rule. Trouble began immediately at the 185-unit facility for veterans, called Airport Homes, near Midway Airport when white squatters refused to allow black veterans to move in. Angry whites denounced Wood and the CHA and insisted that she be dismissed and the body (legally independent of the city and hence free of the perils of Chicago aldermanic pressure) be absorbed into city government. Another confrontation occurred at Fernwood Park on the southwest side of the city when Wood told residents at a public meeting in 1947 that she would welcome blacks and whites to the project. Cantwell wrote to Mayor Edward Kelly (whose political career would be wrecked by the racial disturbances) urging him to retain Wood.

> I wish ... most vehemently to deprecate the efforts to remove Elizabeth Wood from the position which she has held with honor and the efforts to change the status or policies of the Chicago Housing Authority. I know of no agency in government where there has been a more unselfish devotion to principle or where there has been such a scrupulous effort to apply them judiciously.[26]

The following year, however, an act of the state legislature left approval of CHA locations to the city council. This hopelessly politicized decisions regarding public housing. It also put Catholic leaders who did not share Cantwell's moral certitude about the right and wrong in these situations in a difficult position. They knew (and priests like Cantwell often reminded them) that the teaching of their church compelled respect for the rights of persons to adequate shelter and open housing. But Catholic members of the city council also knew that many in their communities, Catholic and Protestant, did not want the projects in their neighborhoods. As a result, Catholic politicians

and Catholic residents of "endangered" neighborhoods did not often concur in Cantwell's moral assessment of housing issues.[27] For them, the question was property values and neighborhood homogeneity. Cardinal Stritch was also somewhat ambivalent on these matters, agonizing as he always did over both sides of the issue. Moreover, further complicating these matters were urban renewal efforts which involved the relocation of people from one part of the city to another.

URBAN RENEWAL

Other urban issues surfaced in the postwar years, initially distinct from but later related to, the public housing issue. In 1947 the State of Illinois expanded the foundations of New Deal initiatives for the rejuvenation of cities begun ten years earlier by establishing a formula for a partnership of private and public resources to reclaim blighted and rundown areas. Urban renewal became an important goal in the urban policies of Chicago in the forties and fifties. Its chief promoters were representatives of the large Chicago downtown businesses, especially Milton C. Mumford, an assistant vice-president of Marshall Field and Company, and Holman D. Pettibone, president of the Chicago Title and Trust Company. Their goal was to arrest the physical deterioration of the downtown and attract businesses and solvent people back to the inner city.[28] Beginning in 1944, they shared their plans with local businessmen and the Metropolitan Housing and Planning Council (MHPC), led by Ferd Kramer, head of one of the largest realty firms in the city. What developed was a combination of private and public efforts that would acquire land, make it reasonable to buy, and then encourage private development. This process would effectively reclaim areas of the city threatened by blight and restore them to productivity and livablity. Everyone would profit.[29]

Mumford and Pettibone spent long hours cultivating business leaders, politicians, and other influential forces in Chicago and initiated a proposal passed by the Illinois State Legislature called the Blighted Areas Redevelopment Act. This law accomplished all the developers' goals. It expanded the powers of the city to acquire property and clear slums. The property could

then be sold to private developers at a "written down" cost. Moreover the decisions on land clearance would be made not by the socially conscious Chicago Housing Authority, which traditionally had the powers to acquire and clear land, but by a new development-minded agency called the Chicago Land Clearance Commission, headed by Ira Bach. A critical part of the 1947 law, which had the support of Mayor Martin Kennelly and Governor Dwight Green, made public housing a tool of urban renewal interests. People dislocated by the projects had to be moved, and decisions about sites for public housing would become even more controversial. If many Chicagoans were leery of public housing, urban renewal was a program that would create an even greater need for these facilities.

The laboratory for Chicago's plunge into urban renewal was the near South Side. Once the site of some of Chicago's finest mansions and still the home of many prestigious Chicago institutions, by the late forties it was threatened by a blight that seemed certain to overwhelm it. Even before the legislation of 1947, the Illinois Institute of Technology (IIT) had begun to reclaim portions of the South Side with an ambitious building program, including structures designed by the German refugee-architect, Mies Van de Rohe. It expanded its holdings from seven to 110 acres by purchasing adjacent real estate as it came on the market. Not far behind was Michael Reese Hospital, which hired a full-time planner, Reginald Isaacs, and began its program of rejuvenation in 1945. Michael Reese worked with the CHA to buy land and relocate people—investing over $600,000 in a private program of development. In 1946 Reese and the IIT formed the South Side Planning Board (SSPB), a private reform group that pushed urban renewal and coordinated redevelopment programs on the South Side. It was through this group that the Catholic Archdiocese of Chicago became involved in urban renewal issues with all their attendant implications.[30]

The potential benefit to the archdiocese for Catholic participation in the activities of the SSPB was considerable, as Stritch's first urban affairs advisor pointed out:

> I personally surveyed the entire area outlined on the enclosed map and note that it embraces all or part of eleven parishes. I called on priests and religious of these parishes and Catholic

institutions to obtain a complete picture of the holdings of the Archdiocese in this area. Obviously to redevelop this area would be of inestimable value to the Catholic parishes and institutions therein. To remove the blight from this slum area and establish good housing for both white and colored would benefit the people morally and in every other way. It would bring new and large congregations to the fine old churches of this area and incidentally increase the value of church property. I believe our Catholic churches would benefit from this program more than any other institution or any business house because our holdings are many and are scattered throughout the entire area.[31]

Moreover, the movers and shakers of the SSPB, IIT and Michael Reese Hospital sincerely wanted archdiocesan participation as well as the cooperation of Mercy Hospital on Prairie Avenue, the largest and oldest Catholic hospital on the South Side. In response to this, Stritch appointed Father Thomas Reed, executive director of the Church Extension Society to serve as his liaison with the SSPB.[32] Although he had no training for the work, Reed lived at old St. John's parish on Eighteenth and Clark, near the proposed redevelopment site, and soon became well-informed on urban issues and the politics of urban renewal. Because of this he was able to serve as Stritch's eyes and ears in Chicago's programs of urban renewal and neighborhood conservation, and was the prelate's main contact with the legion of city, state, and federal officials who were concerned with urban affairs. Through Reed, Stritch contributed substantially to the work of the SSPB. Reed also succeeded in recruiting prominent Catholic laymen such as Blackstone Hotel owner Fred Morelli and Dr. John McNamara of Mercy Hospital for the governing council of the board. With their help and other contributions from the members of the board an executive secretary was hired for the operation along with a small staff.

THE MERCY AREA

Stritch's interests in reclaiming the near South Side were largely motivated by his desire to preserve two major Catholic institutions located there, Mercy Hospital and the Loyola School

of Medicine.[33] Mercy Hospital was one of the oldest Catholic health care institutions in Chicago. It had originally been opened at a site on Michigan Avenue and in 1910 moved to Prairie Avenue. During its history it had alternately affiliated with Rush Medical College, Chicago Medical College, and Northwestern University. In 1919, at Cardinal Mundelein's urging, Mercy broke off from Northwestern and affiliated with the Loyola School of Medicine which had opened in 1910. The affiliation went well, but by the thirties, differences of opinion between the sisters and the Jesuits at Loyola began to unravel the relationship. Moreover, the medical school also began to have serious financial problems.

When Stritch arrived in 1940 he was determined to keep the hospital and the school open and together. His interest in the Loyola School of Medicine led him to take an active part in fund-raising efforts and he hosted an annual dinner that raised thousands each year for the school.[34] In 1948 he also induced wealthy Chicagoan Frank J. Lewis (a regular benefactor of Bishop Sheil) to put up money to help build new facilities for the medical school.[35] So grateful was the school to Stritch that they renamed themselves the Stritch School of Medicine in 1948. Stritch also tried to support the hospital and developed close ties with the mother provincial of the Mercy Sisters, Domitilla Griffin, sister of Springfield bishop James Griffin. When tensions developed between the school and the hospital, Stritch often interjected himself as an honest broker between the two institutions and tried to bring peace.

However, his efforts to keep the hospital and school together faced additional challenge when the area around Mercy began to succumb to blight. When Michael Reese and IIT began their collaboration (prior to the actual founding of the SSPB,) Stritch urged the superior of the hospital community to give the planner, Reginald Isaacs, a fair hearing. "Will you please appoint a committee and ask this committee to get in touch with Mr. Isaacs and go over with him the plan which he has formulated."[36] However, the sisters were not as enthused about the promises of planners and were sensitive to a growing chorus of complaints from doctors and staff who were afraid to live and work in the area. As a result, in 1947 the Sisters of

Mercy announced their intention to move into an expanded modern building on Chicago's near North Side. The proposed complex would be twenty-seven stories tall and have an eleven-story nurses' residence.[37] A huge fund-raising campaign was launched in April 1947 to collect $6 million for the new facility. Stritch reluctantly agreed to be the honorary chairman of the drive and contributed a check of $10,000.[38] However, Stritch's real hope was to keep Mercy on the South Side. Using his personal influence with the Mother, Domitilla Griffin, the cardinal and Monsignor Reed convinced the community to remain on the near South Side with lavish promises that the area around the hospital would be revitalized. To honor promises to the Mercy Sisters and keep Catholic health care alive on the near South Side, Reed made the preservation and expansion of the so-called "Mercy Area" his primary objective in often entangled negotiations of the South Side revitalization project. The sisters were skeptical at first and continued to raise funds for a new hospital.

THE WORK OF THE SSPB: LAKE MEADOWS

Keeping Mercy on the South Side required a host of other complex and interlocking steps which brought about significant archdiocesan cooperation with the planners and developers of the SSPB. Soon after its formation, the SSPB worked to devise a plan of action for the redevelopment of the whole South Side. Within days of the enactment of the 1947 legislation, "An Opportunity for Private and Public Investment in Rebuilding Chicago" was issued by the staff of the SSPB.[39] The report, which listed the Archdiocese of Chicago as one of its sponsors, was aimed at potential investors, and declared the long-term commitment of the IIT, Michael Reese Hospital, and other major institutions to the renewal of the near South Side. Shortly after the report was issued, the New York Life Insurance Company announced it would build an enormous apartment complex in the SSPB area. The procuring of land for this project, called Lake Meadows, took about four years, so it was not until 1952 that ground was broken. Lake Meadows was the flagship for the whole SSPB program. If it succeeded, other plans would succeed; if it failed, it would mean the demise of the whole project. Helping Lake

Meadows succeed was thus linked to Stritch's hopes for Mercy Hospital.

Naturally, the process was not smooth. The year after New York Life announced its plans, the federal government expanded its commitment to housing by enacting the Federal Housing Law of 1949. This legislation offered substantial federal subsidies for such urban renewal programs as those conceived by the SSPB, on the condition that adequate provision be made for the relocation of those displaced. The problem for Lake Meadows, then, was what to do with the people who were displaced by the project. As it was planned, Lake Meadows would not only dislocate slum dwellers, but it also involved the demolition of a number of middle-class dwellings. Virtually all of the displaced would be black. Although New York Insurance planned to allow blacks into its new buildings, it soon became evident that Lake Meadows would be too expensive for many of the former inhabitants of the area.

This realization sent waves of anxiety through the African-American community, fearful of being made homeless in a city that already circumscribed where they could live. Public housing was one way out of the dilemma, and relocation sites, like the nearby Dearborn Homes, became prime options. But public housing was a hot political issue and it was feared that white developers intended to empty the South Side of blacks. This led black alderman Archibald Carey to introduce a resolution in the city council that some viewed as a potential threat to the whole development program. He proposed a ruling that all housing built on land conveyed to private interests by the CHA or the Chicago Land Clearance Commission be made available to occupancy "without discrimination or segregation on account of race, creed, color, national origin, or ancestry."[40] Since this meant integrated public housing facilities, the Carey ordinance threatened to stall the plans for urban renewal, because public housing could not easily be built on a nondiscriminatory basis in all neighborhoods in Chicago. Without adequate relocation sites crucial federal funding would not forthcoming. Single-handedly Carey would have stopped the steamroller of urban renewal dead in its tracks. Catholic leaders viewed this with alarm. Reed wrote to Stritch in early 1949:

> Alderman Carey has before the City Council a proposed ordinance which would legally require a non-discrimination policy in any housing that involved public funds in the assembly of land or in the actual building. Most of the members of our Board believe that Alderman Carey's proposal to force better racial relations by law is unnecessary and certainly is frightening away private capital which is interested in slum redevelopment.

Reed went on to sketch Carey's background:

> He is the son of the well-known Bishop Carey, A.F.M. The Alderman is a minister in charge of the Woodlawn A.M.E. Church. He is also an attorney. Some time ago, he officiated at the marriage of a young couple from our neighborhood. A few months after the marriage he as an attorney obtained a divorce for the woman and shortly thereafter as a minister officiated at her marriage with another party. He is reputed to have an interest in a Negro Life Insurance Company.[41]

With Stritch's permission and encouragement, Reed lobbied Catholic aldermen to defeat the Carey measure and helped secure the closure of Cottage Grove Avenue, a north-south road that bisected the project. When the vote was taken in December 1950 and approved by the city council, Reed wrote to Stritch:

> As reported in the press, the City Council voted 30 to 12 in favor of the New York Life project plans which include the closing of a small part of Cottage Grove Avenue. About two years from now when all the property of this project will be assembled, the City Council will have to vote for the vacation of this part of Cottage Grove and parts of other adjacent streets. This will need a two-thirds majority vote. By that time many of the objectors will be moved to other neighborhoods and the city will have invested so much money into this project that no further effective resistance is anticipated.[42]

Stritch wrote approvingly: "The decision about Cottage Grove Avenue pleased me since it opens the way for a realization of great improvement for our city."[43] It also built support among city council members for the preservation and expansion of the Mercy Area.

THE SEVEN SITES CONTROVERSY

The Carely ordinance was only one of many obstacles that the Lake Meadows project had to overcome. Most especially, as the Carey ordinance scare had demonstrated, it had to provide an acceptable plan for the relocation of those moved out. This hurdle would be overcome with help from Cardinal Stritch. The relocation problem was indeed serious. One study estimated that 16,199 families would be displaced by the Congress Street Expressway, the New York Life Project, West Side Medical Center Expansion, Illinois Institute of Technology expansion, elimination of "alley dwellings," and relocation for new or expanded CHA projects. Relocation housing was built in eight "Courts" projects (Racine Courts, LeClaire Courts, Harrison Courts, Maplewood Courts, Ogden Courts, Archer Courts, Loomis Courts, and Prairie Avenue Courts).[44] Financing came from state funds and matching funds from a voter-approved bond issue in 1947 providing new housing for 1,500 families. The arguments over site selection for these relocation facilities were serious, but sites in white areas were approved when Mayor Kennelly agreed to limit the numbers of blacks who could move into them. However, the "Courts" projects were still woefully inadequate and the need for more relocation housing was evident.

In July 1949 the CHA came to the rescue, proposing construction of 40,000 units during a six-year period with the federal government underwriting the building of 21,000 of these units in the first two years. But where were the sites to be located? CHA board chairman Robert Taylor submitted a list of seven sites that included a mixture of slum clearance land and vacant land around the city. Predictably this aroused the ire of aldermen who fought against public housing in white areas. Once again, the controversy slowed the project and even made New York Life publicly skittish on the Lake Meadows project. Hearings opened in February 1950, and Daniel Cantwell entered the fray, lobbying vigorously for the acceptance of the seven sites. He explained his position in a letter to Alderman George J. Tourek:

> Chicago has a rare opportunity to help solve the housing prob-
> lem for a large segment of our citizens in the housing possible
> under the federal housing act of 1949. The approval, therefore, of
> the seven sites selected by the Chicago Plan Commission and the
> Chicago Housing Authority for public housing is very important
> in the minds of us all.... I am glad to see our ward have a project
> that will be open to all Americans—Negroes and Whites. No real
> American could want anything else. No Christian dare want any-
> thing else. Christ will judge us on how we treat our fellow men.[45]

In an even more dramatic endorsement of the seven sites,
Cantwell issued a statement under the auspices of the Catholic
Labor Alliance:

> Tens of thousands of Chicago families, Negro and White are liv-
> ing in homes that do not meet even the specifications of the U.S.
> Department of Agriculture for breeding hogs, cattle and chick-
> ens.... The Chicago Housing Authority and the Plan Commission
> have selected seven sites, three on vacant land, four on land to be
> cleared. The common good will best be served by approving the
> seven sites as a package. Under no circumstances should the
> vacant sites be rejected. That would deny to low income families,
> Negro and white, some enjoyment of the open spaces, the light
> and air, which God has provided for all of us.[46]

On this issue Cantwell collided with Archbishop Stritch,
who was quite aware of the political controversy the site selection had stirred up. Stritch worried that any hitch in the Lake
Meadows plans could create a backlash against his designs to
keep Mercy Hospital alive on the near South Side. But Stritch
also disliked the forced integration that the CHA relocation plan
entailed, as he commented to Archbishop Aloisius Muench:

> Here in Chicago, we really have a very serious housing problem.
> The city grows year after year, largely from the influx of negroes
> and the slums become wider, and blight touches even the fair
> residential districts. The city, in cooperation with the Federal
> government has a program, but it has not been very successful in
> its execution. There is a great difficulty about putting the pro-
> gram into execution. According to the norm, which I think the
> Federal government imposes, a certain percentage of the housing

facilities must be available to the colored. This, of course creates objections in some neighborhoods to the placing of housing facilities in those neighborhoods. I don't see why they should put any percentage norm on this activity. It seems to me just as unconstitutional to say that 20% of a new housing project must be open to the colored as it is to say that no colored can live in such a housing project. The housing projects ought to be built for all people, and everybody who is eligible for residence in them should be admitted. The large insurance companies and some private corporations are going at the problem in a more constructive sort of way. We are in it up to the neck, because it is so important to us.[47]

Given Stritch's feelings and the work that Reed had been doing with planners and developers, he was surprised and angry when he read in the February 22 edition of the *Chicago Sun-Times* of Cantwell's support for the seven sites. He dashed off a stern letter to Cantwell:

I thought I made it clear that I wanted you, before taking a definite position in these matters, to consult me. You cannot possibly have all my thoughts on them, and it is very easy for you to appear as contrary to my policy. In the future, before you write anything for papers or make any statements on such matters or in any way take part in matters before our public authorities for decision, I want you to consult me.[48]

Cantwell wrote a lengthy letter to Stritch, defending himself and insisting that his support for the seven sites was in a private in-house MHPC document not intended for public consumption:

I did not commit the Church, nor you nor even myself to the seven sites. I did not assume competence to judge them technically....after I pointed out that technically competent persons had after long study approved them, I thought it advisable that the flood-gates of prejudice and selfishness should not be opened in facing this important matter in the City Council. If the sites approved by the experts were to be set aside the reasons should in the interest of justice and peace be clear and above reproach.[49]

In the end the seven sites were defeated, and the ensuing legislation for public housing resulted in a net gain of only forty-seven new units for the city on four inner-city sites.[50] Virtually

all of the sites were on inner-city land or were additions to already existing public housing projects outside the inner city. One would have thought that this ended the matter, but one last hurdle remained.[51]

STRITCH'S INTERVENTION

Even with the approval of the four sites, the Federal Home and Housing Finance Administration still remained unconvinced of the adequacy of the relocation plan and held up approval of the funding. Once again the whole cause of urban renewal in Chicago seemed imperiled. One priest, Father John Ireland Gallery, who was planning for a housing development in his own South Side parish, contacted Stritch and urged him to use his influence with Raymond Foley, administrator of the Housing and Home Finance Agency in Washington, D.C., to secure federal funds for the proposed public housing sites.[52] Gallery wrote:

> So far approval has been withheld, as well as approval of the New York Life (Private) site, mostly because Washington has not been satisfied with Chicago's plans for relocation of present occupants. Part of the impasse is a jurisdictional dispute between federal and city authorities. The local people take the position that the federal men must accept plans that have been agreed on by all here concerned. Foley and Co. feel they must answer to congress if they create a group of American displaced persons, especially when those people will be negroes seeking to enter other neighborhoods.... If you could induce Ray Foley to take action either directly or by setting up a conference on the four sites, you will have broken an impasse that is beginning to look hopeless.[53]

Stritch's contacts with federal housing officials stretched back to the days when Gael Sullivan was the director of the Federal Housing Administration in Illinois. Sullivan had gotten Stritch's brother, Emmett, a job with the agency, and Emmett had kept Stritch in contact with the housing issues of the day. Stritch knew Foley and gladly complied with Gallery's request.[54] When Catholic Charities chief Monsignor John O'Grady came to

town in September 1951, Stritch called on the monsignor to deliver a personal message to Foley asking him to continue the project. O'Grady complied and drafted a memorandum to Foley which requested approval of the housing plans for the city of Chicago.[55] O'Grady wrote:

> It seems to me that from the standpoint of Chicago the only sensible approach to this problem of relocating families that have been displaced by the New York Life Insurance Company project and by other public improvements in the City is the immediate construction of a sizeable number of private housing units for middle-income negro families.[56]

Foley complied with Stritch's request and the public housing was begun, thereby removing the last obstacle to the Lake Meadows project. In 1952 the first spades of dirt were turned over in a project that would be the first of many high-rise towers to line the fashionable Lake Shore of Chicago. Little did many of the residents of Lake Meadows know that they had the cardinal archbishop of Chicago to thank for their new handsome dwellings.

One might have thought that the Lake Meadows triumph with all that it meant for the revitalization of the near South Side would have been enough to keep Mercy Hospital and the medical school in place. Indeed, the sisters even suspended fundraising for a new hospital in 1952 and all seemed to be proceeding according to plan. However, Stritch's work was not done. In 1954 the sisters and Loyola grew impatient with the slow pace of change in the area around the hospital. They then tried a power play of their own and announced a plan to move to the suburb of Skokie, where Loyola had purchased fifty acres of land. Annexation of the Skokie land to the city of Chicago and rezoning took place rapidly. However, Stritch again intervened and Mercy and Loyola remained in place.

However, as soon as external matters seemed to be settled, internal problems between the hospital and the medical school erupted that again threatened continuation at the South Side location. Stritch tried again to patch things over, this time with the help of millionaire and hospital benefactor John Cuneo. But this was to no avail and when Stritch finally left Chicago in 1958,

the feuding between the two institutions escalated. Once again the sisters threatened to leave the near South Side. Egan, now at the head of the Cardinal's Conservation Committee, moved into the dispute and, together with James Doyle, director of the Land Clearance Commission, met with the administration of Mercy Hospital and the sisters. In their discussions, the long-stalled proposal for the Mercy Area were unjammed and the nuns were offered land extending to Michigan Avenue for the price of $250,000, with the assurance that the proposed expressway would run immediately north of them, giving the entire metropolitan area access to Mercy Hospital from every direction.[57] Only half of Stritch's dream for Mercy and the Loyola Medical school could be salvaged. On May 8, 1959, Mercy Hospital and Loyola University jointly announced their decisions. Mercy decided to stay on the South Side and build a new facility with the land Reed and Stritch had acquired for them. Loyola broke away from the rocky marriage with Mercy Hospital and pursued a policy of affiliation with an existing hospital for several years until it eventually built its own medical center on the West Side of the city.

THE CARDINAL'S CONSERVATION COMMITTEE

Stritch's early enthusiasm for urban renewal (especially when it meant keeping Mercy Hospital on the South Side) was eventually cooled by the slow pace with which promises to rehabilitate the Mercy Area were realized. He was also deeply affected by the social problems created by the relocation of people from slum clearance sites to thriving and stable neighborhoods. While urban developers collected their fees and regaled in their splendid accomplishments for the cause of urban renewal, the displaced crowded into neighborhoods that were not ready to accept them. What affected the neighborhoods affected the Catholic Church in Chicago. As a result, although patterns of cooperation with urban planners and developers were maintained, there was a gradual shift in emphasis to neighborhood conservation. Indeed, by the early fifties Stritch was urging the expansion of "subsidized housing" and the removal of "under-standard housing" and he wrote to Cantwell:

Unless Chicago does something and does something in a positive sort of way in the very near future, the flow to the suburbs will continue, and Chicago will find itself in bad shape. All this is not necessary, because many of these areas can be made and preserved as good residence districts with a little planning and a little care. I am very anxious to see the report which is going to be submitted to the Mayor next week on this whole problem.[58]

The "report" he spoke of was the plan to create a city conservation board. Indeed conservation would become the centerpiece of Chicago urban policy.

In Chicago urban pastors were among the first to feel the problems of rapidly changing neighborhoods. From among their ranks would come initiatives in solving the problems of deteriorating neighborhoods. One such pastor was Father John Ireland Gallery, who belonged to a prominent naval family which included two admirals. He was ordained in 1926 and assigned to Monsignor David "Packy" Ryan at St. Bernard's parish on the South Side. When he returned from the Navy in 1946 to take up the pastorate of South Side St. Cecilia's parish on Forty-sixth Street, Gallery remembered Ryan's proudest boast was that he had encouraged restrictive covenants in the housing contracts of the parishioners.[59] A determined, if at times eccentric man, Gallery would pioneer an aggressive stand against urban blight. St. Cecilia's was on the fringe of the black belt in a neighborhood with many wooden frame houses and lower-class whites. Many of the people of the area were renters and a good deal of the land was owned by real estate developers. Upon his arrival, Gallery found high anxiety levels in the parish due to an influx of blacks into the neighborhood. In discussing his worries about the future of the neighborhood with one of his classmates, Monsignor William Campbell of the Catholic University, Gallery was introduced to Monsignor John O'Grady, executive secretary of National Catholic Charities.

O'Grady's interest in housing went back to the thirties, when he lobbied New Deal officials for housing legislation. Moreover, he was an admirer of the organizational tactics of Saul D. Alinsky, whose work he had seen in action during the organization of the Back-of-the-Yards Neighborhood in the thirties.[60] Through O'Grady and Back-of-the-Yards organizer Joseph

Meegan (whose father, Owen, was the janitor at St. Cecilia's), Gallery came to know Alinsky, who helped him organize the West Kenwood Association in 1946.[61] Gallery used the group to press for strict adherence to building code requirements, thereby preventing the doubling and tripling up in houses by incoming blacks. He also urged cleaner and safer neighborhoods, even to the extent of providing garbage cans for persons who did not own them. Gallery boldly marched into the offices of city officials and pressed for slum clearance in his parish. He was able to induce the Chicago Dwellings Association, a semi-private building group, to construct a series of single-family row houses, called Fuller Park Gardens, in 1954.

Ultimately, Gallery was unable to prevent the total evacuation of the area by whites, and by the time he became pastor of St. Christina's parish on the far South Side in 1958, the area around the parish was black. The following year, Gallery's successor, Father Thomas Hosty, sold some parish property for the expressway, and even though St. Cecilia's itself hung on after the Dan Ryan Expressway opened in 1962, its days were numbered.[62] Ten years later the church building was so dilapidated it had to be razed.[63] Nonetheless, at the time, Gallery's efforts were lauded by many as a shining example of community conservation which utilized the parish church as a catalyst for community survival.[64]

O'Grady and Gallery urged Chicago clergy to hold meetings if they were concerned with the deterioration of their neighborhoods and the blight that seemed to accompany African-American migration. Gallery insisted again and again that "Black did not necessarily mean blight," and he urged the priests not to succumb to the same panic which often beset their parishioners. In October 1951 Gallery invited Monsignor Thomas Reed and Monsignor John O'Grady to a meeting which included many of the pastors from blighted areas. Among them were Auxiliary Bishop William E. Cousins, pastor of the rapidly changing St. Columbanus in Park Manor, Monsignor William Byron of St. Joachim's on Ninety-first and Langley on the South Side, and Father Francis Lavin of St. James. Present also were Father James Doyle, Stritch's representative on expressway development, Alderman Robert E. Merriam, chairman of the

housing committee on the city council, and Frederick T. Aschman, executive director of the Chicago Plan Commission. At the meeting O'Grady made clear that the "problem of cleaning slums is not the simple problem which it was thought to be early in our thinking on the subject." The Charities chief pointed out that people who were dislocated were not always eligible for public housing, and "we are becoming acutely aware of the impact of slum areas upon other parts of the city." O'Grady called for a coordination of public agencies, FHA, CHA, CLCC, CDA, private builders, financiers, and the people themselves to solve the problems. O'Grady, Reed, and Merriam agreed that the job "required a maximum of coordination and that the city must give official recognition to a conservation program."[65]

Gallery used the opportunity to share the success of the West Kenwood Association. He recounted his efforts to stop the spread of panic among the white people by stemming the spread of blight. He urged strict enforcement of the building code to prevent multiple-family dwellings, the development of a sound community program, and extolled the advantages of the neighborhood (proximity to work and recreation). He concluded by stating that there were two essential considerations contributing to the Association's hope for success. The first was to talk about race relations as little as possible—this with the conviction that the key to a solution of the problems of transition areas lay in the development of sound neighborhood units and thereby race difficulties would resolve themselves. The second was to develop a full and integrated program of neighborhood conservation by bringing together elected officials, public agencies and city departments, neighborhood civic groups, newspapers, and individuals.[66]

In 1952 Mayor Kennelly had appointed a special commission headed by city housing administrator James Downs to study conservation. It issued a report to the mayor in November 1952 urging strong city support and coordination of agencies to deal with neighborhood conservation. The result was the enactment of the Illinois Housing Act of 1954. Under section 220 of the law, each municipality was empowered to establish a Community Conservation Board to determine the appropriateness of declaring certain areas conservation areas. If

this were done, the residents of that area would be permitted to avail themselves of liberalized rehabilitation mortgages and thus stabilize and upgrade their neighborhoods. These efforts at community conservation had already been anticipated by the Catholic pastors of Chicago.

Monsignor Reed was enthusiastic about conservation work and on October 31, 1952, he wrote to Stritch:

> On the subject of "The Pastor and Neighborhood Conservation" I have mentioned in earlier reports that studies were being made on this problem by various civic and private agencies, the results of these studies will not appear until probably the early part of 1953. In the meantime however, much thought and experimentation has been devoted to this problem and I join in the opinion of several others that this problem should be brought to the attention of many of our pastors to acquaint them with the problem and the results so far of the studies and experiments conducted to meet this challenge. This is important because of the rapid spread of blight throughout large areas of the city. Monsignor John O'Grady, Monsignor John Fitzgerald, Monsignor William Byron and the Reverends John I. Gallery, John Gleeson, James Doyle and others would be willing to conduct a meeting on this subject for approximately 40 pastors whose parishes are directly in the path of blight.[67]

Reed's suggestion was approved, and a meeting was called at the Lake Shore Club for November 26, 1952. Under Stritch's signature a letter was sent inviting pastors from threatened areas. "Strong and adequate family life," Stritch wrote, "cannot be maintained without concern with the damaging effects of inadequate housing and deteriorating neighborhoods." He continued: "Our concern with the spiritual, social and economic aspects of community life is shared by public officials...."[68] In addition to the clerical participants, Reed invited Downs and Aschman, together with D. E. Mackelman, deputy coordinator of the Plan Commission, and Saul Alinsky of the Industrial Areas Foundation. In his speech to the assembled pastors, ghost written by Reed, Stritch insisted that near blight areas "can be changed. They can be saved." He concluded his talk:

I would like to have you consider this problem very thoroughly. We are in a position to do a great deal toward building up neighborliness and self-help in our neighborhoods. Naturally there is another phase to our pastoral problem. As things are going now, we are building a new archdiocese on the perimeter of Chicago. This is a very heavy burden. It would not be what it is, if we only try to save Chicago, save Chicago from itself, save Chicago from some of its greedy citizens, working the thing out in a plan. We can not only reclaim some of the blighted areas ... but we can prevent other areas from becoming blighted.[69]

In April of the following year, a follow-up conference was held at one of the largest parishes on the South Side, St. Sabina's Parish at Seventy-eighth and Throop. Its founding pastor, Father John Egan (no relation to the Cana head), had built a magnificent plant and had established an athletic and recreational program that drew youth from over ninety parishes.[70] Since 1952 Father John A. McMahon had been pastor, having come from St. Charles Borromeo, a West Side parish in the throes of racial transition. McMahon saw the same thing happening at St. Sabina's as the city's black belt moved inexorably south. The April 16, 1953, meeting was attended by Reed, Downes, Monsignor George Casey (who had taken a personal interest in the question of changing parishes), O'Grady, and leaders from assorted community organizations, including Fred Henderson of the Southtown Planning Association, Julian Levi of the South East Chicago Commission, Joseph Meegan of the Back-of-the-Yards Council, and Saul Alinsky of the Industrial Areas Foundation. While the general topic was a discussion of conservation efforts on the South Side, another item for discussion was a piece of pending legislation, explained by Julian Levi, involving penalties for zoning violations.[71] Levi urged Reed to encourage the pastors to lobby their representatives and senators on behalf of this legislation. It was the first time that Levi would be introduced to Catholic circles.

In the wake of the St. Cecilia and St. Sabina's meetings, the prominent pastors concerned formed a steering committee to establish an Archdiocesan Conservation Committee, formally called the Cardinal's Conservation Committee. The steering

committee included Reed, Monsignor John D. Fitzgerald (now the pastor of Ascension parish in Oak Park), Monsignor William Gorman of Resurrection parish on the West Side (chaplain of the city fire departments), Father John Ireland Gallery, Monsignor Vincent Moran of St. Philip Neri parish, and Father Martin Farrell of St. James parish. This group set to work learning about successful neighborhood conservation programs. They then launched an educational campaign designed to acquaint the pastors and parishes in changing neighborhoods with the nature and extent of the problems facing them.

At these meetings Reed encouraged conservation efforts while keeping Stritch informed about the situations he encountered. One outcome of these meetings was a conservation program spearheaded by Father John Quinn Corcoran of St. Mel-Holy Ghost parish on the West Side. Because of Corcoran's work with the Holy Name Society of this huge parish Reed urged the priest to use existing Holy Name groupings within the parish to form a community organization that would preserve the community. Corcoran responded positively and helped form the Garfield Park West Community Organization, which, at its peak, enrolled five thousand members.[72] Corcoran worked tirelessly with businessmen to stem blight by insisting on the maintenance of building codes, compelling unsavory businesses to leave, and encouraging white residents not to panic at the approach of blacks on the West Side. Corcoran's work was typical of the kinds of groups the Cardinal's Conservation Committee inspired.[73] Father Thaddeus Neckerman of Sts. Peter and Paul in South Chicago, Father John R. Gleason at St. Columbanus in Park Manor, Servite Father Jerome DePensier of the Basilica of Our Lady of Sorrows on the West Side, Monsignor William Murphy of St. Carthage Church on the South Side, and Monsignor Joseph Cussen of Our Lady of the Angels Church also formed conservation groups to stem urban blight.

Conservation organizations were often successful in preserving neighborhoods threatened by deterioration and decline. But they also were suspected by some priests (Cantwell, for one) of being "fronts" for the old neighborhood protective associations that tried to keep blacks out.[74] Indeed, when Monsignor

John Egan took over the administration of the Conservation Committee, one of his first targets was the City Conservation Board. Egan's insistence on neighborhood integration led him to change the tactics of the Cardinal's Conservation Committee and insist on more racial integration than earlier community organizers had done.

As it urged community organization, the Cardinal's Conservation Committee also continued private dialogue with influential city officials to bring about slum clearance and the conservation of selected neighborhoods. One important project was on the near South Side: Father Martin Farrell of St. James parish on Twenty-ninth and Wabash proposed the building of low-income row-housing on land adjacent to the parish. The St. James project received many promises of support from private developers and public officials. Even though there were differences, Catholic officials were especially careful not to publicly antagonize or alienate city officials. This was evident in Stritch's reaction to a pamphlet entitled "The Church and Neighborhood Conservation in Chicago," published by Monsignor John O'Grady under the auspices of National Catholic Charities. O'Grady used Chicago as an example of positive action in behalf of critical urban issues, but when he singled out some problematic areas between Church and urban developers, Stritch had them excised from a preliminary draft of the text.[75] "I think," he wrote Thomas Reed, "we are not doing the right thing if we direct criticism against the authorities. Our work is to try to cooperate with the authorities and try to make proper representations to them. It would be very much better, it seems to me, to do this in conferences and conversations and not to bring out the fact of a real divergence in a public pamphlet."[76]

EXPRESSWAY BUILDING AND THE CHURCH

One instance of church and government cooperation was the negotiation of rights-of-way for the rapidly expanding expressway system in Chicago. Expressways were indispensable arteries of commerce and communication, but they also reshaped urban neighborhoods, splitting some in two and even

destroying others. The original highway projections for Chicago had been developed in the thirties. When the war was over, the State of Illinois assumed the responsibility for planning and building some of its own roads, but in the fifties federal funds became available for a massive interstate highway system. Three major highways came to be built in the Chicago area: the West Side or Congress Street Expressway, the South Side expressway (called the Dan Ryan), and the Northwest Expressway (later called the Kennedy). In the mid sixties a road extending southwest of the city (the Stevenson) also jutted out from the downtown. Each of these projects involved tremendous amounts of money, complicated land assembly deals, rights-of-way, and land clearance.

The direct impact of this building program on the parishes seemed minimal. In all, only five parish plants were completely obliterated by the advent of expressways. (One of them, Holy Guardian Angels was destroyed twice.) The more significant problem were the parishes directly affected by the encroachment of the expressway in their territorial boundaries. Twenty-five parishes were affected in this manner. Old parishes with fairly well-defined boundaries were often bisected or even trisected by the building of expressways. Even though the numbers of houses moved might have been minimal, the expressways set up geographical barriers which were psychological roadblocks to parishioners. Moreover, the presence of a noisy expressway with its noxious fumes, congestion, and the alteration of traffic patterns by the presence of on and off ramps made urban properties less valuable and caused people to move. Even more, the displacement resulting from freeway expansion was extensive.

Once expressway building picked up steam in the fifties, Stritch tried to deal with it as he had urban renewal, by appointing a priest to oversee the matter. His selection here was Father James Doyle, who also served (ironically) as the archdiocesan director for displaced persons coming into the diocese from Iron Curtain countries. Swamped with work from his other responsibilities, Doyle was unable to give expressway issues the same attention Reed gave to urban affairs. As a result negotiations with expressway planners were often undertaken by individual priests or ethnic groups who had specific goals in mind.

The indomitable John Ireland Gallery, for example, used his influence of his family name and city hall contacts (as well as dogged persistence) to compel a shift in the direction of the Dan Ryan Expressway. When he learned that a portion of his parish (land between Wells and Wentworth Avenue) was in the path of the newly planned expressway, Gallery managed to convince city planners to spare the church. Motorists today still angle around the "Gallery Bend" on the Dan Ryan around Forty-fifth Street.[77] Three other bends were made in the expressway projects: two on the West Side expressway and one on the North Side. The West Side alterations were made by Monsignors William Gorman of Resurrection parish and John D. Fitzgerald of Ascension parish, Oak Park. Gorman insisted on a bend in the expressway to prevent the road from cutting the parish in two. Fitzgerald was successful in diverting a proposed off ramp into his Oak Park parish, thereby maintaining the neighborhood's security and reducing its congestion.[78]

The most dramatic exercise of Catholic power to change an expressway involved the rerouting of Northwest Highway through the property of the mother church of Chicago's Polonia, St. Stanislaus Kostka. Angry Polish Catholics wrote to Stritch demanding his help in preserving the church building and the parish. Stritch mobilized the resources of the Holy Name Society in what was probably its last great lobbying effort. Stritch wrote to Monsignor Edward Kelly, director of the Archdiocesan Union of Holy Name Societies, and ordered him "to have your organization ... pass a Resolution fittingly expressing their opposition to the ... rerouting of this highway and to send a copy of it to the Governor of our State and the Mayor of our City."[79] Ever sensitive to the Poles, Stritch took the matter to the governor himself. The action was effective. The city Department of Public Works reexamined the plan and secured a relocation of the Chicago and Northwestern Railway east in order to preserve the majority of the church's property.[80] A section of the church property and the school buildings was sliced away, but the parish was handsomely recompensed with the sum of $1.2 million. This they used to rebuild the elementary school and the high school on the other side of the church. However the proximity of the expressway contributed to the decline of the neighborhood and eventually the parish high school closed.

DISILLUSIONMENT WITH THE PROMISES OF
URBAN PLANNERS

Gallery, Fitzgerald, and Reed were well known to city offi-cials and their influence was often successful in achieving goals mutually beneficial to the church and developers. However, not all these parishes had pastors with the connections of Gallery, Gorman, Fitzgerald, or the Holy Name Society. Lack of clout killed Holy Guardian Angels parish, an Italian parish on the West Side, which was directly in the path of the Dan Ryan. When new land was purchased for the parish on the near West Side at Cabrini and Blue Island Avenue, a new church was built for the transplanted community in 1959. However, in 1963 another expansion progam, this time by the University of Illinois, resulted in the destruction of the new Holy Guardian Angels Church, even though parishioners waged a bitter fight spearheaded by Father Italo Scola, the pastor of the parish, and Florence Scala, a prominent laywoman.[81] Other parishes affected by the expressway's inexorable march through their boundaries found themselves so bereft of parishioners that they were even-tually compelled to curtail operations, close their schools, and finally close entirely, or consolidate.

Some urban renewal programs wiped out parishes as well. The University of Illinois Medical Center expansion on the West Side eliminated St. Charles Borromeo parish, despite the efforts of Father Leo Coggins to preserve the handsome church and thriving school. He attempted to have housing built for the hos-pital workers, but those efforts came to naught when city slum clearance and housing authorities told Coggins that his six-block project was "too small" to merit serious consideration.[82] Not long after Coggins was transferred to St. Raymond of Penafort parish in Mount Prospect, St. Charles was closed and it was razed in 1968. Nearby St. Jarlath parish suffered the same fate the following year.[83] In 1941, when the state legislature des-ignated a three-hundred acre tract near Cook County Hospital as a Medical Center District, nearby Holy Trinity parish was consolidated into the Chicago Medical Center and became known as the Cardinal Stritch Foundation.[84] Housing projects rarely closed parishes but certainly changed their makeup. St.

Philip Benizi parish on the near North Side, actually closed as a result of the expansion of the Cabrini Housing project, which changed the once heavily Italian neighborhood into a largely black area.[85] Indeed, one parish, Our Lady of the Gardens, was created to serve the enormous Altgeld Gardens housing project on the far South Side of the city.[86]

Sentiments ran high for urban renewal among city officials, urban boosters, and real estate officials; and by 1956 the pace of urban renewal had picked up new steam with the advent of Richard J. Daley. But after years of uncritical support for the work of developers, suspicion had settled in among younger priests like Father Leo Mahon and Monsignor John Egan that the needs of displaced people and the poor were not receiving proper attention. Eventually, even Stritch grew frustrated with the situation and called for more effective action:

> When we instituted action for Chicago neighborhood conserva-
> tion and reclamation, we realized that a principal effort must be
> stimulating to action many groups. We envisioned a project
> which could become a reality only if we had the cooperation of
> other groups. In fact, we were so intent on achievement that we
> put aside any thought of public recognition of our efforts.
> Realistically we saw entrenched opposition, mere lip service, and
> strange apathy. Where there should have been intelligently
> planned programs of instant action, we were confronted with
> hindrances more troublesome than open opposition.[87]

The "hindrances" Stritch complained of were the delays in the redevelopment of the Mercy Area and of the St. James parish project on Twenty-ninth and Wabash. Even though city planners gave Reed every assurance that both projects would see completion, officials of the Chicago Land Clearance Commission and others began to drag their feet.[88] O'Grady, who became involved in the matter, reported to Reed in 1957 after appearing before a congressional hearing with Chicago Housing Coordinator James Downs:

> I did raise the question with them [Downs and Alderman Robert
> Murphy] before they went on the stand about the St. James
> Project, and they assured me that the contracts had been let and

let and they were going to start building immediately. I told them if nothing was done, I might think of exposing it for the record, but they assured me I had nothing to worry about.[89]

However, the assurances to O'Grady were meaningless. The Mercy Area had to wait until the late fifties, and the St. James project fell by the wayside, victim of internal politics in the Chicago Land Clearance Commission and the opposition of Catholic philanthropist Frank J. Lewis, who did not want low-income dwellers near the Lewis Maternity Hospital.[90]

By the late fifties, Catholic leaders were growing exasperated by these unfulfilled promises. The go-along-get-along tactics of Reed, Gallery, and Gorman were soon to be supplanted by a tougher and more aggressive attitude toward urban affairs represented by Father John Egan.

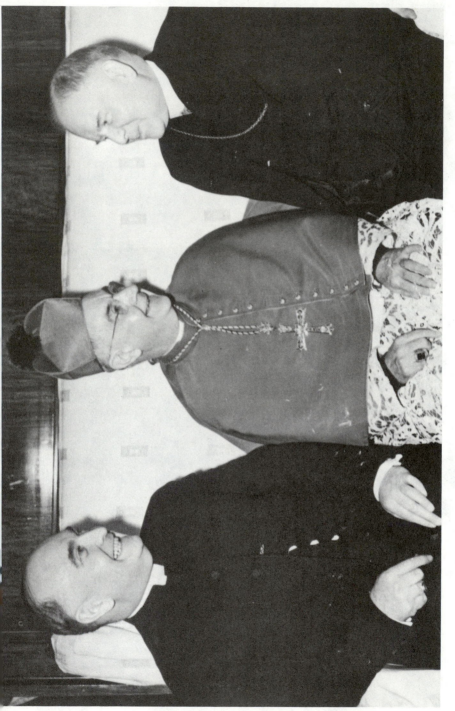

Archbishop Samuel A. Stritch enroute to his installation in Chicago flanked by Bishop Bernard Sheil and Bishop William O'Brien

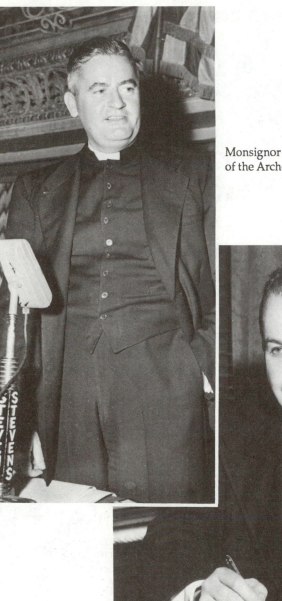

Monsignor George Casey, vicar general
of the Archdiocese of Chicago

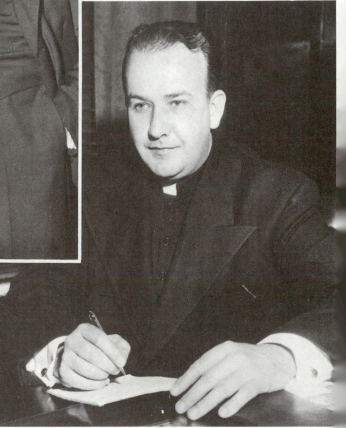

Monsignor Edward Burke, chancellor of the Archdiocese of Chicago

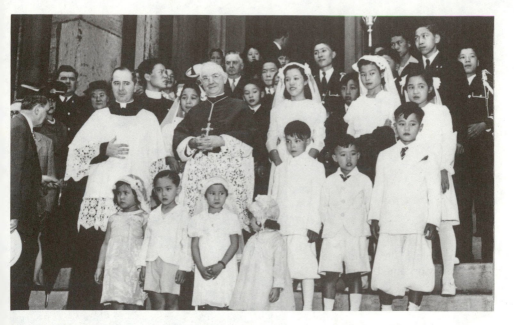

Stritch presiding at the baptism of Chinese children in Chicago

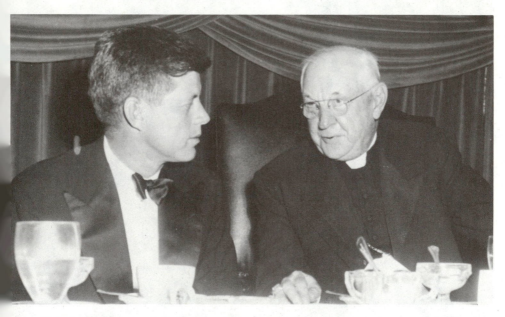

Stritch with Senator John F. Kennedy at a banquet to dedicate the opening of the Lt. Joseph P. Kennedy, Jr. School for Exceptional Children in Palos Park

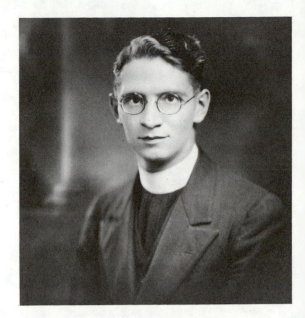

Reynold Hillenbrand as a
newly ordained priest

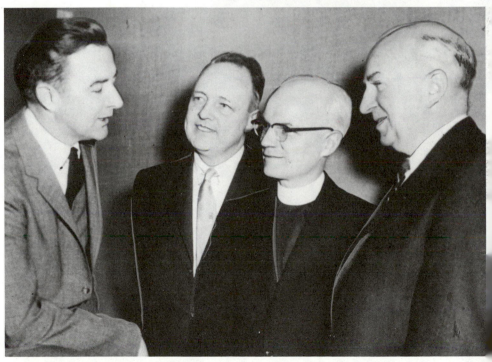

Left to right: Minnesota Senator Eugene McCarthy with CFM leader Patrick Crowley,
Monsignor Daniel Cantwell, and John Nuveen

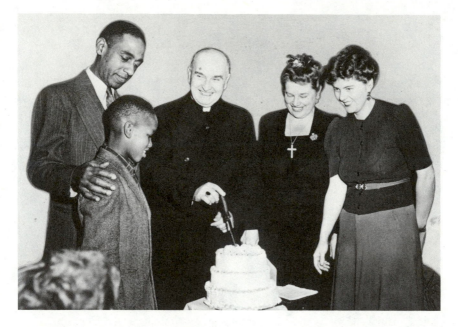

Bishop Bernard Sheil with John Yancey, Catherine De Hueck, and Ann Harrigan

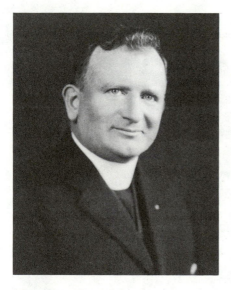

Monsignor Daniel Byrnes, pastor of Visitation Church

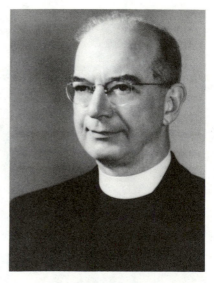

Father Joseph Richards, one of the first diocesan priests to work among Chicago's black community

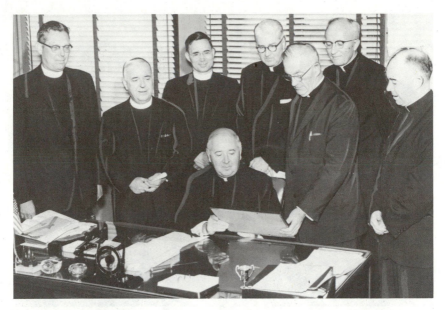

The Cardinal's Conservation Committee of the Archdiocese of Chicago.
Monsignor Thomas Reed, seated. Left to right: Father Martin "Doc" Farrell,
Monsignor Richard Kelly, Monsignor Harry Koenig, Monsignor Vincent
Moran, Monsignor William J. Gorman, Monsignor John A. McMahon,
Monsignor John Egan

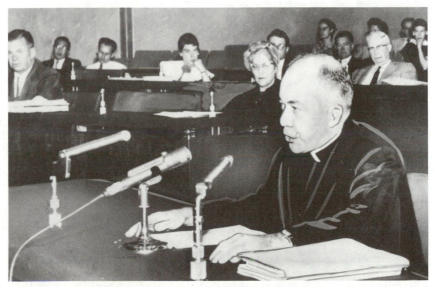

Monsignor John Egan testifying before the Chicago City Council regarding the
Hyde Park-Kenwood proposal

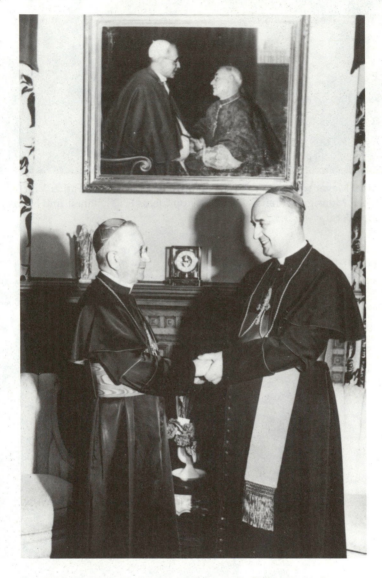

Archbishop Albert G. Meyer and Apostolic Delegate Amleto
Cicognani on Meyer's installation in Chicago

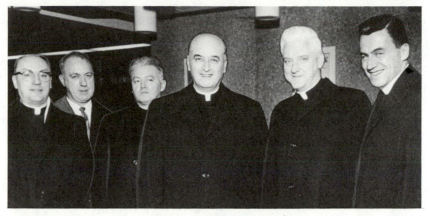

Cardinal Meyer with (l. to r.) Monsignor Donald Masterson, Father Vincent McAleer, Monsignor Francis Byrne, Bishop Cletus F. O'Donnell, and Monsignor Clifford Bergin

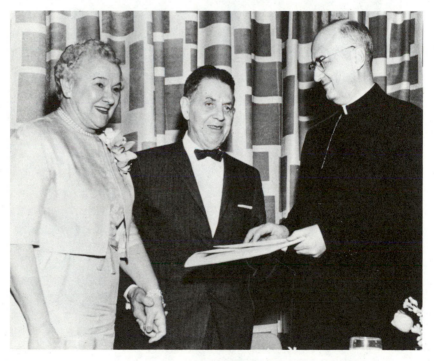

Meyer presents an award to administrator George Klupar as Mrs. Klupar looks on

7

Community Organizing and Professional Concerns

Sentiments ran high in Chicago for urban renewal, strongly supported by a coalition of church and city officials, urban boosters, and real estate agents. But it was an inherently unstable alliance with each group having a different set of objectives. As far as the Church was concerned, moral and economic issues revolving around the reshuffling of people caused by urban renewal projects were central. What did these newcomers do to stable urban neighborhoods, which were the crucible of Chicago Catholic life? What kind of justice was being done to those who were forced to relocate? When it became evident that public housing was not going to solve the problems caused by dislocation, and that neighborhood conservation organizations were sometimes a front for racial protective associations, Catholic leaders, especially those concerned with social justice, grew restive and broke away from the urban renewal coalition.

REMOTE ORIGINS: HELPING THE HISPANICS

This new phase of urban activism developed with the archdiocesan work among Puerto Ricans. During the fifties Puerto Rican emigres had begun to come in large numbers to Chicago, many of them recruited by the Castle-Burton employment agency, for service as domestics.[1] Church officials, like Stritch,

did not make distinctions between Mexicans and Puerto Ricans; they were simply all Spanish-speaking. Because of the number of Spanish-speaking in his diocese, Stritch developed an intense interest in their welfare, a concern which intensified when he became chancellor of the Church Extension Society and chairman of the American Board of Catholic Missions. Both organizations sent millions of dollars to Hispanic home missions in the Southwest. Moreover, he maintained regular correspondence with Archbishop John J. Cantwell of Los Angeles on the subject of Mexicans in the United States, and supported the efforts begun in the late 1920s by Archbishop Robert Lucey of San Antonio and Father Raymond McGowan of the NCWC to develop an effective ministry for Spanish-speaking Catholics in the Southwest.[2]

In 1943 Stritch took a trip to western Texas and New Mexico, and what he saw appalled him.

> There is a dearth of schools, settlement houses, children's clinics and sanitary housing. The incomes of most of the families are below the subsistence level, and they are forced to live on inadequate diets. The social status of the mexican [sic] population is thoroughly unjust and they are treated as an underrace.... The proselytizers are active among them and are doing very much harm among the young.[3]

Stritch suggested that "it would be helpful if Archbishop Cantwell, Archbishop (Leo) Byrne and Archbishop Lucey would consult together and invite all the Bishops of the Southwest to a Conference on the Mexican problem."[4] Stritch broached this at the meeting of the bishops in 1944, and it resulted in the formation of the Bishop's Committee on the Spanish-Speaking, which urged greater cooperation between the bishops and the American Board of Catholic Missions in behalf of the struggling Church in the Southwest.

Stritch's concern for the "Mexican problem" was not confined to the Southwest. Since the 1920s large numbers of Mexicans had come to Chicago, finding work in the railways and steel mills of the industrial city. Here they settled in one of three separate Chicago neighborhoods: the near West Side, where they worked with the railroads; the Back-of-the-Yards, where they worked in meat packing; and South Chicago, where

they worked in the steel industry.[5] A small number of migrant workers even appeared regularly to work in the declining number of truck farms in the dwindling farm communities of the Archdiocese of Chicago. Because they were Catholic, Stritch felt a paternal responsibility for their welfare, as he confided to one correspondent:

> I do keep in touch with the group of Mexican and Spanish-speaking Catholics here in Chicago. I am much interested in them and we want to try and throw our arms of protection around them. They are Catholic and they need some recognition.[6]

The primary missionaries to Hispanics were the Claretian Fathers at St. Francis of Assisi parish, who also reached them via storefront chapels and makeshift facilities. Later they branched out from St. Francis and opened Our Lady of Guadalupe Church on East Ninety-first Street. As he had done the black ministry, Stritch generously subsidized the Claretian Mission and on Christmas 1948 one of them wrote gratefully:

> Thanks to God and to Your Eminence, the spiritual problem of The Mexican Colony in Chicago has been solved. The ever increasing attendance at Holy Mass and at the Sacraments forced me to put two more Masses with sermons in Spanish in the Sunday schedule. In a short period of three years I have revalidated over five hundred marriages contracted before a Justice of the Peace or a Protestant Minister. The Youth problem too has been solved especially since we have opened the Gym and Youth Center. Also St. Francis School is in the best of shape with an attendance of about 430 Mexican children.[7]

In response to the growing need for centers in the forties, Stritch opened a Spanish-speaking mission called the Vicariate of the Immaculate Heart in the Back-of-the-Yards.

The need for a more extensive Spanish-speaking ministry developed when large numbers of Puerto Ricans entered the archdiocese, settling in the South Side's Woodlawn neighborhood. By 1953 there were twelve to fifteen thousand Puerto Ricans in Chicago, and their numbers were projected to increase by ten thousand per year.[8] Until the mid-fifties, the only organized work among the Puerto Ricans had been done under the auspices of the CYO by Sheil's personal secretary, Monsignor

Peter Meegan. However, when Meegan was driven from Sheil's side by Mrs. Wiltgen, responsibility for the Puerto Rican ministry had somehow fallen into the hands of Sheil's non-Catholic chauffeur, Gunnar Larsen.[9]

The neglect of this group soon came to the attention of Father Leo Mahon, a newly ordained curate at Woodlawn's Holy Cross parish.[10] After Mass one Sunday, Mahon was approached for spiritual help by a group of Puerto Ricans who attended the parish church. Mahon did not know Spanish but offered to assist the young men and went first to a local Opus Dei house in Chicago, on the assumption that someone could speak Spanish. Opus Dei refused to help, and Mahon turned to a group of Young Christian Workers near his parish. Here he found two willing recruits to work among the Puerto Ricans, Lester Hunt, director of the popular University of Chicago radio program "University Round Table," and Nicholas von Hoffman, who also worked at the university.

With a handsome grant of $10,000 from Cardinal Stritch, Hunt and von Hoffman and Mahon formed the Woodlawn Latin American Committee and combed the neighborhood, assessing needs and trying to keep the community together. After the collapse of Sheil's CYO empire, Stritch formed the Cardinal's Committee for the Spanish-Speaking in 1954 and appointed Father Mahon as its director and Father Gilbert Carroll as his assistant. Like many former Sheil enterprises, the work with the Puerto Ricans was put under the umbrella of Catholic Charities. Mahon and Carroll learned Spanish and provided religious counsel and social organizations such as the Caballeros de San Juan and a spiritual, evangelical group called Hijos de la Familia de Dios. Mahon's interests in Hispanic ministry intensified as time went on, and he became one of the catalysts for opening of the Chicago archdiocese's mission of San Miguelito in Panama in the early sixties.[11]

THE ALINSKY CONNECTION

His interest in the Puerto Rican community would bring Stritch into direct contact with Saul Alinsky and the new

methodology for urban affairs. Alinsky was no stranger to the Catholic Church or to the Archdiocese of Chicago. He had been a close associate of Bishop Bernard J. Sheil, who helped him establish his community organizing operation called the Industrial Areas Foundation and made many important fund-raising contacts for him. He enjoyed close friendships with many Chicago-area priests, such as Abbot Ambrose Ondrack of St. Procopius Abbey in Lisle and the priests of the Back-of-the-Yards. He also counted Monsignor John O'Grady of National Catholic Charities as a close friend.

It was O'Grady who had heard of the work of Hunt and von Hoffman and set up a dinner meeting for them and Alinsky at the Blackstone Hotel in late 1953. Present also was Father John Egan of the Cana Conference, who had met Alinsky several months before through philosopher Jacques Maritain. During the course of the dinner, the acerbic Alinsky baited von Hoffman mercilessly about his lack of expertise in working with the Puerto Ricans and the meeting soon degenerated into a shouting match.[12] As Alinsky later explained it (probably to cover up his rudeness toward the bright young von Hoffman), he was testing the mettle of the young man in order to hire him for the Industrial Areas Foundation.

Egan was deeply impressed with Alinsky and introduced him to Monsignor Edward Burke, who in turn presented the organizer to Stritch. For all his tough-guy bravado and disdain for the powerful, Alinsky was properly deferential to the prelate and Stritch took a liking to him. What probably attracted Stritch to Alinsky more than anything was the organizer's highly detailed and extremely candid reports. Stritch's utter fascination with information, especially about the city of Chicago, led him to commission Alinsky and the IAF to study the Puerto Rican situation in Chicago in preparation for the establishment of a community organization. The agreements between the two were informal, although Alinsky did draw up extensive memoranda for Stritch. As von Hoffman and Hunt poured in their data and analysis of the Puerto Rican community, Alinsky discovered Puerto Ricans all around the city. He urged that Stritch allow him to "study ... communities where Puerto Ricans are now settling...."[13]

This led to the commissioning of two other reports by the Archdiocese of Chicago—one dealing with the near North Side, and another about the Grand Avenue corridor. The near North Side study was undertaken "for the purpose of developing those circumstances whereby peoples of all races and creeds can live and work together in a harmonious, equal and integrated pattern."[14] The area (bounded by North Avenue on the north and the Chicago River on the south, and on the west by the north branch of the Chicago River) had a population of over ninety thousand and stunning differences in lifestyles, characterized by sociologist Harvey Warren Zorbaugh in a classic 1929 study as "The Gold Coast and the Slum." The report to Stritch in 1956 was filled with informative details about every aspect of the life of the area, including the six Catholic churches (the Cathedral was one of them) that were part of the study. Although the study revealed little support for a strong community organization in either the North Side or the Grand Avenue area, it piqued Stritch's interest for more.[15]

The final IAF study commissioned by Cardinal Stritch in 1955 was a work on the racially troubled neighborhoods of Chicago's south and west sides. At Alinsky's urging, Stritch released Father Egan from his assignment to the Cana Conference in order to work with von Hoffman as an intern for the IAF. The study was to be an intensive education for Egan. He and von Hoffmann scoured the neighborhoods, speaking to ordinary citizens, visiting social spots, and speaking with real estate developers. In 1956 Egan finished his work and went back to the Cana Conference but with a deepened interest in the work of the city and hands-on experience of Alinsky's confrontational style. In 1958 Stritch decided to upgrade the Cardinal's Conservation Committee by making Egan its full-time executive secretary. Egan was not a trained urbanologist, but his work with Cana and his association with Alinsky convinced him of two things: the Church could be a very powerful social force in the city of Chicago if it could only mobilize itself for action; secondly, dealing with the complexities of arcane politics in the city and among developers required people tough, smart, savvy, shrewd and informed. Under Egan's leadership, the Conservation Committee assumed a more adversarial stance toward develop-

ers and city officials and became one of the most important information-gathering and lobbying agencies for social reform of any American archdiocese.

Egan was openly skeptical of the conservation approach that city and church officials promoted as the answer to neighborhood problems. Like many others, Egan believed that local conservation organizations were often fronts for racial exclusion. Moreover, conservation powers were often used to demolish urban dwellings without the attendant responsiblity to provide replacements for those dislocated. Consequently Egan's first target was Chicago's Community Conservation Board.

In a memo to Stritch shortly after he took over, Egan complained that the board "has managed to spend nearly a million dollars in administration without accomplishing anything."[16] Moreover, efforts to goad the Conservation Board to more vigorous action fell on deaf ears. Egan was even more frustrated when he met with Mayor Daley and pressed him to appoint Catholic choices Robert Cronin or Paul Reynolds to a vacant post on the Conservation Board. Daley promised to follow up on the suggestion but did nothing. Egan urged Stritch to "encourage Mr. Daley to sit down from time to time with Msgr. Burke, Msgr. Reed and Msgr. Egan and listen to some of the things they have to say."[17] However, by this time Stritch was already packing his bags for Rome, and the matter lapsed. Therefore, when the University of Chicago revealed plans to remove housing in its area, Egan was stung to action.[18] Egan's trial by fire would come when he challenged the University of Chicago's plans for redevelopment of the Hyde Park–Kenwood communities because they did not make adequate provision for the relocation of twenty-thousand poor and low-income people whose dwellings they intended to demolish.

THE FIRST CAMPAIGN: HYDE PARK–KENWOOD

The area around the University of Chicago was south of the downtown in a community known as Hyde Park. Once a fashionable suburb, it had been a prime location until the forties, when the movement of blacks southward had caused neighborhood blight. Multiple occupancy of single-family dwellings,

crime, and decay created social problems that threatened the safety of those attending the university. Initially, the university sought to stabilize the neighborhood with the formation of an effective community organization known as the Hyde Park–Kenwood Community Organization. This body had an intellectual commitment to the notion of interracial living but soon found that it was unable to stanch the flow of whites from the neighborhoods or prevent the overcrowding that led to blight. By 1949 it was decided that tougher measures would be necessary if the university was to survive.

In 1951 Robert Maynard Hutchins resigned as chancellor of the university and was succeeded by Lawrence A. Kimpton. Kimpton was dedicated to preserving the neighborhood and worked closely with an affiliated organization, the South East Chicago Commission, whose executive director was Julian Levi. Using contacts in the state legislature and the Metropolitan Housing Commission, Levi secured the passage of a law in 1953 which allowed the condemnation of buildings, not necessarily dilapidated but in danger of becoming so. Moreover, the South East Chicago Commission, again at Levi's instigation, secured an amendment to the 1941 Neighborhood Redevelopment Corporation Act which brought areas designated as conservation areas under the power of eminent domain. With these two legislative arrows in its quiver, the University of Chicago began to make ambitious plans to deliver its neighborhood from the encroachments of blight and fight off any attempt to place unwanted public housing in the university environs.

The first of these conservation projects, called Hyde Park Redevelopment Projects A & B, proposed in 1954, were designated to raze a square block of the most dilapidated section of the area. Initially, Reed and the archdiocesan representative on the Hyde Park Community Council, Father Edmund Godfrey, pastor of St. Thomas the Apostle Church in Hyde Park, supported the plan, which included a new park adjacent to the parish property. Reed reported to Stritch:

> The Reverend Edmund Godfrey, Pastor, is in favor of this project. He does not wish to make a public statement on it for the very good reason, he does not want to antagonize any parishioners

who may have to be relocated.... After discussing this project briefly with Your Eminence ... I obtained your authorization to express the approval of this project by the Archdiocese.[19]

Later, in July 1954, Reed appeared before the Chicago Park District, public officials, and members of the South East Chicago Commission to recommend the razing of the block, with the proviso: "[that] the South East Chicago Commission would show acceptable plans for the adequate and humane relocation of the people in the block providing them with dwelling units that meet with generally accepted standards."[20] The plans were approved, and the redevelopment took place. The housing plan, however, was never announced. Stritch and Reed felt betrayed.

As a result, when a more comprehensive urban renewal plan was announced by the university in early February 1958, with indequate housing provisions, the stage was set for a battle royal between the Archdiocese of Chicago and the university. The old skirmishes over religious indifferentism and anti-Catholic bigotry were nothing compared to the knock-down-drag-out fight that emerged over urban policy.

The University of Chicago plan of 1958 demanded the demolition of over seven hundred structures and the relocation of four thousand families, or twenty thousand people, over a five-year period. In all, nearly four thousand dwelling units would be lost permanently. The biggest losers would be the poor and elderly inhabitants of the areas, whose homes would be leveled and who could not afford better housing. The Cardinal's Conservation Committee of the archdiocese had long been aware of the university's plans through regular information from Father Leo Mahon and others whom Egan knew from the Cana Conference. As they discussed the situation, it became evident that this would be the Lake Meadows project all over again, with displaced persons spilling into adjacent neighborhoods, with vague, unfulfilled promises that housing would be available. But before these promises could become a reality, neighborhoods would be inundated with newcomers, thereby undermining the efforts of those who were valiantly trying to retain some order. Moreover, since a portion of the financing for the renovation would be covered by federal grants and local

revenue, this expensive project threatened to consume a large amount of the city's precious bond money. Egan was ready to do battle.

When Egan brought the Hyde Park–Kenwood Plan (as it was called) before the members of the Cardinal's Conservation Board, he urged stiff resistance, and a heated discussion ensued. Many of the older members, especially Father Gallery and Monsignor Gorman, had resented Egan's appointment in the first place and opposed his insistence on confrontational tactics as counterproductive. They hoped, as in past difficulties, to settle the matter privately with city officials. But the mood had shifted and Egan won support for a more vigorous plan of action from no less than Monsignors Thomas Reed and John D. Fitzgerald, who had been active in earlier policies. Even more importantly, Monsignor Edward Burke, Egan's patron in the chancery office, signed on as a supporter of a firm policy. Through Burke, Cardinal Stritch's support was assured; although by the time the battle was joined in 1958, Stritch would be en route to Rome. Critical support also came from Father J. M. Kelly, editor of the *New World*.

The Church rolled out its heavy artillery in this battle. The survival of schools, churches, and charitable institutions was inextricably linked to the stability of urban neighborhoods. Not only did these buildings represent millions of dollars in investments, but even more, incalculable spiritual attachments. The Hyde Park–Kenwood Plan, they argued, was a prime example of an urban renewal plan that might make one neighborhood look good but would spread blight and overcrowding into other areas of the city like a ripple effect. Even more, there were issues of justice and charity that piqued the conscience of Egan and others. Most of the displaced were poor and black who were powerless against a big university with its political connections. Moreover, as Arnold Hirsch has pointed out (but without the full theological impact that is intended), Egan and his associates viewed the city as an organic entity.[21] All seventy-five communities of the city were designed to work together as parts of the one body called Chicago. Permitting any one community to follow its own progress selfishly at the expense of others—particularly the poor—was unthinkable.

At Egan's urging, the *New World* began a series of critical articles on the Hyde Park-Kenwood proposal soon after it was announced in early 1958. In one editorial Father Kelly accused the plan of attempting to preserve a "shining new island" in the midst of an urban sea of woes.[22] In subsequent articles the *New World* kept up a barrage of criticism. On May 2, 1958, Father William F. Graney asked: "Where are the 20,000 to 30,000 displaced by demolition to be relocated?"[23] One week later Graney articulated the central Catholic argument against the plan in an editorial entitled "Common Good Takes Precedence over the Rights of Individuals." Graney stated: "Public welfare demands adequate provision for churches, schools, recreational facilities, or even less necessary advantages for a community such as parking or shopping areas. Public authority must carefully weigh these necessities and advantages against the present needs for housing in our city before solid buildings are demolished."[24] On June 11, 1958, the Cardinal's Conservation Committee issued a declaration criticizing the "isolated city planning" and the "lack of housing opportunities for people in the middle and lower income groups," and recommended four alterations in the proposal: land clearance only as needed, affordable housing in Hyde Park for "families of small and intermediate income," clarity on the criteria for rehabilitation, and a keen eye on the effects of the plan on the overall city housing supply.[25] Soon after the issuance of the statement, Ferd Kramer, former chairman of the Metropolitan Housing and Planning Council, accused the Committee of "doing a great disservice to Chicago" by opposing the Hyde Park–Kenwood plan.[26] Others accused the Church of opposing the urban renewal plan because it was trying to prevent the influx of blacks from the Hyde Park neighborhood.[27]

INTERNAL OPPOSITION

Vigorous opposition from developers and the University of Chicago was presumed, but criticism of Egan's stance on Hyde Park–Kenwood emerged from a quarter least expected, the ranks of the Hillenbrand-inspired social activists. Most disconcerting of all was the defection of Cantwell, who agreed with

Egan's goals but viewed the use of power politics with distaste. In a strong letter to Egan, Cantwell wrote:

> For years we—and I certainly mean the collective pronoun to mean you—have been trying to build up an image of the Church in human life differing from what went before us and from what still generally prevails. We deliberately abandoned the notion that the Church gets its work done by pushing its weight around and by using secular power.... Why, I ask myself, were all these positions set aside when The New World and the Cardinal's Committee began the campaign about Hyde Park.... We could not have selected a worse possible set of circumstances.... In Hyde Park we have confronted a very knowledgeable, sensitive, and perceptive group of people with a most disagreeable image of the Church.... I strongly suspect that the New World and the Cardinal's Committee were desirous of creating an awareness of their existence and attracting attention. I have not the slightest quarrel with these objectives.... My problem is with the methods employed....[28]

Even more troublesome to Cantwell was the perception of many social-minded Catholics that opposition to the Hyde Park project was only a veiled maneuver to keep blacks from moving into all-white neighborhoods. This attitude was expressed in a letter to Catholic Interracial Council President R. Sargent Shriver from Ben Heineman, chairman of the Chicago and Northwestern Railway System: "The position which he [Egan] has taken and the manner in which he has taken it has been in my opinion, expressly designed to encourage racial conflict. Moreover, it is widely believed that his underlying motivation is to impede the flow of negroes into the south west side."[29] Shriver reported the letter to Cantwell (with Heineman's reduced financial contribution to the work of the Catholic Interracial Council), and Cantwell responded sympathetically to Heineman's complaint:

> It is my opinion that the Church in this instance, has made a grave blunder, and has been acting in a manner that inevitably will do much harm to the Church and to the community at large.... the confusion ... stems both from the fact that the racial

overtones of the New World editorials would give any sensitive and informed person grounds for believing that we were trying to keep Negroes from moving into other neighborhoods in Chicago and that for this reason we have been urging a limitation on demolition in areas currently occupied by Negroes.[30]

The disagreement among the liberals became public in the summer of 1958 when Ed Marciniak wrote an editorial for *Work* decrying the opposition to the Hyde Park project and urging its completion. When the editorial was picked up by the daily newspapers and used to discredit the archdiocesan position, Marciniak received an irate phone call from *New World* assistant editor, J. M. Kelly, criticizing him for issuing "a statement without consulting with him and advising him of it." He then threatened that if the Catholic Council on Working Life and the Catholic Interracial Council continued their opposition, they could no longer count on publicity from the *New World*.[31] If Kelly's warning was not enough, Burke phoned Cantwell about opposition to the "official policy" and said in a follow-up memo to Cantwell: "It seems to me that any organization we permit to use our name should be under our complete control. Certainly Marciniak did not help us by his statement."[32] If Cantwell's dissent was not enough, Egan also felt the wrath of the most prestigious Catholic voice on the University of Chicago campus, Professor Jerome Kerwin, who also weighed in with his opposition.[33]

As disconcerting as this must have been, Egan stuck to his guns. When the plan was formally debated before the city council in September 1958, Egan drafted his testimony along the lines of the June 11 statement. He began by making it clear that no matter who dissented from the official position, "The Catholic archdiocese cannot approve this plan as it now stands."[34] Egan's invocation of the authority of the Catholic archdiocese so outraged the *Chicago Tribune*, a staunch defender of the plan, that the newspaper's official welcome to Archbishop Meyer was followed by a lengthy article deriding Egan for placing "Catholic members of the city administration and of the city council under some pressure to decide a political question in accordance with the views of their religious leaders," and lambasting fears of neighborhood deterioration as "exaggerated."[35]

The climax of the battle was Egan's testimony before a crowded city council chamber in October where, in blunt language, he condemned the plan as unjust and unfair to the poor. Egan responded forcefully to the charges that he was representing a "vested" Roman Catholic real estate interest [churches and schools] and nothing else:

> The vested interest of the Archdiocese of Chicago is human beings. Everything we do is pointless without them. Our churches, schools, hospitals, and institutions of every kind have no other purpose but to serve man and thereby serve God. It does not matter if our institutions return a profit, if our properties are protected from the slums' corrosive effects but turn away from the service of human beings. Man, his welfare and happiness, is the be all and end all of the Archdiocese of Chicago's entire effort in every field of action it enters on. That is our vested interest; I have been sent here to protect it and speak for it.[36]

"Remember," Egan lectured the council, "you are not voting on a plan to build something; you are voting on a project to tear something down."[37] Nonetheless, Levi had done his homework well and had secured the support of key aldermen and Mayor Richard J. Daley. With only minor modifications in the plan, the city council voted overwhelmingly to approve it and in short order it was also approved by the Housing Home Finance Administration in Washington.[38] Egan was badly outmaneuvered and abandoned in the Hyde Park–Kenwood debate, but he retained his office in the administration and lived to fight another day.

MEYER'S COMING: A NEW START

The booming guns of the Hyde Park–Kenwood debate were heard in distant Milwaukee and in the first weeks after his 1958 appointment to Chicago, Archbishop Meyer met with Egan and was assured that he did not have to get involved in the Hyde Park issue. Meyer had spent a lifetime keeping out of "political" matters and was relieved that his first days in Chicago would not be given over to doing battle with city and private authorities. However, the days of his isolation were

drawing to an end. The Chicago environment precluded noninvolvement by the archdiocese in the internal affairs of the city. Meyer got an inkling of this from a letter O'Grady wrote to him shortly before he became archbishop of Chicago. It reflected well the frustration Chicago priests and he himself felt with city officials on the urban renewal issues:

> They [Conservation Committee] have made great progress in spite of great obstacles. One of the greatest is the continuous opposition from the local government. We've had in Chicago as in other cities, a feeling on the part of the government officials that they could do all the thinking and planning for their local communities. They really did not want any strong, dynamic voluntary organizations. They did not mind as long as the organization confined itself to the making of speeches and the passing of resolutions. They tried in every way possible to control the thinking and planning of the priests and the people. I have seen this effort at meeting after meeting.[39]

With the prodding of men like O'Grady, Cantwell, and Egan, Meyer's cautious approach to urban affairs soon gave way to curiosity and then a commitment to action. He spoke regularly with Egan and, early in 1959, arranged for the priest to give him a no-holds-barred tour of the city. Egan did this with careful attention to the big developments as well as urban neighborhoods and the people on the street. After that day, Meyer's caution was not completely overcome, but he came away even more aware that Chicago's complex urban problems were deep and convinced that the Church had a substantial interest and right to be active in urban affairs. As archbishop, he had a duty to lead in this area.

There was nothing like a sense of duty to move Meyer into areas where he was temperamentally uncomfortable. He began consulting urban sociologists like Father Joseph Fichter, S.J., whom Egan brought to his attention, and read the carefully crafted study of the Church in Chicago written by Belgian urban sociologist, Father Francois Houtart.[40] Houtart had come to Chicago in the fifties at the invitation of Bishop Sheil. He resided at St. Gall's parish on the South Side while he conducted an intensive sociological investigation of the impact of the Church

on the city. The results of his work were first heard in a series of lectures he delivered at the Sheil School of Social Studies in the early fifties and later in a lengthy report that was published in the international sociological journal *Compass*.[41] Houtart was amazed at the vibrancy of the Chicago church and the effectiveness of its social welfare and educational institutions. But he lamented that the Church's impact on the political, economic, and moral climate of the city was less than its potential. Houtart's work was sent to interested pastors by Monsignor Reed, even though it drew some mild criticism from Stritch.[42] Meyer's active curiosity gave Egan an opening he had never found with Stritch, whose interest in urban issues was real, but more diffuse.

Recognizing the gravity of Chicago's urban issues, Meyer authorized Egan to upgrade and professionalize the staff of the Conservation Committee. In 1959, with Reed's help, Egan restructured the committee, staffing it with a rotating membership of pastors and an expanded professional staff.[43] Symbolic of the new approach of the body (and reflecting the fact that Meyer was not yet a cardinal), Egan had the name of the committee changed to the Archdiocesan Conservation Council, and a year later the more professional-sounding Office of Urban Affairs (OUA). Egan was soon in business in offices on 720 North Rush Street.[44]

THE OFFICE OF URBAN AFFAIRS

Under Egan, the Office of Urban Affairs became a whirlwind of activity. Egan added Michael Schiltz to the staff of the OUA in the fall of 1960, to compile statistics and maps of the archdiocese. One of the first things Meyer requested from Egan was a map of the archdiocese. Schiltz produced the maps with the help of Peter Beltemacchi, a young disciple of Father Andrew Greeley at Christ the King parish. The mapping project was followed by a set of population projections for the archdiocese. Schiltz also did work for McManus at the school offices.[45]

In order to encourage homegrown talent, Egan urged Meyer to approve Father Andrew Greeley's plans to study sociology at the University of Chicago in 1960. Greeley's permission

to go to "Moscow Tech," as it was derisively referred to in the chancery, went a long way toward bridging the chasm that had existed between the institution and the archdiocese since the days of Mundelein. Greeley was one of many priests who were permitted to attend the university and study sociology.

Still another project under the auspices of the Office of Urban Affairs was the publication of a series of articles entitled "The Urban Crisis—A Christian Concern" that appeared on the pages of the *New World* in the spring of 1961. Many of the articles were written by Jesuit sociologist Joseph Small of Loyola; and there were also pieces by community organizer Thomas Gaudette, housing specialist John M. Ducey, and zoning expert Thomas W. Tearney.

The new approach that Egan brought not only involved a greater adversarial stance to city officials and urban planners, but also included the building of new coalitions with like-minded members of other denominations. Interdenominational cooperation had taken a hard blow in Chicago since the Catholic banning of the Evanston conference. But the passing of Stritch and the advent of the more ecumenical-minded Pope John XXIII created a new climate for joint ventures in Chicago. Egan forged close contacts with Dr. John Harms of the Church Federation of Greater Chicago and Rabbi Richard G. Hirsch of the Union of American Hebrew Congregations. Together, the three compiled a study package entitled "Religion, Community Life and Chicago's Housing" for dissemination and discussion.[46] From April 26 to 29, 1960, the participants met at the Congress Hotel to discuss the issues raised by the study guide. This major ecumenical meeting was the first of many similar gatherings to be attended by Chicago Catholics, climaxing with a major conference on religion and race in January 1963. Typically, Meyer was hesitant in these areas but later embraced them strongly.

Egan's relationship with Meyer was always formal and professional, but Meyer genuinely appreciated Egan's efforts to help him learn about the city and drew on his expertise in drafting a statement read in the prelate's name before the United States Civil Rights Commission. The commission had been formed by President Eisenhower and included among its members Notre Dame University President Theodore Hesburgh,

C.S.C. As the committee traveled around the country, it elicited testimony from prominent civic and religious leaders. In New York, Francis Cardinal Spellman had appeared before the committee. When the group came to Chicago, they requested a statement from Meyer, but he was still uneasy with the idea of speaking too forcefully about issues he was still learning. At Hesburgh's suggestion, he directed Egan to draft a statement and then carefully edited it. Egan appeared before the committee in the name of the archbishop in May 1959 and proposed the formation of community organizations among blacks to empower them to preserve their neighborhoods. Although this testimony would get intertwined with that of Saul Alinsky, who delivered an impassioned plea for racial quotas in neighborhoods, it acquainted Meyer with the work of community organizing according to the principles of Saul D. Alinsky. Community organizing would become the centerpiece of Egan's urban strategy. Alinsky's confrontational style of community organizing provided a methodology for the new aggressiveness of Chicago Catholic urban policy.

COMMUNITY ORGANIZING

The migration of the blacks into the southwest corner of Chicago continued unabated throughout the fifties. Blockbusting, white panic, and threats of violence prompted two of the leading clergymen of the area, Monsignor John S. McMahon of St. Sabina's and Monsignor Patrick Malloy of St. Leo's parish, to take steps to arrest the deteriorating situation.[47] From his days at the changing West Side parish of St. Charles Borromeo, McMahon had seen how easily an unorganized neighborhood could fall prey to the forces of panic. He was one of many Chicago priests to take Monsignor O'Grady's ideas on neighborhood conservation seriously, and he was dead set against racial segregation.[48] Just before Stritch left for Rome, McMahon asked for permission to use parish funds to secure the services of the Industrial Areas Foundation in organizing the neighborhood. Alinsky reluctantly agreed to help, and dispatched von Hoffman and two other full-time organizers to comb the area.[49] Before long a plan for organizing the commu-

nity was devised. To implement the plan, Alinsky demanded money and a public committment from the pastors of the area. Those two items could only be supplied by the active support of the archbishop of Chicago.

When Meyer arrived in late 1958, Egan and McMahon laid the plan before him and asked if he would secure the financial and moral support of the pastors of the area. This was a daunting task. The pastors of the Southwest Side were among the toughest of the old Irish barons and would not come together easily in so controversial a project as an Alinsky-style community organization. At issue was a call for a "fair practice code of community life," whose purpose would be the elimination of discriminatory practices which prevented economically stable black families from renting and purchasing homes. This code would be a "yardstick" for determining the true commitment of any community organization or improvement group to authentic Catholic social teaching—a clear challenge to "clean-up-paint-up" neighborhood conservation organizations that were actually designed to keep blacks out.

Because he was new to the archdiocese, Meyer expressed some reluctance about Egan's and McMahon's request, but nonetheless called a meeting of the pastors concerned on January 6, 1959, at Christ the King rectory in Beverly. Egan reassured Meyer, who was worried about the issue of "timing":

> I am presuming that at the conclusion of the meeting you will desire to make a few remarks. In this regard I know that the several pastors who have worked so diligently week after week during the past year to build up the organization and make it successful ... would be heartened by a few words by you. At the same time the pastors who have adopted a "wait and see" attitude may be encouraged to offer their talents, time and prestige to the enormous work that lies ahead.[50]

Meyer listened carefully to the presentations by McMahon, Egan, and von Hoffman about the proposed community organization and concluded the meeting by granting his approval to the undertaking.[51] The January meeting at least temporarily mobilized Catholic support, and by April a meeting of forty-five community leaders took place at which it was agreed to establish

a community council. In May, these individuals convened a large public meeting at which a temporary organization was formed. In August 1959, the IAF completed its work in the Southwest Community and withdrew from the organization. In October 1959 the Organization for the Southwest Community (OSC) was officially formed at a communitywide congress.[52]

Despite its auspicious beginnings, support for the OSC among Catholic pastors was erratic at best. Once Meyer became absorbed in the work of the Vatican Council, he delegated much responsibility for "domestic affairs" to Auxiliary Bishop Cletus O'Donnell and Egan. By 1963 the OSC was floundering. In a tough memo to Alinsky, von Hoffman spelled out the problems succinctly:

> I think it is very important to bear in mind that the situation in these parishes is totally different from that obtaining on the Northwest side. Egan, of course, knows this but he sometimes forgets it. Egan, nor Clete O'Donnell, nor the Chancery Office, nor Meyer, cut the kind of ice on the Southwest Side that they cut on the Northwest Side. The sort of pressure that has yielded money from all those parishes on the Northwest Side would not yield anything like the same amount from the Southwest side. Of course, in this regard, I think it should be pointed out that at no time has the Cardinal or those under him put the same pressure on the Southwest Side pastors that has been put on the Polish pastors on the Northwest Side. On his single visit to the Southwest Side in connection with the OSC you will recall that the Cardinal's words were very gentle indeed. Naturally, they were an endorsement but the same kind of ante-up spirit was just not present in what he said. With certain noble exceptions, the pastors out on the Southwest Side are practically a caricature, a cartoon of the sins of omission and commission of the Irish Roman Catholic clergy.[53]

Egan concurred in von Hoffman's assessment and lamented the clerical indifference that hurt the OSC. In 1964 he besought Meyer:

> If the need were not so great, I would not pursue this subject at this time, when you have so many other things on your mind,

but the OSC does need the support of the pastors now more than ever. I note that you will be speaking at St. Cajetan Church on Sunday April 19, and a strong word from you on that occasion will go a long way.[54]

Ultimately, the OSC was unable to effectively manage neighborhood integration. The point of no return came in the summer of 1965, when a young white man named Frank Kelly was fatally shot by a black youth while standing in the parking lot of St. Sabina's. After the slaying, the neighborhood began to rapidly empty of whites. The OSC eventually folded in 1970.[55]

NORTHWEST COMMUNITY ORGANIZATION

The community organization with which von Hoffman compared the OSC was the Northwest Community Organization (NCO). The Northwest Community had at one time been the bastion of Chicago's Polonia. But already in the fifties the situation was changing. "This area," Reed wrote, "is being affected by the super highway program. There has been a large immigration including a number of Puerto Ricans and a large movement of the older residents, particularly of Polish and Italian ancestry, to new suburban areas. The problems of these parishes are generally the same."[56] The encroachment of the Northwest Highway had taken many people out of the community. But not everyone was willing to roll over and play dead for the forces of development. Already in the early fifties, the parishioners of Holy Innocents parish on Armour Street had banded together to resist an urban renewal project that would have demolished housing. They found one of their assistant pastors, Father Anthony Janiak, ready and willing to help them organize and fight city hall. Other pastors, such as Father Umile Broccolo of Holy Rosary on Western Avenue, urged the formation of community organizations to assure neighborhood stability. In early 1960 Alinsky was invited to help organize the Northwest community. Once again Egan approached Meyer, asking the cardinal to use his powers of moral and personal persuasion on the pastors of the community. The result was a historic meeting of all twenty-two pastors of the area, chaired by Cardinal Meyer.

Meyer not only encouraged the work of community organization but commanded the pastors to open their parish coffers to fund the first year of the community organization.

Despite Meyer's support for the NCO, he had mixed feelings about associating with the blunt and irreverent Alinsky. At the same time he was assisting in the organization of the NCO, Alinsky attempted to set up a community organization for the people of the Archdiocese of Milan, Italy. In response to a query from Vatican functionary Monsignor Paul Marcinkus about the character of the community organizer, Meyer responded:

> I have no personal acquaintanceship with the gentleman mentioned. I do know however that those who have talked to me about him have some very serious doubts in their mind and would most earnestly recommend that the Holy See be most cautious in dealing with him.... It may be observed that he seems to speak rather freely of a close personal relationship with His Holiness himself.[57]

Despite his suspicion of Alinsky, Meyer did give the critical support needed to fund the NCO, which opened shop in December 1961. Veteran organizer Thomas Gaudette assisted in its formation and Father Anthony Janiak played a significant role in it. Indeed, Janiak became a one-man crusader, often clashing with conservative pastors and public officials. In one dramatic incident, Janiak staged a sit-in at the offices of the La Salle National Bank, which held the mortgages for slumlords and the operators of seedy taverns in the community area. Janiak's action resulted in modest efforts to clean up the offensive businesses and decaying properties.[58]

Unlike the OSC, the NCO never had integration as its primary goal, simply because no one could have stopped the influx of Puerto Ricans. Because of this, the NCO is still alive.

THE WOODLAWN ORGANIZATION

One church-supported community organization that did succeed was the Temporary Woodlawn Organization (TWO)— the first all-black community organization in the United States. The Woodlawn area, immediately south of the University of

Chicago, had a population of about sixty-five thousand in 1960, 80 percent of which was black. Almost half the housing was substandard and rents were higher than the citywide average. Over 12 percent of the community was unemployed, and almost 25 percent received some form of public assistance. The Catholic Church of the area, Holy Cross on Sixty-fifth and Maryland, had long been designated for "colored work" and was the home of activist priests Robert Doyle and Leo Mahon.

In 1956 Father Martin ("Doc") Farrell was transferred to the pastorate of Holy Cross. From previous assignments he knew firsthand of the ills of the community: the slumlords who charged exorbitant rents for hovels, the refusal of banks to lend money to blacks to improve or purchase homes in the area, the overcrowded schools. Farrell and two Presbyterian ministers, Charles Leber and Ulysses S. "Buck" Blakely ("Buck and Chuck" as von Hoffman would jokingly refer to them), began meeting to seek solutions to the problems of the area. Their efforts reinvigorated an existing but moribund community organization by establishing new committees to deal with neighborhood problems. They hoped to sensitize the residents of the neighborhood to the potential for conservation projects such as sidewalk repairs, better street lighting, and arresting the deterioration of buildings in the old neighborhood.[59]

In late June 1958, Farrell keynoted a well-attended public session with Commissioner J. Paul Holland of the Community Conservation Board at McCosh School auditorium, at Sixty-fifth and Champlain. After hearing Farrell describe the plans he and the ministers had drawn up for the area, Holland left the meeting "amazed and pleased with the group's unity," and stated: "No sound building in this area will be torn down."[60] Encouraged by the momentum of the meeting and with Holland behind him, Farrell helped to organize the Woodlawn Block Club Council, whose purpose was to devise a conservation plan for the area. In addition to maintaining the good housing stock, Farrell urged the group to rid the community of "the 20 percent of the neighborhood ... made up of illegal conversions, shabby hotels and objectionable taverns."[61]

However, Farrell knew that to make a lasting impact on Woodlawn's serious problems would require a highly effective,

action-oriented community organization. To secure this he began making regular pilgrimages to Alinsky's IAF offices, urging Alinsky to bring his techniques to Woodlawn to create a community organization for blacks. But Alinsky dismissed him, claiming that the residents could not raise the money he needed to fund the organizational efforts. If they couldn't raise the money, Alinsky argued, they did not have the kind of spirit necessary to do battle with city and private interests. Farrell, used to doing battle on the question of integration, was undeterred by Alinsky's often blunt rejections and kept pressing the organizer for help. What eventually changed Alinsky's mind, however, was not the pleas of a sentimental priest, but the possibility of doing battle with the University of Chicago. When the university announced plans in 1960 to begin slum clearance in preparation for a South Campus expansion into the Woodlawn area, which involved widespread demolition of all types of housing and the displacement of hundreds of Woodlawn residents, Leber, Blakely, and Farrell were outraged. They felt especially betrayed since the University of Chicago proposed to use the same conservation board policies that Commissioner Holland had assured them would never be used to destroy the neighborhood. Farrell and his two cohorts formed the Woodlawn Pastor's Alliance and descended on Alinsky, determined to persuade him to give the residents of Woodlawn what Hyde Park–Kenwood had lacked: a decent community organization to fight the university and the city. Alinsky agreed, and Farrell immediately set to work raising the funds the organizer demanded to begin the operation.

To Farrell's delight, Cardinal Meyer felt confident enough of his grasp of the issues to enter the fight against the University of Chicago. This gave Alinsky the financial and moral base he needed to move into the situation. Burke and Egan set up a meeting between Alinsky and Meyer, wherein the archbishop offered $50,000 from Catholic Charities for the fledgling organization. Egan, who was present at this meeting, heard Alinsky warn Meyer that what was about to happen was going to be very controversial. Meyer simply pointed to the crucifix in his office and quietly assured Alinsky: "The man on that cross was controversial."[62] In addition to the grant from the archdiocese,

matching funds flowed in from other foundations and the Presbyterian Church. With these monies, the Temporary Woodlawn Organization began in early 1961, as residents mobilized to protest the university's expansion plans, as well as the overcrowded schools, the high rents for substandard buildings, and other assorted ills.

The involvement of the archdiocese did not deter the University of Chicago in the slightest. They had bested Egan in Hyde Park–Kenwood and felt they could easily summon public sympathy again for their cause and stir up resentment toward the Church. An alternative community organization was co-opted by university officials, called the Associated Clubs of Woodlawn. It functioned as an umbrella organization for all who opposed the IAF efforts. The university newspaper, the *Chicago Maroon*, accused Catholic officials like Egan of importing the Industrial Areas Foundation into Woodlawn as a "hate group" and once again attempted to portray Catholic resistance as narrow interest group politics and secretly antiblack. One official of the Lutheran Church, for example, decried the formation of the Woodlawn Organization as "an attempt by Monsignor Egan ... to do something rather specific and rather desperate to preserve Catholic congregations in Woodlawn."[63] Later, five Woodlawn area ministers publicly disassociated themselves from the IAF-sponsored organization efforts.[64] At the end of June, the *Christian Century* attacked IAF efforts and accused the Catholic Church and Cardinal Meyer of encouraging the organization of Woodlawn to keep blacks from moving into white neighborhoods. For proof, they gave a malignant twist to an address Meyer had delivered the previous autumn to his priests on the issue of racial justice:

> Cardinal Meyer said: "We all realize that there are many practical problems facing a pastor in a changing neighborhood— rapidly falling income, suddenly empty classrooms, vacant pews in the church and high maintenance costs continuing." Will somebody rise and say that this reference also is to Negro churches and not to integrated churches? What we cannot understand is how the Roman Catholic church bridges the gulf between statements like those made at the clergy conference and

the strategy being followed in Woodlawn, between papal encyclicals which bear on Social Christianity and the Back-of-the-Yards Council, between support for the outstanding work of the Catholic Interracial Council and support for the sort of politico-economic organizations which are created by the Industrial Areas Foundation.[65]

Meyer was undeterred by the criticism and kept up his support for the Woodlawn group. Despite the efforts of the South East Chicago Commission and the University of Chicago, by March 1962 a firm alliance of ninety-seven community groups was formed into the Woodlawn Organization, which swung into action and mobilized opposition to the University of Chicago. This stopped the planned development in its tracks. Later, with the advent of "Black Power," the organization became a model of community activism nationwide and one of the models for Lyndon B. Johnson's Community Action Program (CAP). Despite a tumultous and financially shaky history, the organization still exists today.

CONCLUSION

Egan's tactics and Meyer's support provided a thrilling moment in Chicago Catholic history. It was a moment very much in the forefront of the churning activism that would sweep American society in the sixties. But in the long run, the aim of the policy—that is, more stable neighborhoods and successfully integrated communities—failed. White Catholics simply moved out of the city into the suburbs. This sapped many of these community organizations of vital leadership. Moreover, as in the case of the Organization for the Southwest Community, the support of priests was erratic at best. The power base of Chicago Catholicism had moved away from the urban centers to the suburbs. Community organizations fell into disarray as urban blight moved inexorably into neighborhoods struggling for existence. By 1989 so many of the grand old parishes of the West and South Sides were closing and consolidating that the *Official Catholic Directory* entry for Chicago included a list of those parishes that had closed.

In late 1989 Cardinal Joseph Bernardin began the sad task of closing urban parishes and schools that no longer fit the chancery's criteria of viability. Small urban parishes continued to exist, and the various white enclaves and regentrified areas of the city continued to have a vibrant parochial life. But the era of the large urban parish, with an army of sisters staffing a large, thriving school and a half-dozen black-cassocked curates in attendance on a lordly monsignor, were over. In the struggle to preserve the old neighborhoods by means of a distinctively Catholic appeal to the common good, the forces of "solidarism" gave way to individual gain and the lure of suburbia.

8

The Challenge of Race:
Stritch, the Uncertain Trumpet

"We gave them quite a show," chuckled Samuel Stritch after his first formal contact with Chicago's black community.[1] Catholic Week of the American Negro Exposition had been replete with all kinds of music and demonstrations, and the cream of the city's black Catholic elite were well represented, including Dr. Arthur Falls, member of the executive board of the Chicago Urban League, and James Dorsey, a prominent black Catholic attorney from Milwaukee. Hovering behind the scenes was the chief convert maker among blacks in Chicago, Father Joseph Eckert, S.V.D., whom Stritch had met in April 1940 at a meeting of midwestern clergy engaged in the "colored apostolate."

"I am most anxious," Stritch later wrote to Father Eckert, "to do all in my power to further the Apostolate of the Church among our Colored Catholics. The work which you and your confreres are doing in Chicago is admirable and gives me great hopes for the future."[2] For Samuel Stritch, the conversion of African-Americans to Catholicism was his highest priority in any kind of racial ministry. This would remain his position throughout his eighteen years in Chicago. But the shifting sands of racial relations in Chicago and the nation at large highlighted other needs that Stritch would find difficult to confront from 1940 to 1965.

249

CHICAGO AND THE RACIAL ISSUE

Although blacks had been living in Chicago and its environs from the very origins of the city (indeed, one of the original settlers of Chicago, Jean Baptiste Pointe du Sable, was a black from Santo Domingo), the core of Chicago's black population was added during the Great Migration of 1915-1918.[3] In 1910 approximately 44,000 black residents comprised 2 percent of the city's 2,185,000 inhabitants, and more than half of them lived outside a small black ghetto.

World War I's demand for labor and the shutting off of European immigration compelled Chicago's industries to recruit black laborers from the South. Fed up with Jim Crow legislation and attracted by the prospects of better living and working conditions in the North, blacks, by the thousands, followed the route of the Illinois Central Railroad and arrived in Chicago from the rural South. African-American migrants moved into the old areas near the center of the city, mainly on the South Side, where they rapidly filled the limited number of housing units in established "negro" neighborhoods. As World War I ended they started to push the ghetto outward along its borders in the first great expansion southward between South Parkway and State Street. By 1920 Chicago's African-American community was 110,000 strong or 4.1 percent of the city's population. A growing population cramped into limited living quarters was a recipe for violence.

These tense conditions exploded in a horrendous race riot in 1919 when black strikebreakers were imported to replace striking white workers seeking higher pay and better working conditions. This left 39 dead and 519 injured. The 1919 riot was one of the worst outbreaks of racial violence in the North and left a permanent state of tension between whites and blacks in the city of Chicago. Moreover, white Chicagoans, fearful of the decline of property values, determined to maintain racial segregation in housing by systematically bombing the homes of blacks who moved into white neighborhoods or of whites who sold to them. Indeed, a house was bombed every twenty days in Chicago between July 1, 1917, and March 1, 1921.

In the 1920s, as we have seen, white real estate interests in Chicago undertook a new approach to keep neighborhoods free

of blacks—the racially restrictive covenant. This was a mutual, written agreement among property owners in a given area by which each signatory agreed not to sell or lease his property to a black nor let a black live on it, except as a *"bona fide"* servant. By the 1940s as much as 80 percent of all white residential property in Chicago and the suburbs was covered by the blanket of restrictive covenants.

Although the depression slowed the rate of African-American migration to the city, the numbers continued to increase. By the beginning of the depression the black population jumped to 233,903. World War II also brought another large migration of black labor badly needed for war production. By 1940 the city's black population was 278,000, or 8 percent of the city's total. By 1950 it rose to 492,000 persons, or 14 percent of the city's population. Between 1950 and 1960 the black population increased by 65 percent, from 492,000 to 813,000. Meanwhile, in the same period (1950–1960), there was a decline in the white population. For the first time in its history, the city's total population decreased by 70,000 residents. By 1960 blacks comprised 23 percent of all Chicagoans. With every surge of the African-American population the swelling population pushed the limits of the black belt farther south, west, and north. The main area of black settlement was an upside down L-shaped strip of land running from Sixty-seventh Street to Chicago's Loop, and then jutting out to the west between the Chicago-Burlington and Quincy Railroad, South Sixteenth Street and the Chicago and Northwestern Railroad, and Kinzie on the northwest. Regardless of their social status or economic condition, African Americans were kept within the confines of these streets as long as possible. City officials and other civic leaders did little to ameliorate conditions in the black belt. Moreover, blacks were barred from jobs in white areas and prohibited from using public facilities by a de facto segregation that was every bit as rigid as the segregation of the southern states.[4]

CATHOLIC RESPONSES

The first recognized ministry to black Catholics began in the basement of Old St. Mary's Church in the downtown. Archbishop

Patrick Feehan (1829–1902) recruited Father Augustine Tolton, the first ordained black priest in the Chicago archdiocese, to minister to the struggling community. Tolton helped to establish St. Monica's Church on the South Side in 1893 and labored indefatigably until his premature death of sunstroke in 1897. St. Monica's was the main gathering place for the tiny black Catholic community of Chicago, served by white diocesan priests until 1917, when Archbishop Mundelein requested the services of the Fathers of the Divine Word to serve black Catholics. Even before the tragic race riot of 1919, Mundelein was intent on maintaining St. Monica's exclusively for African Americans.[5] The Divine Word Fathers pastored St. Monica's, aided by the Sisters of the Blessed Sacrament, who arrived at the parish in 1913. When St. Monica's burned in 1924, Mundelein consolidated the parish with the older South Side Irish parish of St. Elizabeth.

After the race riot of 1919, Mundelein even more firmly insisted that black Catholics attend St. Monica's and later St. Elizabeth's Church. The man who set the standard of ministry to African Americans in these parishes was Father Joseph Eckert, S.V.D., a German immigrant who regarded the rapidly growing black area of Chicago as a mission territory. He aggressively sought out black children to attend the parish school and actively proselytized the parents to become Catholics. Eckert achieved phenomenal success and a quickening of black Catholic life on the South Side made necessary an expansion of facilities, which included a high school and plans for a hospital.[6] In 1932 Eckert was appointed head of St. Anselm's parish on Sixty-first and Michigan, another old parish on the South Side whose neighborhood had become predominantly black. Eckert took the nearly dead parish and within a couple of years had it up and running with a thriving parish school staffed by the Sisters of the Blessed Sacrament. The sisters also opened one of the areas's first high schools for African-American Catholics at the parish.[7] In eight years Eckert baptized over 1500 converts.[8] Following closely on the accomplishments at St. Elizabeth's and St. Anselm's was Corpus Christi parish on Forty-ninth and South Parkway. It too had begun around the turn of the century as an Irish parish with

a magnificent Italian Renaissance church. The parish had at one time been so prosperous it was able to donate money for one of the theology buildings at St. Mary of the Lake Seminary. By the end of the twenties, however, the neighborhood was black and the diocese handed the parish over to the Franciscan Friars, who operated it for a time as a retreat center, and then reopened it as a parish in 1933. It became a lively hub of black Catholic life with a large grade school and a thriving high school.[9] On the West Side of the city, a small contingent of black Catholics were ministered to by the Jesuits of Holy Family Parish at St. Joseph's Mission. This tiny chapel opened in 1933 under the direction of the saintly Father Arnold J. Garvy, S.J.[10]

Mundelein considered these efforts sufficient to tend to Chicago's growing numbers of African-Americans. But prescient observers like Monsignor Reynold Hillenbrand noted that such policies were bound to be insufficient to meet the growth of the black population. He wrote to pioneer Catholic interracialist Father John LaFarge, S.J., who had visited the seminary: "I fear you come to Chicago too seldom and we must take every occasion to bring the Negro problem before the seminarians of Chicago. Our local situation is becoming more acute each year."[11] Hillenbrand spoke accurately. The seminarians he prepared for ordination would devote much of their priestly ministries dealing with the effects of these demographic shifts, either by staffing parishes in all-black areas, or coping with massive suburban growth, in part sparked by white-flight. Between 1893 and 1940 only ten parishes were affected by the expansion of the black population into all-white neighborhoods. In 1950 the number of parishes affected was thirty-eight, and by 1960, seventy-six.[12] This represented millions of dollars in real estate and the voluntary relocation of several hundred thousand Catholic men, women, and children. Moreover, the increasingly insistent demands of blacks for access to white Catholic institutions such as schools, hospitals, and fraternal organizations— demands echoed by their white supporters—called on Catholics to put into effect the teachings on social justice that they had espoused so vigorously during the thirties. Mundelein did not live to see it. Samuel Stritch and Albert Meyer did.

STRITCH'S POLICIES

Cardinal Stritch was least well-equipped temperamentally and philosophically to deal with this aspect of change in Chicago Catholic life. Stritch was indelibly southern in his attitudes on racial issues. He displayed this in private conversation, when he would refer to blacks as "niggers." Once, he accused one of his Milwaukee priests of leaving his quarters at a Catholic high school "unfit for a nigger."[13] Chancery official and later Bishop Cletus F. O'Donnell was once ordered by Stritch to "give this nigger a good tip" in reference to a railroad porter who had carried the archbishop's luggage on board a train.[14] In a letter to his chief theological adviser, Stritch wrote from Hobe Sound, Florida: "Do not choose the winter climate of Florida if you have some deep thinking to do. Here you take on the habits of the colored folk and do as little as is consistent with being alive."[15]

Other than the conversion of blacks to Catholicism, Stritch was generally ambivalent on racial matters. He moved reluctantly to attack racial discrimination in his archdiocese then only under the pressure of demographic, social, and political events. Intellectually and theologically, he believed in equal rights for the "colored," but his "gut-feelings" on racial attitudes never totally changed. This was exemplified in 1957, the year before his death, when he upbraided a pastor who compared black migration into his parish to the Soviet invasion of Hungary, but he also warned the bishop of a neighboring diocese against the perils of interracial mixing, which he called "mulattoism." In part, because of his reluctance to speak and act, sad incidents of racial discrimination occurred in parishes, schools, and other Catholic institutions, such as hospitals, with regularity during his eighteen years in Chicago.

At the outset of his administration, Stritch did not even deal directly with racial matters but handed them over to Monsignor George Casey for disposition. For example, in 1942, at Holy Angels Church on the South Side, blacks were not permitted to seat themselves in the center pews. One black Catholic complained:

> While waiting for Mass to begin an usher came to me and asked me to move on the far side of the Church because the pew I was

sitting in was for white only.... I have always been taught that the Church was "God's House" and that everyone was welcome. *He* wouldn't ask me to sit out of view of everything because my skin is dark.[16]

Stritch handed the matter over to Monsignor Casey, who replied to the woman:

I wish to assure you that no discrimination is intended by this regulation. Certainly the good order and the common good require certain regulations and such regulations are not intended to be discriminatory.... I am given to understand that from one hundred to one hundred and fifty Colored people attend the various Masses at Holy Angels on Sunday. By far the majority of these find no inconvenience and do not consider the existing regulation as discriminatory. I am sure that you will feel better about this whole matter if you follow the practice of the majority.[17]

Stritch's laissez-faire policy on racial issues became even more pronounced when he dealt with groups formed to identify and counteract racial discrimination. For example, in 1941 Dr. Arthur Falls wrote to Stritch:

On more than one occasion, efforts have been made in Chicago to develop an active Catholic Interracial Group which would be able to make a distinct contribution to the program of interracial cooperation.... I therefore should like to request that Your Highness consider the possibilities of a Chicago Catholic Interracial Council, developed under your auspices....[18]

Stritch replied in a noncommittal way: "I am pained to learn from your letter that here in Chicago there is some difficulty in securing for our Colored brothers the recognition of their rights. I am sure we all want to make a Christian justice and a Christian charity the prevailing norm in our community action."[19] But words of justice and charity notwithstanding, Stritch was wary of any group that might potentially stir up racial troubles. Earlier that year, when a group of cloistered Dominican Sisters wanted to open a convent for "colored Catholic girls," Stritch turned them down saying: "the opportune moment has not arrived for the erection of a contemplative convent for colored girls and women in this Archdiocese."[20] The "opportune moment" would never arrive.

VISITATION: A BASTION OF SEGREGATION

Stritch also did very little to curtail some of the most fla-grant racism in the parishes. Such was the case of a bastion of racial segregation, at Visitation Parish at Fifty-fifth and Halsted Street on Chicago's South Side. Visitation was a proud old Irish parish founded in 1886 at Garfield Boulevard and Peoria Street.[21]

In June 1932 the Irish-born Monsignor Daniel Byrnes assumed the pastorate and became a virtual czar of the South Side Irish Catholic community. He began a tremendous building program during the depression and made Visitation one of the premier parishes of the archdiocese. In 1936 the parish school registered 1,441 children, and 637 girls attended a parish high school which dated back to 1915. Scores of Visitation's young men went to the seminary and hundreds of its daughters entered the convent. In 1939 Byrnes instituted a colossal May Crowning ceremony that annually closed down busy Garfield Boulevard and became a community institution. Byrnes's pow-erful influence helped in the formation of the Garfield Boulevard Improvement Association, one of many community groups dedicated to cordoning off the neighborhood from the incursions of the black belt. This organization actually held its meetings in the parish hall and regularly sponsored "paint-up-clean-up" committees which monitored the condition of prop-erty in the area with an eye to keeping out blacks by insisting on proper upkeep of housing stock. Father Martin Farrell, a son of the parish, later characterized Byrnes as "a good man, right on just about every subject but one."[22] Farrell meant race relations. Farrell recalled how Byrnes could give a sermon without men-tioning blacks or race issues. For example Byrnes would say: "I was walking down the boulevard the other day and I noticed that some of those houses on such and such a street needed some repair."[23] Everybody knew what he was saying: keep the neighborhood clean or blacks will move in.

Byrnes was a power in his community and beloved by his people. When he died of a heart attack in 1952 ecclesiastical and civic dignitaries flocked to the church to pay their respects.[24] Without a doubt, Byrnes was at the heart of efforts to prevent blacks from moving into the neighborhood. This was painfully

evident when its parishioners played a role in the Peoria Street riots which took place in the neighborhood. In a letter of protest to Cardinal Stritch, Arthur Falls wrote:

> It would not be correct to state that only Catholics have partici-pated in these recurring evidences of group hatred, but certainly Catholics have been most active in them and frequently have been in positions of leadership. The last riot was clearly a reflec-tion of the anti-Negro and anti-Jewish attitudes which for years have characterized the clerical and lay leadership of Visitation Parish.[25]

Only later, in the wake of the 1949 Englewood riots, again spawned in the Visitation district, did Stritch direct his secretary, Monsignor John Fitzgerald, to put a stop to the antiblack activi-ties.[26] But, apart from this, Stritch refused to deal forcefully with Byrnes and Visitation. Edward Marciniak tried to put a good face on the matter in a letter to a black leader, "Even the Cardinal hasn't been able to do anything about him."[27] More-over, the Dominican Sisters were cowed into silence by his strict insistence on racial segregation. When Sister Gustave Olson dared to question the racially discriminatory admission policies of the parish school, she was promptly shuttled off to a new mis-sion.[28] Byrnes's successor, Monsignor Richard Wolfe, proved to be almost as intransigent as his predecessor. A native of the South Side and former pastor of Old St. Patrick's, Wolfe took immediate steps to reassure the parishioners by having the parish bulletin of his appointment read: "Father Wolfe comes to Visitation not as a stranger but as a friendly neighbor, *who knows and respects the great spirit and traditions of the people who compose Visitation Parish.*"[29] Wolfe would be as big an obstacle to integra-tion as was Byrnes. The Visitation situation would fester until the time of Cardinal Meyer.

SCHOOL SEGREGATION

In addition to problems in parish worship, blacks found resistance from white Catholics when they tried to integrate Catholic schools. Again, Stritch did little to remedy the situation. Schools were an important part of black interest in Catholicism

and an important tool for proselytizers such as the Divine Word Fathers. In a study commissioned by various Protestant church groups titled, "Catholic Penetration of the Negro Community," black researchers Horace Cayton[30] and Frank Dorsey pointed out that, to blacks, "the first and most compelling feature of the Catholic Church was its system of schools that offered a superior Christian education."[31]

The established black parishes, St. Elizabeth's, St. Anselm's, and Corpus Christi, all had thriving schools for black children. It was the movement of black children into all-white schools on the South and West Sides that caused problems. As in the case of parish membership, it was Cardinal Mundelein who had originally laid down the policy of racial segregation in the Catholic schools of Chicago. White pastors in changing neighborhoods regularly directed black children to "colored schools," usually at some distance from their homes. The growth of the black population on the West Side, in the vicinity of the Jesuit-run Holy Family Church, an old parish at Roosevelt Road and May Street, was a case in point. In the thirties blacks had begun to move into the neighborhood with the building of the Jane Addams Housing Project. To cope with the numbers of black Catholics, the Jesuits reopened St. Joseph's School, under the leadership of Father Arnold J. Garvy. Father Elmer A. Barton, S.J., the pastor of Holy Family, attempted to keep his school all white despite the increasing numbers of blacks who wanted to go to Holy Family School. One such parishioner was Spencer A. Wilson, who complained to Stritch:

> In May of this year, I moved my family from the South Side to the West Side, residing in the parish of Holy Family Church. This Church is located at Roosevelt Road & May Streets. My family and I have been hearing Mass there on Sundays. Monday evening, August 16, my wife and I approached Father Barton ... and expressed our desire to enroll our youngest son in the elementary school.... He explained to me, that I must enroll my child in St. Joseph's School which was for colored children and near my residence. I asked him why there should be separate schools and separate churches in the same parish since we were all Catholics, English speaking people, and Americans. His reply

was that the temperament of the white parishioners would not permit the mixing of the two races, although he would be perfectly willing to have them mixed.[32]

Stritch waltzed around Wilson's complaint with a "just give it time" sermon:

> Our holy religion sums up all its moral teaching in the word "charity" and we must work until finally we have removed certain stubborn social facts which militate against the wide exercise of Christian charity. Much has been done, and if we work with understanding zeal, the whole thing will be done in the not too distant future. I know that the presence of this social fact is a temptation to impatience, for I myself am impatient at it. The colored man, without in any way losing pride in his race or advocating the melting of it into the general population, must be accorded his rights, and his dignity must be respected. Let us pray that the thing we are trying to do will speedily be done, and let us not spoil the speedy coming of it by an emotional approach to the solution of a great problem.[33]

Holy Family would remain segregated until the sixties.

In another incident in 1944, even the complaints of State Senator Christopher C. Wimbish protesting segregation at Holy Cross School in Woodlawn elicited no action from Stritch.[34]

A SUBTLE POLICY SHIFT

However, before the end of the war Stritch's conscience began to give him trouble about the racial issue. In 1943 he received a vehement complaint from a woman named Ernestine Martin. He shared this with Monsignor Joseph Morrison:

> I had a surprising letter today from some lady in Indiana, who is much wrought up over the admission of the colored girl from your high school into St. Mary's in Holy Cross, Indiana. Indeed were my southern prejudices as alive as in the most rabid southerner, I could not ever have taken the position which she takes. I think that I have answered her in a way that will let her know that I am fully in sympathy with the action of the Sisters at the college.[35]

To Mrs. Martin he had replied:

> I cannot understand how there could be any difficulty over the admission of a colored girl ... it would be very strange if a Catholic institution too far forgot Christian charity as to refuse to do what other schools of the same level are doing.[36]

In the summer of 1944 Stritch received a letter on the same topic from Mother Mary Samuel Coughlin:

> We have been asked by a priest who has charge of negroes whether our Trinity High School will admit negro girls as students. My spontaneous answer would be "Yes." Possibly we would lose a few students if we admitted negro girls; but we would be willing to suffer that for the principle. However, the residents of Oak Park and River Forest [communities adjacent to the high school] see objections to having negroes at Trinity High. They would probably wish to move out into these two suburbs; and if negroes bought property, the valuation of the property of the white residents would be lessened.... I wonder why the Lord made some people black and some people white—or, did He?[37]

Stritch wrote back: "I do not know of any other decision that is possible in the case which you present ... when you have room you will not make any racial distinctions in accepting girls. The problem is very difficult and all that we can do is to try and be Christians."[38]

What had brought about this change? Perhaps the virulence of Mrs. Martin's racism and the spontaneity of Mother Samuel's willingness to integrate the school shook something loose in Stritch. In any event, policies dealing with racial matters began to quietly shift after 1945. Beginning in 1945, Stritch overturned the segregation policy of his predecessor and permitted black children to attend schools that had previously welcomed only white children. The first school to feel the effects of this new policy was Holy Angels School on the South Side. Stritch went to great lengths to assure the success of Holy Angels, graciously subsidizing the parish with archdiocesan funds and securing the services of the Milwaukee-based School Sisters of St. Francis to replace the Sisters of Mercy who withdrew from the school. Stritch pleaded with Mother Corona Wirfs, head of the community:

Our problem is that we want to take a very large number of colored children into the school. We have the facilities and in time can have also a High School. The Sisters of Mercy teach the school, but they simply cannot give us Sisters for our enlarged work.... This is indeed a mission work. God is blessing our efforts for the colored. Would you consider taking this school? I know your love of souls and I am hopeful that you will say "Yes."[39]

Wirfs approved and Holy Angels became one of the premier sites for the education of black youth on the South Side. The policy change seemed so effective that even the outspoken black daily, the *Defender*, added Stritch to its 1950 Honor Roll of those breaking down racial barriers in Catholic institutions.

RACIAL INCIDENTS CONTINUE

But there were limits to Stritch's new racial policy. Except for a statement about discrimination in Catholic hospitals, Stritch never made his desegregation order a matter of the public record through a letter to all the priests, or at a clergy conference. The result was that incidents of blatant discrimination continued. Father Francis Quinn of St. Ambrose parish on Forty-seventh and Ellis Avenue was an example. In early 1946 former seminarian Robert Heywood and a friend had written Stritch regarding a sermon Quinn had preached on the feast of the Epiphany in which he boasted, "There isn't a colored family in my parish," and rejoiced that for twenty years the parish had maintained its all-white status. Heywood and O'Laughlin wrote a sharp letter to the pastor and ruefully noted: "As you preached your ill-disguised racism, we couldn't help but wonder how the dark-skinned King who brought his gifts would have felt on this Epiphany 1946, if he had approached the Church of St. Ambrose."[40] Heywood and O'Laughlin also wrote to Stritch, who promised to "look into this matter at once."[41] But apparently nothing was done, and in late June, Quinn preached another sermon that was taken down and repeated verbatim by a disgruntled black parishioner to Stritch:

The Niggers have taken over Corpus Christi church, Holy Angels and St. Anne's and now they are trying to take over this church;

but if it's left to me, they will not. Every time I park my car I'm afraid a Nigger will stab me in the back. Just last week a Nigger from Shakespeare school snatched a white woman's purse and when he was questioned he had snatched several other purses. What's the matter with you white people? Are you yellow? Now all Nigger lovers go back and tell the Niggers what I said.... Our forefathers from Ireland came over here and prepared the way for us in this church and the Niggers are not going to run us out.[42]

Other parishioners added their voices to the black woman's complaint.[43] Stritch instructed Casey to call Quinn and "tell the pastor at St. Ambrose to be careful and prudent in what he says from the pulpit. If he really made the statement attributed to him, he is only causing more trouble for us here in Chicago."[44] When questioned by Monsignor Casey about his intemperate pulpit oratory, Quinn retorted:

I did denounce lawlessness among the colored here in Kenwood. I, for one, cannot sit back while our women are raped and beaten.... The next letter of complaint from the negress will be a complaint that I have no negroes in my school. Isn't that just too bad. I cannot begin to care for my white children. When the day comes that you compel me, that will mark the end of St. Ambrose.... I know this is a problem for the Chancery Office. I know it is hard to decide. It would be much better to sleep on it a bit longer. If you don't you will find them demanding a colored Auxiliary Bishop for Chicago. I have some pretty decent colored in the parish. They are very much in the minority. The riff raff nigger I cannot tolerate any more than the riff raff white of which Kenwood has plenty.[45]

Finally, Stritch directly intervened in the St. Ambrose case, when Rosalie Kirtley, a black Catholic woman, attempted to register her son Ronald in the parish school. When Quinn refused admission to the child, Stritch finally wrote to the pastor:

The boy is a Catholic boy of your parish. Clearly he is a child of your flock and has a right to enter your school. In admitting Catholic children of your parish into your school there may not be set up a standard of race or color. You are the pastor of all

your people. Merely because the child is a negro is no legitimate excuse for refusing him admission.[46]

Quinn reluctantly complied with Stritch's request, but warned the Cardinal that the encroachment of blacks meant "St. Ambrose will be no more."[47] In 1956 Quinn resigned his pastorate and retired to St. Paul, Minnesota. St. Ambrose was, by that time, nearly all black.

Another incident occurred in far-off Lake Forest, where the former editor of the *New World,* Monsignor T. V. Shannon, used a Sunday sermon to display his racism. A young woman from Milwaukee wrote to Stritch about her visit to Shannon's parish:

> He mentioned the rioting in Cicero and said: "A dreadful thing." He then recalled when he built a two million dollar establishment in Highland Park with this statement: "I said then, as I say now, God bless and keep the colored people—out of *my* parish." Next he quoted someone as saying "When dealing with an inferior race we must either marry them or shoot them," "Well," he said, "We aren't marrying them," again a chuckle.[48]

Stritch replied to the young woman: "I shall take up the matter of what you say in the letter with the priest who made these remarks." But, he hoped, "that you get a chance to see some of the really outstanding work which is being done in parishes where there is no distinction whatsoever between colored and white."[49] But, as in the case of Quinn, Shannon's remarks continued. There clearly was no penalty for racism in the Archdiocese of Chicago.

As late as 1956 Father Henry Matimore, pastor of St. Clotilde's parish on the South Side, could write a Christmas letter to his flock comparing the white flight taking place in his parish boundaries to the flight of the Hungarians from Soviet tanks in the ill-fated revolution of 1956.[50] Only when the black newspaper, the *Defender,* picked up the story was Matimore corrected by Stritch:

> Now, Father, you know your theology. It is not necessary for me to tell you that you have made a very grave mistake in this letter.... We are not concerned about the color of people but we are concerned with their souls.[51]

CATHOLICS AND RACIAL VIOLENCE

The racist attitudes of some members of the Chicago clergy reflected the mood of the people in the parishes, who feared greatly for their property values and the viability of their communities. Typical was a letter from James E. Beemster to the Catholic Labor Alliance, protesting the Alliance's support for the building of a public housing project on 130th Street. He clearly spelled out the reasons for his disagreement and the impact it would have on the Church:

> The attitude you take that no depreciation of values should result by encroachment of the colored may be all right for theorists and college professors but experience has proven that such depreciation does take place. We have in this community approximately eleven Catholic schools and churches in addition to many other churches of other denominations.... What will happen to these churches if the colored people move in on us? You will find several of them closed up. Don't kid yourself.[52]

Even the racially tolerant Robert Heywood understood the attitude and expressed it in a letter to Quinn of St. Ambrose:

> We understand very well that the practical reason for the exclusion of Catholic negroes is your desire and that of your parishioners to retain the prosperity and well-being of your parish—its church, convent, schools and utility installations. We understand well enough than an influx of an impoverished population would reduce the income of your organization, disturb its behavior and manners, and impair somewhat the physical facilities for pastoral services.[53]

Beemster and Heywood had put their fingers on one of the major dilemmas of postwar Chicago: when blacks, in desperate search of decent housing, moved into white neighborhoods, their presence provoked vigorous, and sometimes violent, white opposition.

From the time of the Detroit riot of 1943 until well into the 1950s, there was a steady stream of racial incidents in Chicago "at the seams of the black ghetto in all directions."[54] The worst disturbances were at public housing projects. Six serious riots

occurred: the Airport Homes housing project (1946), Fernwood Park housing project (1947), Park Manor (Seventy-first and Lawrence, 1949), Englewood (Fifty-sixth and Peoria, 1949), Cicero (1951), Trumbull Park (1953), and Calumet Park (1957). All of them included significant participation by Catholic laity and, sometimes, the approval of Catholic clergy. In virtually all of them Cardinal Stritch kept silent or issued bland noncommittal replies in private correspondence.[55]

The first such incident occurred late in 1946 when several black veterans attempted to move into a public housing facility on 60th and Karlov known as the Airport Homes. White squatters moved into the empty homes to prevent a black move-in, and mob violence erupted at the site. In an effort to calm tensions Commissioner Thomas Wright of the City Human Relations Committee and Third Ward alderman Ralph Metcalfe sought help from local clergymen, including Father Michael Fennessy of St. Nicholas of Tolentine Church, who promised to put one of his curates on the problem.[56] Two other Catholic priests came out to the project as well. "The reception they got," Father Daniel Cantwell wrote later, "was not strictly liturgical. They were lucky to get out of the neighborhood without having their car overturned."[57] Appeals for help in quelling the disorder came to Cardinal Stritch from Arthur Falls, who telegrammed the prelate requesting help in mobilizing "dynamic Catholic leadership supporting [Housing] Authority stand for equal opportunity all citizens."[58] Stritch did not reply to Falls's telegram but did reply to a teacher who "eagerly look[ed] forward to a clear statement from the Catholic Church of Chicago, denouncing these crimes against humanity."[59] Stritch replied:

> Anybody living in Chicago ought to know my stand for justice and charity in race relations.... You may be sure that keeping within my competence I am doing my utmost in the inculcation of Christian principles in community living.[60]

Racial turmoil erupted two years later in the Park Manor Community between Sixty-seventh and Seventy-ninth Streets on the South Side. Black families had begun to move into the area in 1945 and 1946 and were driven out by hostile crowds who threatened them and vandalized their property. One group

monitoring the "racial integrity" of the community was the Park Manor Improvement Association—one of many community groups dedicated to keeping blacks out and included in its membership a number of Catholics. Edward Marciniak of the Catholic Labor Alliance had taken aim at the association in 1944 in an article in *Work* which was reprinted in the *Chicago Sun*. His criticism of their "united effort to keep Negroes out of the community" prompted an angry response from a Park Manor resident:

> I've been wondering just where you live or how close to your home are the colored. There isn't any community in Chicago where a negro family moved in that within a short time homes are devaluated to a small fraction of their original cost. I know, because I have had the experience twice and I don't want it again. The next thing our clergy will preach is inter-marriage with negroes.... Frankly, I believe that your article is about the best invitation to a race riot yet. When that time comes you can only blame yourselves.[61]

Incidents of arson, vandalism, and property destruction began in 1945 in Park Manor and picked up momentum throughout 1948.[62] The unsettled conditions affected the neighborhood's St. Columbanus parish on Seventy-first and Prairie, whose pastor, Monsignor William Gorman, had to be removed because of his inability to deal with the changing situation. In 1946 he was replaced by Father William E. Cousins, who in March 1949 was consecrated auxiliary bishop of Chicago. The steadily escalating violence in the neighborhood raised concerns on all parts, but left the priests of St. Columbanus curiously passive. When representatives of the Catholic Labor Alliance approached Father William Chawk, an assistant at the parish, to see if Cousins would give permission to distribute the periodical *Work*, Chawk said "he did not think it would go over very well with the people in the parish." "Because of the race question?" the worker asked. "Yes," he said.[63]

On the very day Chawk was speaking with the CLA representative the worst violence in Park Manor erupted on Seventy-first and Lawrence when mobs stormed the home of black residents, Mr. and Mrs. Roscoe Johnson. The Johnsons, who happened to be Catholics, were made prisoners in their home and

feared for their lives. One of the assistants at St. Columbanus visited the Johnsons, and a police escort had to be arranged to get him in the door. Cantwell commented sadly about the crowd at the Johnson home: "Outside the building were the people who called the priest 'father.' They would have lynched the Johnsons if they had the chance."[64] Later tensions developed over the admission of black children to the Catholic school in Park Manor. Cousins, in imitation of Stritch, avoided public comment on the violence, but worked behind the scenes to reconcile the warring parties and readily admitted black children to St. Columbanus School in the 1948–1949 school year.

At the end of 1949, racial and anti-Semitic violence erupted on Peoria Street in the Englewood neighborhood of Visitation parish. When a black couple came to visit the home of Mr. and Mrs. Aaron Bindman, a Jewish family on Peoria Street, rumors spread that blacks were moving into the neighborhood and the Bindman home was attacked by large mobs. Once again outraged citizens wrote to Stritch asking for some kind of public statement:

> I know you are familiar with the anti-Semitic and anti-negro riots that took place on 55th and Peoria Streets. I am sure you know the part that the Church of the Visitation played in instigating these riots. It has been brought back to us by reports from civic defense agencies in the city of Chicago that particular Parish Church has embarked on a career of "purifying the neighborhood." It was also pointed out that Rev. Burns [Byrnes] of the Visitation Church has a history of being anti-negro.[65]

Stritch deflected the issue at hand with reference to previous statements:

> I think it is very clear from my actions and statements that I abhor and condemn anti-semitism and any discrimination in our community against fellow-citizens because of race or color. Time and time again I have made this fact very clear and in my work it has been the governing principle of my actions.[66]

Stritch took public action only in the summer of 1951 when the western suburb of Cicero, a community of 70,000, exploded into racial violence, causing international headlines. Harvey

Clark, a Chicago transit worker, and his family attempted to become the first blacks to reside in Cicero, setting off a racial riot in the all-white, largely Eastern European community. The press silence which had characterized the outbreaks at Airport Homes, Fernwood, and Peoria Street gave way to massive coverage that was heard around the world. Mobs of young persons stormed the Clark home, destroying their possessions and battling with Illinois State Guardsmen and local police called in to restore order. Many of these young rioters were Catholics from one of the nine parishes in the city or from nearby Berwyn. William Gremley, the public affairs director of the Commission on Human Relations and a member of the Catholic Interracial Council, wrote a devastating article in the Jesuit weekly, *America*, entitled "The Scandal of Cicero." Gremley pointed out how the rioters wore: "sweaters with school names or crests on the back, Knights of Columbus lapel pins and rings, scapulars or other medals seen through an open shirt ... some fairly definite physical symbols of Catholic faith."[67]

Stritch was so alarmed by the violence and the bad press that he sent a special letter to all the pastors of the area, insisting they preach a sermon on racial justice. Other Catholics, embarrassed by the Cicero riot, issued independent statements condemning the violence. In late July, a group of twenty-nine residents of Cicero, Berwyn, Forest Park, and South Oak Park addressed a letter to their neighbors, urging them to examine their consciences in regard to the Cicero race riots.[68]

After the National Guard had restored order to the troubled suburb, the American Friends Service Committee and the Catholic Interracial Council formed a joint committee to investigate the conditions in the Cicero-Berwyn Area. Civil rights activist Bayard Rustin and Catholic Interracial Council member David McNamara combed the area interviewing pastors and community leaders about the riots and what needed to be done to prevent further violence.[69] McNamara found that the reactions of the clergy mirrored the prevailing attitudes of the community and reported to Father Cantwell:

> Between September 13 and October 10 I visited the eleven
> churches in question and talked to ten pastors and two assistants

... two pastors and two assistants displayed what I considered to be reasonable attitudes regarding the Cicero riot and race relations in general; Five pastors displayed attitudes ranging from disinterest to annoyance. Three pastors displayed attitudes of hostility, in varying degrees.[70]

Following on the heels of the Cicero riot were the disturbances at the Trumbull Park Homes, a 462-unit facility of the Chicago Housing Authority located between 105th Street and 109th Street, and Oglesby and Bensley Avenue on the far southeast side of Chicago. The housing development was located in the all-white community of South Deering and had been built in 1938. They fell under the racial composition rule established by Secretary of the Interior Harold Ickes in the thirties. Even when these rules were struck down in 1947, they continued to be observed at Trumbull Park. In 1952 a dark-skinned Argentinean family attempted to move into the neighborhood and was driven out. In July 1953 Mr. and Mrs. Donald Howard, light-skinned blacks, and their two children moved into an apartment in the project on South Bensley Avenue. When the news spread through the community, mobs gathered outside the Howard home and began pelting it with bricks and rocks. Violence escalated throughout August and September; nonetheless three more black families moved into Trumbull Homes. The acts of violence, harassment, and vandalism which ensued made South Deering a virtual police state as officers moved into monitor the movements of those going in and out of the troubled neighborhood. Much of the opposition to the black move-ins was generated by the South Deering Improvement Association and the National Citizens Protective Association, many of whose leaders were Catholics.

A particular scene of disorder was at the only Catholic Church in the community, St. Kevin's, on 105th and Torrence Avenue. Since Mrs. Howard was a Catholic, representatives of the American Civil Liberties Union and the Council Against Discrimination visited Father Raymond Pavis, the assistant pastor at St. Kevin's, about the prospects for Mrs. Howard coming to Mass. Pavis assured the visitors that he would welcome Mrs. Howard and telephoned to tell her so. Soon after the visit, Pavis

publicly welcomed the Howards to St. Kevin's and urged his parishioners to avoid mob violence. Mrs. Howard and her sister and mother attended the Mass in late 1953 without incident.

The Howards did not return to Mass until early January 1954. At that point antiblack incidents began when stones were thrown at their car. Early in the summer of 1954 troubles began in earnest at St. Kevin's. More black Catholic families had moved into the Trumbull Park Homes and registered their children at the parish school. The pastor, Father Michael Commins, promised to conduct a personal campaign for tolerance in the parish with sermons, literature, and personal calls. Even as he made this pledge, on July 18, 1954, one black woman, attending 8:00 Mass at St. Kevin's, Mrs. Charles Falls, was struck over the head with an umbrella by Mrs. Sophie Ferrera. Commins deplored the violence on the church steps as "very un-Christian like." Nonetheless, violent incidents on parish property continued. As black Catholics showed up for Mass in squad cars, they were often attacked or harassed by white parishioners, many of whom were leading members of the South Deering Improvement Association. By the end of 1954 conditions seemed to improve, and Cantwell wrote to Stritch:

> I thought you would like to know that five of the Negro Catholics living in Trumbull Park housing project attended Mass yesterday at St. Kevin's. It was accomplished without any unfortunate incident.... This successful first step toward normal Catholic parish life would, I thought, please you and add to the joy of Christmas. Here in the building we offered some of the prayer and fasting of Ember Week for peace in Trumbull Park.[71]

But Cantwell was premature in his hopes for a return of "normal Catholic parish life." Racial incidents resumed and escalated in 1955. One Sunday six blacks attended Mass at St. Kevin's, guarded by police. The pastor begged for an end to the harassment and violence, while outside his parishioners formed a mob and shouted racial epithets as the blacks emerged from the service. The Catholic Interracial Council made valiant efforts to defuse tensions by passing out literature on the situation, visiting the black Catholics in the project, holding meetings with the pastor and assistants, and briefing Cardinal Stritch and other Catholic dignitaries on the situation.[72]

The Trumbull Park disturbances lasted nearly four years. As the tension continued unabated, members of the CIC and other civil rights activists, like CORE co-founder Homer Jack, began to grow impatient with Stritch's silence. In March 1956 Jack published an article in *Christian Century* entitled "Test at Trumbull Park," openly criticizing Stritch's silence:

> Throughout this affair the Roman Catholic archdiocese of Chicago has been a disappointment. Anyone who read the special Christianity issue of *Life* magazine must have been impressed with the efficiency of this, the world's largest Catholic diocese. Why then can't it be effective when a problem like Trumbull Park looms up? Perhaps a non-Catholic expects more from the Roman organization than he should.... Yet one cannot read of the courageous stand taken in tense racial conflict by the archbishops of St. Louis and New Orleans without wondering why Cardinal Stritch, head of the Chicago archdiocese, has failed to assume leadership in this instance. Why has he refused to come out publicly when some of his concerned laymen have implored him to do so? The cardinal's silence is more ominous than the bungling of some of his priests.[73]

Edward Marciniak published a spirited defense of Stritch, noting his work in the area and his support for the Catholic Interracial Council. However, the need for some clear statement was increasingly necessary.[74] Finally, in June 1956, at the time he announced the formation of the Committee for the Spanish-Speaking, Stritch also spoke out against the Trumbull Park violence. The *Defender* praised Stritch for breaking "his long silence on the Trumbull Park atrocities." But it wondered "why the church had not been more forthright previously in its actions since the community in which Trumbull Park is located is predominantly Catholic."[75] Later that year Stritch heard a tape recording of some of the reactions to his message by black Catholics in Trumbull Park and promised an even clearer statement of principles. But, as so many other of Stritch's promises, the statement was never made. Until the end, Stritch never could bring himself to join his theoretical sense of the need for racial justice with his inner convictions about interracial relations. He replied to a question from Bishop Martin McNamara of Joliet about appearing at an NAACP program with Protestant ministers:

In our condition in these northern States there can be no argument from prudence to excuse us from taking a firm stand on according the negro his full rights and opportunities in social and political life. There is no civil law impeding such action. The argument that some Catholics may give up the practice of their religion cannot be sustained by facts. The fact that when a negro moves into a neighborhood the white move out and thereby do an injury to parishes is based on the false assumption that white are forced to move out.... In the Church there must be no distinctions of race or color. This means in church attendance, in schools and in our activities. It also includes hospitals and all our institutions. We must be catholic.

But, after having said this he concluded the letter:

While I would not deny a negro all his rights and opportunities, I foresee that even when our problem is happily resolved, there will be neighborhoods largely negro and largely white. I cannot conceive that any negro or any white looks to the solution of the problem through mulattoism.[76]

SUPREME COURT DECISIONS AND THE CIVIL RIGHTS MOVEMENT

Stritch was even less reconciled to the notion that legislative or judicial means ought to be employed to enforce racial change. He had worked quietly for the defeat of a permanent Fair Employment Practices Commission in the Illinois State Legislature in 1945, a piece of legislation that had been introduced several times. When it went down again in 1945, Bishop James Griffin of Springfield worried about the damage to the Church's reputation among blacks:

The F.E.P.C. Bill died in the Senate during the week. A colored representative from the south side and who was a Catholic, was quite bitter against Father Barrett of the Hospital Association for appearing against the bill.... The colored gentleman—pardon the word—did make the distinction between the Church and the individual. His attitude was one of hurt feelings rather than condemnation.... True, there were many other features in the bill

which were not good, but Father Barrett should have made the distinction more emphatic and thereby saved the alienation of many of these colored people from the Church.[77]

Stritch dismissed the concern:

In the matter of the F.E.P.C. Bill I think that things have gone just as we expected. The whole thing put us on the spot and I think that Church Authority has come out very well. Individual priests have appeared on both sides. Where the mistake was made I think is that as you say the distinction between the intent of the legislation and the particular provisions of this Bill was not made clear. All of us are for what was intended. Some differ regarding the particular provisions of this Bill. Among those who feel that there were provisions in this Bill which were not wise at this time or perhaps at any time were those who had a great love of human rights and human freedoms.[78]

When the Supreme Court began deliberations on the issue of racial integration, Stritch was deeply concerned. In late April 1954, he received a letter from Archbishop Gerald O'Hara, apostolic nuncio to Dublin and bishop of Savannah, Georgia. O'Hara had received news about the *Brown* vs. *The Board of Education* case from his auxiliary bishop, Francis Hyland. Hyland had heard rumors that the Court was going to strike down compulsory segregation, and he worried about its impact on Church schools and other institutions. O'Hara had written back to Hyland and insisted "we cannot do anything that would involve the loss of souls" and "we cannot do anything that would create in the minds of the Negro population the false idea that the Church is opposed to their enjoyment of every legitimate human right." But O'Hara recognized as well that the admission of blacks into Catholic schools would make "many parents, even those who rank as devout Catholics," withdraw their children. Indeed, O'Hara seemed willing to tolerate the continuation of segregation. He concluded:

I think it can be truthfully said that the Colored people in Georgia know where you and I stand on this question. We would like to see the Colored admitted to all other schools, but we know that due to the mentality of the people of the South, even of our

own Catholics, this would have, as I said before, the result of emptying our White schools and bringing about little by little the loss of many souls. I myself lost friends fifteen years ago when I permitted Colored patients to be admitted to the Cancer Home. Devout Catholic men and their wives turned against me and have remained hostile ever since.[79]

Stritch responded to Hyland at O'Hara's request:

My information is that the hearing of the case had been completed and that the Court is studying it and preparing its decision. Let us be hopeful that the decision will be prudent and helpful! For the present, certainly it seems to me that the proper thing to do is to avoid making any statement on the matter. What if the decision demands great changes? Knowing all the facts, I think that our position should be quietly and without any statement to accept it.[80]

In the meantime the Court issued the *Brown* decision and Hyland wrote to Stritch:

It will be no news to Your Eminence that the decision is not being received very well in Georgia by the people generally and particularly by those in public office. Certainly the Church should be the leader in promoting justice and charity in all their forms, but it seems to me at present that we shall have to await developments on the State level, both to avoid "scandalizing" our White Catholics and to safeguard the greater and more permanent interests of our Colored people.

Hyland confided to Stritch, "Needless to say, I am not at all certain that my present position is the correct one, all the more so because in recent months some of the Bishops have become extremely 'righteous' on the subject of segregation. Almost overnight, it has become both a 'sin' and a 'heresy.'"[81]

Stritch, who had recently returned from the canonization of Pope Pius X, and after a conversation with O'Hara, wrote to Hyland:

I think there are some interpretations of the Supreme Court decision which are a bit exaggerated. As far as I can see, in the decision the reference is to public schools and not to private schools.... All

in all, my advice is to wait out the storm and then to reach decisions which will be in conformity with what can be done towards the ideal in the circumstances which prevail.[82]

In the end there would be no doubt Stritch would follow the decree of the Supreme Court. The following year in a letter to Clair Driscoll, lobbyist for the Illinois bishops, regarding a bill before the Illinois legislature implementing the desegregation order, he stated: "Since the United States Supreme Court decision fixed the norm for public schools, this proposed legislation is aimed at Catholic and private schools. We shall follow the norm and do it without hesitation."[83]

In a letter to Archbishop Muench he wrote:

There is no good reason for segregation in our country. However, we have to face a fact. There has been segregation and there has been segregation over a great many years. In many areas, the colored population has not had its rightful opportunities in education and probably because of a lack of these opportunities there are differences that have to be faced. The whole question is whether in certain areas to try to do this thing over night or do it gradually over a period of time.... Eventually segregation will disappear.... There just isn't any chance of maintaining segregation as a long time practice any more in this country.[84]

But he always felt that enforced integration was the wrong approach and said as much to an FBI agent assigned to monitor the Chicago black situation. This man reported to Director J. Edgar Hoover:

You might be interested to know the greater majority of Cardinal STRITCH's comment concerned the integration problem in the Chicago area. It was his personal opinion, given in a confidential manner, that while "some progress" had been made, he felt it was totally on the surface. He said there was no violence of any kind when Negroes moved into an all white parish neighborhood but that in a very short time the whites just moved out.... It is his feeling ... that when the real tests of integration come they will not be in southern cities but instead will be in northern cities such as Chicago. His feeling on this matter is based on the fact that the Negro group as a whole is a matriarchy with the mother

of the family acting as the stabilizing influence in their normal southern homes but that when the group moves to the north usually it is the father and eldest male children and consequently there is no family solidarity or stability to the group. The Cardinal plans to conduct a confidential experiment to see if in one such Negro-crowded parish they could start a program which will inculcate some family responsibility with the male children.[85]

CATHOLIC HOSPITALS

One bright exception to Stritch's reticence in racial matters was his condemnation of racial exclusion in Catholic hospitals. Only two hospitals admitted African-Americans in the Chicago area: Cook County General Hospital and Provident. There were twenty-five Catholic hospitals in the Archdiocese of Chicago in 1940 and only three were owned by the archdiocese (St. Vincent's, Misericordia, and Lewis Maternity).

Forging an archdiocesan policy related to racial admissions was difficult, since the hospitals, like other religious-order-dominated institutions of the archdiocese, had successfully resisted the centralization tactics of Cardinal Mundelein. Mundelein had appointed Father John W. Barrett as his representative to the Catholic hospitals in an effort to rein them in, but most of the hospitals ignored him and went about their own business. Soon after coming to Chicago, Stritch met with Barrett and the priest impressed on Stritch the need for more coordination in the hospital situation. At Barrett's urging, Stritch formed an Archdiocesan Catholic Hospital Council, consisting of representatives of the Catholic hospitals of the archdiocese, and insisted on annual meetings. Barrett informed Stritch:

> In the case of a few of the hospitals of the Archdiocese, I should like to see them a little more conscious that the Director of Hospitals is the Representative of the Archbishop in matters of interpreting diocesan policies in the work of coordinating our vast resources in the hospital field.[86]

Because these hospitals were virtually autonomous of the archdiocese, they were free to exclude blacks or segregate them if

they did admit them. And this is exactly what happened in Chicago. Catholic hospitals that operated in changing neighborhoods often had a color line or racial segregation in their wards, if they admitted blacks at all. The effect of this policy sometimes had fatal consequences. A typical example was the case of Mrs. Maude Johnston, a black woman with chronic heart problems.

Mrs. Johnston was an exemplary black Catholic. In 1912 she had entered St. Monica's School with the first twelve black children. In 1929 she helped establish a chapter of the Federation of Colored Catholics in Chicago, and in 1932 she had assisted the establishment of St. Joseph's Mission on the West Side. In the late thirties she aided Father John F. Ryan in founding Holy Name of Mary parish on the far South Side. In 1943 Mrs. Johnston offered to donate blood to the Red Cross blood bank and was informed that she had a serious heart condition. She received some treatment from the Mercy outpatient clinic, but when she suffered a severe heart attack on the night of January 28, 1944, she was urged by her doctor to enter a hospital. Her husband took her to nearby Mercy, where she was informed that she could not be admitted and would have to go to the all-black Provident Hospital. She refused to go and was taken instead to County Hospital, where she very nearly died. When she was recovered her strength, Mrs. Johnston wrote to Stritch:

> Reporters from two newspapers [the *Defender* and the *Bee*] have been trying to see me concerning the story of discrimination in the hospital, and I only want to say that it is a good thing that it is to me that this happened, because I would not release the story to the press.... I bring these facts to you because this whole experience has shaken my faith, and of course, my husband has stopped going to church. My non-Catholic relatives—I don't know what to say to them. The women of the parish, who also have been very active in church work for many years, are greatly incensed. I try to discourage them from doing anything rash, but, you know, we can take just so much.[87]

Soon after the Johnston incident, Stritch leaned on Mercy Hospital and secured a lifting of the racial ban; however, blacks continued to be denied maternity care at Mercy Hospital, and

black patients were housed in the oldest section of the hospital, nicknamed "the Black Hole of Calcutta." At times, male and female patients were kept in the same room without any screens or privacy.[88]

Another hospital in the area, Lewis Maternity, also had a racial exclusionary policy. With a generous grant from Catholic benefactor, Frank J. Lewis, Lewis Maternity had begun in the 1930s to prevent Catholic young women of poor means from going to secular hospitals, where they might receive birth control information. Lewis served the population of the near South Side, but excluded blacks from admission. However, the nature of Lewis's financial contribution to the hospital was a one-time affair, after which the institution was expected to make it on its own. By 1943 the hospital began to experience serious shortfalls and had to be subsidized from archdiocesan funds. In 1945 the Sisters of Providence, who administered the hospital, wrote to Stritch:

> As Your Excellency is well aware, the number of patients at Lewis Memorial keeps decreasing continually, and the income likewise, so that the Sisters have been obliged repeatedly to ask for help from the Chancery Office to make up for an insufficient budget ... we are wondering whether we should not be rendering Your Excellency a service in offering to withdraw our Sisters from an establishment whose patients could most likely be absorbed easily by other maternity or general hospitals of the city of Chicago.[89]

Stritch responded: "Mr. F. J. Lewis tells me that he is prepared to do much just as soon as conditions will permit for the hospital. I think it would be a mistake at this time to make the decision which you request."[90] Stritch had been working to preserve the hospital for some time. In 1941 he had coordinated a major upgrading of the services offered by the hospital and tried to keep it from raising its prices. One concession he agreed to was allowing poor Protestant mothers to register in the Catholic hospital, but, in approving this, he wondered if "such a procedure might also awaken the now dormant question of whether Negro mothers should be admitted."[91]

The question did not remain dormant long, and as a way of securing the financial stability of the institution, Stritch, in a

confidential memo, pushed for the admission of blacks to Mercy and Lewis hospitals:

> I think that there is a great need for a general maternity hospital on the south side that will admit negroes. Despite my efforts, Mercy has a colored line. Providence [sic, Provident] Hospital cannot meet the demands.... I envision Lewis as a maternity hospital patronized largely by negroes. We would of course not admit this to the public. How fine it would be to take care of these mothers! Mr. Lewis in the past has been against making Lewis in fact practically a hospital for negro mothers. I shall see him in Florida and shall persuade him. If we abolished without reservations the color line, we could raise the rates and set up the proposed departments.[92]

Lewis eventually did open up to black OB patients but kept them segregated. This was the best Stritch could do.

Discrimination against blacks in hospitals persisted well into the fifties. The interracial group at Friendship House sent Stritch a full report in 1955 charting evidence. The report charged: "Out of a total of fifteen Catholic hospitals in the Chicago area from which we were able to secure information (there are 22 in the area in all), only one, Alexian Brothers Hospital, admits patients on the basis of need and does not segregate."[93] The report went on to describe two types of hospitals: those which admitted negroes only on an emergency basis or on OB referral and segregated them, and those which admitted negroes only if they had a private room available at the time. Blacks had been hired in service positions, but in the professional ranks there was a noticeable lack of staff appointments for black doctors, and in only a few hospitals were black registered nurses found.[94]

This indictment of Chicago Catholic hospital practice, damning as it is, was less direct than the blunt speech given by Dr. A. M. Mercer in January 1950, when he became president of the Cook County Physicians Association. Mercer flailed Catholic opposition to national health programs as a subterfuge to continue their policies of racial exclusion.

> Negro Catholics have no personal rights to lose when it comes to their health. They cannot enter a Catholic hospital like other

Catholics. They *can enter* provided they submit in humility to segregation and discrimination. Even if they are willing to submit, they cannot be treated by a physician who is not white. It seems to me that we are barred purely on racial grounds, because most Catholic hospitals have white doctors of both the Protestant and Hebrew faiths on their staffs. A white atheist doctor has a much better chance of joining their staffs than a qualified Negro doctor.[95]

Stritch, who as we have seen had an abiding interest in health-care issues, supported a study day on the topic of race issues and Catholic hospitals sponsored by the Catholic Interracial Council and Friendship House. Father Barrett attended the meeting and spoke of the problems he encountered trying to convince the sisterhoods and the medical staffs of Catholic hospitals to accept black patients. The following year another conference was held and Stritch himself attended. He delivered a strong speech—one of his few forceful public comments on an issue of racism within the Catholic community:

As far as the care of the sick in our hospitals, on what right principle can we base our decision? How can we kneel before our blessed Savior on the Cross with His arms outstretched for all, and limit our charity and limit our ministration to any particular group. Charity embraces all and where these ugly distinctions obtain they have been justified on the grounds that the privately controlled hospital had to have patients, and has to have a proportion of patients who are pay patients in order to enable it to do its charity, and it cannot so extend its charity that it will become impossible to do any charity.... But ... it can look at man just as God looks at man, and without making distinctions of any sort.[96]

Cantwell was so elated with the speech that he wrote to Stritch:

Please permit me to say that the talk you gave yesterday at the hospital conference was magnificently clear and inspiring. I am sure that no one can have the slightest doubt about what you want done in our hospitals. It remains for us to try to create among the administrators a strong inner desire to implement these Christian principles and above all to reach the staff members more effectively.[97]

True to his word, Cantwell used Stritch's strong public statement to move on Catholic hospitals. After a city ordinance was passed in 1956 precluding racial exclusion from hospitals, members of the Catholic Interracial Council dutifully visited every Catholic hospital to insure compliance.[98]

CONVERT WORK

For Stritch, the conversion of blacks to Catholicism was clearly his highest priority. This interest went back to his earliest days as a priest in Tennessee. As a bishop he continued to pursue this interest. He had written to Bishop Joseph Hurley in 1943: "Ever since I have been going to Florida, and that is more than twenty years, I have been longing for some work among the colored in that state."[99] He had earlier stated to Monsignor T. V. Shannon, who frequently sent him statistics on the growth of the black population in Chicago: "I was very much interested in the information you gave me in your letter on the decrease in the white population in Chicago in the decade 1930–1940. I do think that one of our great works for religion in Chicago at this time is a more intense effort for the conversion of our colored people. Last week it was a joy for me to confirm 250 colored adults at Corpus Christi Church."[100] In many ways, he had assumed national leadership in championing the cause of black conversions. In his role as chairman of the Chicago-based American Board of Catholic Missions, he had championed strong financial support for convert work in the South. He wrote to Cicognani:

> I think we can do even more. When we send out to the Bishops of the dioceses in which there are large negro populations asking them to submit their usual requests for grants from the American Board of Catholic Missions [ABCM], I can ask them to tell us in some detail about their Negro Missions. I know that they use a great deal of money which they get from our Board for the Negro Missions. I shall try to gather together a very good report and give you a copy of it, so that you may send it to the Holy See.[101]

In August 1946 the Board of the ABCM "decided to do something in a special way for the negro missions of the

South."[102] In September, Stritch appeared before a meeting of fourteen bishops of southern dioceses at the home of Archbishop Joseph Rummell of New Orleans and urged the prelates to make a special study of the needs of the Negro missions and present petitions to the ABCM. The bishops lunged at the proposal and launched into a wide-ranging discussion of many areas of the black mission.[103]

Stritch had also been instrumental in forming the Catholic Committee of the South (CCS).[104] The Catholic Committee of the South would become a major impetus for the work of black conversion and school integration. In 1946, Stritch had reported to Cicognani that one of the top priorities for successful conversion work was "negro vocations to the priesthood."

> It was the unanimous opinion of the bishops that a beginning be made to provide negro priests for the negro missions in their dioceses.... Presently in the South the only opportunity a Catholic colored boy has of being a priest is offered by the Fathers of the Divine Word Seminary in Bay St. Louis. It does not stand to reason that all aspirants to the priesthood want to become religious.... Everybody was convinced that an ultimate solution of the negro mission problem involves the training of colored diocesan priests.[105]

BLACK PRIESTS FOR CHICAGO

In his own diocese Stritch had already accepted one young black man as a candidate for the priesthood, Rollins E. Lambert. Lambert was born in 1922 in Chicago. A bright student, he was educated at Senn High School on the North Side and received a partial scholarship to the University of Chicago, where he studied political science in the hope of entering the diplomatic service. His religious upbringing had been as a Christian Scientist, but in 1941 a Catholic coworker had taken him to the Easter Pontifical Mass, where he was deeply attracted by the beauty of the Latin liturgy. His attraction to Catholicism was reinforced by contacts with the Calvert Club of the University of Chicago and the solicitude of Professor Jerome Kerwin of the Political Science Department. Kerwin sent him to the Dominican House of

Studies in River Forest for instructions in Catholicism and on December 24, 1941, Lambert was baptized. He received his First Communion from the hand of Archbishop Stritch at the Midnight Mass.

In 1942 Calvert Club chaplain Father Joseph Connerton requested that Lambert be admitted to St. Mary of the Lake Seminary. From 1942 to 1949 Lambert studied at the seminary, serving for a time as a personal secretary to Monsignor Hillenbrand. He was ordained to the priesthood in 1949, and Monsignor Joseph Morrison, chaplain of the Catholic Interracial Council, preached at his first Mass. He was sent to the West Side St. Malachy's parish, the site of the successful apostolic efforts of Fathers Joseph Richards and Martin Farrell, where he taught courses in religion and Negro history at the small high school set up on the fourth floor of the parish school building. Lambert was intelligent, urbane, and cautious, a perfect "first-case" for black diocesan clergy. The young priest carefully avoided any of the "hot" issues concerning race that were beginning to surface in the archdiocese at the time. As Lambert later expressed it: "I felt as the only black priest I had to set an example of being a hard-working and conscientious assistant."[106] Lambert's work as an assistant and later chaplain of the Calvert Club of the University of Chicago eventually won him a place in the work of the United States Catholic Conference, where he signed on as an advisor on African Affairs for the Conference's committee on International Peace and Justice. Lambert would be followed in the seminary by two other black seminarians, George Clements and Kenneth Brigham.[107]

THE CONVERT MAKERS

The clearest sign of the priority Stritch assigned to the work of the black apostolate was his willingness to deliver his most precious assets to the work: priests. Two men, in particular, became the pioneers of black conversion work in the Archdiocese of Chicago, Martin ("Doc") Farrell and Joseph Richards. Farrell had been reared on the South Side at Visitation parish, a community he would later characterize as "a bastion of segregation."

Richards likewise was a product of the South Side. Growing up at Visitation parish, Farrell had observed Monsignor Byrnes's efforts to keep blacks out of the area with his "clean-up/paint-up" sermons and, as a pupil at De LaSalle High School, had innocently questioned why the Christian Brothers did not admit black pupils. Richards did not have similar experiences but had once hoped to be a missionary. Both men were drawn to black work during their seminary years after a meeting with Joseph Eckert, S.V.D. These interests were encouraged by the rector, Monsignor Hillenbrand, and Josephite Father Joseph Gilliard, who somehow heard about the young seminarians and visited them at Mundelein.

Toward the end of his life, Mundelein was beginning to have second thoughts about his racial policies and approved the idea of allowing diocesan priests to work among the blacks. Usually diocesan priests turned a parish over to religious orders, once it had become black. Soon after their ordination in 1938, Farrell and Richards were assigned, with Father John Brown, to the once prosperous St. Malachy's parish on the West Side of Chicago. The parish was in a state of decline as whites were moving out to make way for a growing black enclave that would soon become the dominant group in the neighborhood. To that point the only place for black Catholics on the West Side was St. Joseph's Mission on Fourteenth Street, an offshoot of Holy Family parish. Farrell and Richards would change that.

Both of the young priests were filled with good intentions about working with the "colored," but neither of them knew exactly what to do. Farrell and Richards soon turned to the nearby Divine Word Fathers for help in missionary techniques to work with the blacks and learned from them the importance of the Catholic school as an instrument of evangelization. A trip to Harlem, to observe the work of St. Charles Borromeo parish, introduced them to effective techniques to convert blacks to Catholicism.

Farrell and Richards began roaming the streets of the neighborhood (walking the pastor's Irish setter) and inviting black children to come to the school. Afterwards the two priests unabashedly went door to door, personally inviting people to come to the parish and send their children to the school. In the

1938–1939 school year, both were surprised to see the numbers of black children who showed up for registration. The use of the Catholic school as an instrument of evangelization soon became the hallmark of their successful ministry among the blacks of Chicago. A high school for African Americans was begun in the forties that emphasized black culture and history. (This was the school where Father Rollins Lambert taught Negro history.) Black sociologists Horace Cayton and Frank Dorsey pointed out the importance of the schools to blacks along with the schools' importance in securing conversions. They characterized the number of black conversions to Catholicism as a "trickle," offset by the steady flow of new Protestants into the city. "But," they warned, "this trickle could become a mighty stream if the Church pressed forward its educational work among Negroes and integrated them into its parishes and institutions."[108] Farrell and Richards did everything in their power to have the Cayton and Dorsey prophecy come true.

As a condition for admission to the school, parents had to promise to take instructions in the Catholic faith and attend Mass faithfully every Sunday. Farrell later attested that convert classes were never under eighty persons. Although Richards and Farrell would later be criticized for "coercive" tactics, the response from African-American parents and children was overwhelming. The convert classes consisted of thirty lessons, given twice a week, and offered three times a day to accommodate different schedules. Eventually a special catechism devised by Father William Cogan was used for these lessons. One priest would give the formal instructions; another would conduct private interviews, meeting with all of them an average of three times apiece. Based on the material from these interviews, the priests came to know their parishioners well enough to invite them to become Catholics. Records of all these people were kept, as well as checks on Mass attendance and marriage cases. Chancery officials like Monsignor Romeo Blanchette of the Archdiocesan Tribunal were kept constantly busy with the flow of marriage cases submitted to them by the priests in the "negro apostolate."

Initially, Catholic chancery officials were skeptical of the work of the two priests. But, as time went on, amazing results

began to show which convinced even the most reluctant that good things were happening in a West Side neighborhood given up for lost.

In subsequent assignments, Farrell and Richards were able to replicate the success story of St. Malachy's. After eight years at St. Malachy's, Richards was sent to Holy Angels parish. The parish had once been the home of Auxiliary Bishop Alexander McGavick. After McGavick's departure for LaCrosse, Father Maurice J. McKenna was appointed pastor. During his twenty-two-year pastorate, the neighborhood directly west and south of the parish changed, and he tried as best he could to keep blacks out of the parish. It was he who insisted they sit in the aisles during Mass. When McKenna died in 1945, he was succeeded by Father James Duffin, who asked Stritch if he could have Richards as his assistant. When Richards arrived, the parish was nearly dead. Only a handful of parishioners attended Mass, and the school had only ninety-five students, taught by four Sisters of Mercy. Richards immediately began by taking a census of the parish and followed it up with home visits.

During his years at St. Malachy's, Richards had become a self-taught demographer and studied the concentrations of blacks in various areas of the city. He argued that churches in black areas need not be given up for lost, but could be rejuvenated with the right combination of priests and nuns. Stritch gave them a contingent of School Sisters of St. Francis headed by Sister M. Hortensia Stickelmayer, a veteran of twelve years of working with blacks in Yazoo City, Mississippi. Under Stickelmayer and Richards school enrollment skyrocketed to 1300 pupils and over three hundred were under religious instruction. The numbers of Masses and parish organizations shot up considerably, and twenty-eight nuns worked in the school. Summer sessions were introduced which drew more sisters freed from regular assignments. CYO-type vacation schools flourished, with nuns and seminarians leading black youths to city parks for recreational programs. So large did the school population grow that Duffin undertook $600,000 in improvements on the buildings.

The success of the Holy Angels operation was infectious, as many of the seminarians that worked all summer at Holy

Angels volunteered for "Negro-work" once they were ordained. Stritch bragged to Cicognani: "I have positively no difficulty in getting priests interested in this work, and ... I ... propose to put more of my own priests in this mission work. I think it will be good for them and it will be good for the work."[109] True to his word, Stritch allowed any priest who requested to work in black parishes.

Richards revitalized parish life in many other ways. He concocted elaborate ceremonies to impress and overawe his black neophytes, and imitated the enlivened preaching and teaching of the Baptist ministers that blacks had known in the South. (Richards once confided to Father Jake Killgallon that he believed good pulpit oratory would have his parishioners "feeling the flames of hell scorching their asses!")[110] Parish organizations blossomed. Soon the PTA was one of the largest in the archdiocese. A Blessed Sacrament Society was set up for the women, a Holy Name Society for the men, Big Brothers for the young men, and a Young Ladies Sodality. Pre-Cana and Cana Programs were in place, as was CFM. But, by and large, Specialized Catholic Action did not make much of a dent in black communities. One of the most popular programs sponsored by Richards was an endearing children's choir known as the Little Angels. In 1957 Richards succeeded Duffin as pastor of Holy Angels and continued there almost until his death in 1976.

A year or two after Richards left St. Malachy's, Farrell was transferred to St. James on Twenty-ninth and Wabash. Working with Father Francis Lavin, Farrell opened the moribund Catholic school to black children and replicated many of the successful techniques he and Richards first tried at St. Malachy's. Farrell's parish was in the midst of much of the urban renewal zone of the near South Side, and he worked assiduously on housing projects and was eventually drawn into the civil rights movement.

The philosophy and approach of these men was simple: changing neighborhoods provoked three reactions on the part of white priests. One was a desperate attempt to retain the dwindling numbers of whites; a second was assuming an air of resignation that the place would close; a third embodied a strong missionary outreach to convert blacks to Roman Catholicism.

Obviously Farrell and Richards took the third option. In their estimation, African-American immigration did not have to be disaster for the Church, because blacks, despite their southern Protestant heritage, could and would become Catholics. In the perilous conditions of urban life, Farrell and Richards believed the Church could extend a helping hand to black children and their parents by providing a quality grade and high school education. By placing black children on equal footing with white children, the blacks would be in a better position to demand the rights that racist society had denied them. Neither man had much use for the interracialist approach which attempted to cajole whites into "conceding" rights to blacks.[111] However, despite the differences in tactics with the interracialists, the conversion efforts of Farrell and Richards were shot through with the confident Catholic spirit of the age: natural law had dictated that racism was wrong; therefore it was the duty of every faithful Christian to actively combat it. Questions or doubts about this basic position did not surface very often.

Farrell and Richards encountered opposition in their work, especially when they attempted to find places for black students in Catholic high schools. School problems were frequently referred to them because of their reputation for friendliness to black students. Unable to do anything about the situations themselves, their main recourse was to archdiocesan officials and often to the archbishop himself.

CONCLUSION

The knotty racial issues of the forties and fifties found ambivalent and less than forceful leadership from Cardinal Stritch and were largely dealt with by the Catholic Interracial Council and the priests in black convert work. The advent of the Civil Rights Era would bring a new tenor to the work of racial justice in the Archdiocese of Chicago. A new archbishop would build on the foundation of his predecessor.

9

Chicago Catholics in the Civil Rights Era

No more vivid difference marked the administrations of Stritch and Meyer than did their handling of the race situation. Stritch's priority was to convert black Chicagoans to Catholicism. He was less enthusiastic about interracial organizations, although he did tolerate interracial activists to operate in his archdiocese. Meyer, by contrast, turned a more favorable eye on those Catholic groups that favored racial integration, such as the Catholic Interracial Council and Friendship House. Moreover, he was considerably more firm in dealing with instances of racial discrimination. The differences between Stritch and Meyer, on this issue, were almost like night and day for Daniel Cantwell, who remarked, in 1959: "Happily we have in Archbishop Meyer the most aggressive leadership that we have ever enjoyed."[1]

THE CATHOLIC INTERRACIAL COUNCIL OF CHICAGO

The philosophy of these interracial organizations was best expressed by Daniel Cantwell. "The question of better race relations in the future," Cantwell wrote in the first issue of *Work*, "is to a very great extent a problem of communicating—between those whites who respect the negro's essential equality and dignity and those whites who do not."[2] This would be the work of

289

the largest of the interracial organizations, the Catholic Interracial Council, and a smaller group at Friendship House.

The Catholic Interracial Council (CIC) was the brainchild
of Father John LaFarge, S.J., who had organized the first of these
committees in New York in 1938.[3] LaFarge wrote extensively on
the moral and social implications of racism and committed himself to uprooting it in the Catholic community. LaFarge's program involved organizing committees of lay Catholics from
professional fields who would educate people in the principles
of interracial justice and change Catholic attitudes about blacks.
Given the controversial nature of this work, LaFarge became
adept at stroking the hierarchy. Even Stritch approved of LaFarge,
and had once written him:

> May I say that I have been much pleased with your writings dur-
> ing these times on the Negro question. You have a balance and a
> thoroughness in your study of this question which is so pleasing
> after reading some of the emotional thinkers. I am sure that you
> are doing a very good work and doing it well.[4]

The formation of the Catholic Interracial Council in Chicago
had taken time. Early groups, such as the Federated Colored
Catholics, and articulate black professionals, such as Dr.
Arthur Falls, had lobbied for organized groups of black Catholics to combat racism within the Church and press for black
rights in the city. But even they were slow in coming. Even
though the Detroit race riot of 1943, sent shock waves through
major metropolitan centers in the north, nothing happened on
the Catholic front in Chicago to deal with the problem of
racism. An editorial in *Work* feared for Chicago: "For there is
going on in the United States a subterranean race war which
only needs some nettling or an ill-advised rumor to bring it out
in the open."[5]

Cantwell called for the formation of a Catholic Interracial
Council as early as 1943, but not until early 1945 was he able to
organize an independent group of lay Catholics for this pur-
pose. This included Illinois Appellate Court Judge Roger J.
Kiley, Alderman George D. Kells, attorney (later Judge) John P.
McGoorty, attorney Augustine Bowe, and black labor leader
John Yancey. These men began meeting in each other's homes

and later, as the group grew larger, in quarters provided by Monsignor Joseph Morrison of Holy Name Cathedral.[6] The fruits of their discussions were collected in a brief report proposing the formation of a Catholic Interracial Council in Chicago. In late September 1945 these men applied for formal recognition and Morrison presented the matter to Stritch. Morrison praised the men in a way that allayed any fears Stritch may have had about them: "You know most of these men to be good and serious Catholic men, ready to bow to the voice of authority, and I make so bold as to request you to grant them the privilege of an interview with you in the near future, so that they may receive the benefit of your counsel, the approval of your high office and fruits of your own experience in this worthy cause."[7]

Their goals were spelled out clearly. In the preamble of their constitution they proclaimed: "The purpose of this organization is to achieve a spiritual unity between people of different races so that in their dealings with each other they will be actuated by the Divine Precepts of Charity and Justice."[8] To implement this goal, the Catholic Interracial Council determined to operate as a fact-finding and educational body to "educate and mold public opinion, particularly the opinion of Catholics in matters calling for the application of the Catholic principles of interracial justice."[9] Stritch wrote back to Morrison:

> I thank you very much for sending me the report of the men who, under your supervision, have been studying during the last nine or ten months the whole question of securing for our minorities the full enjoyment of their rights in our community. I am intensely interested in doing everything within my power for the realization of the principles of our democracy in the treatment of minorities. I shall be glad to see these good men and I would appreciate it much if you would come with them to see me.[10]

Stritch met with the men and, after making some minor alterations in their constitution, formally approved the organization. But he was not eager to attach his name or the prestige of the archdiocese to it too closely. He insisted that they report to him on their activities, especially when they took a public stand on "sensitive" matters. Stritch's concerns in this matter were heightened in response to the actions of one member of the

group who approached the white pastor of a black parish and introduced himself as a representative of "The Cardinal's Interracial Committee." Cantwell hastened to apologize for the misnomer and reassurred Stritch:

> For, the Council as we have envisioned it, is not a highly central-ized body determining diocesean [*sic*] policy, which would be an absurdity, or telling parish priests what we would like them to do, which would be both irreverent and unrealistic.... It is my opinion that it has not been advisable and is not yet advisable to bring more priests into the discussions as regular participants. From my experience it tends to slow the discussion of the laymen and in that way to slow the progress of the group, for the pur-pose of the discussion is the mutual formation of the men in understanding, respect and charity.[11]

Stritch was happy that the proposed organization was not going to be strongly centralized and urged Cantwell to seek more advice from priests, but warned him not to overburden those engaged with black convert work. Moreover, he wanted no competition with the convert work, which was his chief priority:

> I think that the organization should be rather small. I would not like it to branch out into a lot of subdivisions. It should be some-thing in the nature of a Conference and not of a central organiza-tion with a lot of branches. Certainly we must keep in mind the great value which will come to us from the advice of priests. There seems to me to be a reason why we should *not* ask the priests in our colored mission work and should be free from any sort of other activities which may interfere with their work. From long years of experience I know how frequently the priest finds himself frustrated if he is identified with something out-side of his work.... The work of your organization can contribute to the success of his work, but the two things should not be iden-tified.[12]

Cantwell made revisions in the constitution of the Catholic Interracial Council and Stritch wrote him:

> We have an important work to do in our missions for the colored. Thank God they are progressing. No one thing pleases me more than what is being done in these missions for souls. We have

done very much for them and our program includes some very important things in the near future. It has been possible for us to do a great deal in breaking down stupid prejudices.

Stritch offered an additional word of caution about the activities of this group:

We want of course carefully to analyze situations and to avoid uncontrolled emotion in the solution of them. There is a work of education and it will not be accomplished in a day. Exaggerations which in the end may be violative of the rights of individuals must be avoided or they would not be in the benefit of any group.[13]

Soon thereafter, the newly formed Catholic Interracial Council took up residence in a small office at 3 East Chicago Avenue owned by Holy Name Cathedral. Stritch did not micromanage the affairs of the CIC and it began to mount educational and fund-raising programs that kept it afloat. Conferences and study days on racial issues, as well as an annual Communion breakfast which featured a prominent speaker became important parts of its programs. Catholic high schools, especially those operated by the School Sisters of St. Francis, often welcomed them warmly. They also sponsored black children who wished to attend Catholic high school, thereby confronting the predominantly white high schools students with the moral implications of the race question. This policy also revealed which high schools deliberately excluded black pupils. They sponsored high school interracial days that sensitized white Catholic students to racial issues. On a variety of fronts the CIC was quietly pushing back the frontiers of racial toleration in Catholic institutions and in the larger community.

The Catholic Interracial Council also became the eyes and ears of the the Church in coping with various outbreaks of racial violence. CIC "investigators" were sent to Cicero in the early fifties to discover if Catholic attitudes on race relations could be changed by the clergy. The CIC also functioned as an independent Catholic voice on race-related legislative matters before the city council and the state legislature, and as advocates of black Catholics who were victims of discrimination.

Cantwell was central to the organization and his quiet leadership of the CIC won him the city's brotherhood award for his role in quelling tensions at the Airport Homes and Fernwood riots. This gave the Council an added measure of respect in the community. Cantwell vigorously opposed back-room tactics using church "clout" to effect outcomes, preferring instead the strong medicine of moral exhortation. Because of this he did not hesitate to speak out publicly when he felt it could aid in altering attitudes. Indeed, Cantwell did some of his best writing and lecturing in explaining the Catholic position on race relations. Cantwell's thesis on segregation equipped him with the raw data for on-going research into the state of racial relations in Chicago. His first article, "Race Relations—As Seen by a Catholic," appeared in the *American Catholic Sociological Review* in December 1946.[14] In 1952 Cantwell authored a widely distributed pamphlet entitled "Catholics Speak on Race Relations." Published by Fides Press, it consisted of a compilation of statements by bishops and theologians refuting common errors on racial issues.[15] In July of the same year the Claretian publication *Voice of St. Jude* published Cantwell's "Catholics and Prejudice."[16]

By 1952 the CIC's activities had expanded to the point where it was able to hire its first full-time executive director, Lloyd Davis. Davis, a black, enhanced the visibility of the CIC primarily by his interest in fund-raising events and by bringing onto its board such important Catholic laymen as R. Sargent Shriver, president of the Kennedy-owned Merchandise Mart and chairman of the Chicago School Board. Davis masterminded the production of an annual benefit show for the Council, showcasing the contributed services of Catholic and black entertainers. The success of this benefit allowed the work of the CIC to continue and enjoy a better financial base.

Even though programs picked up, however, membership grew slowly through the early fifties. This changed when interracialism received a tremendous boost after the *Brown* decision of 1954, the Montgomery Bus Boycott of 1955, and the Little Rock incident of 1957. Indeed, these stunning events lifted racial relations to the status of a moral issue in the public eye, a development eminently pleasing to Cantwell and those who followed him.

CHANGES IN THE CATHOLIC INTERRACIAL COUNCIL

The new state of civil rights issues mandated new directions and strategies for the CIC, and the Chicago Council would move into a position of national leadership in this area. Cantwell initiated a series of meetings with John Egan, Walter Imbiorski, Russell Barta, and Edward Marciniak to discuss the future of the movement. "For myself," he wrote in a memo to his coworkers and friends, "I want to be sure that I am in touch with actuality, that I am really aware of the spirit and mentality of the men and women of our time, that its real perplexities and problems find me sensitive and receptive and not preoccupied with issues no longer vital and commanding."[17]

With the rising tide of civil rights activism, the CIC had to be ready to take advantage of the changing national mood. The members of the Chicago Council proposed a major unification of Catholic Interracial Council operations around the country in 1957, resulting in the formation of the National Catholic Conference for Interracial Justice (NCCIJ) at a convention at Loyola University in Chicago in late August 1958. The NCCIJ became a major stimulus and coordinator of Catholic participation in the civil rights movement and was symbolically headquartered in Cantwell's Chicago, not in LaFarge's New York. In 1959 the youthful Matthew Ahmann was chosen as executive secretary of the new organization and played a central role in the racial policies of the Catholic community of Chicago during the Meyer years.

Ahmann was a native of St. Cloud, Minnesota, and a graduate of St. John's University. In 1952 he came to Chicago and served as business manager of *Today* magazine, the periodical of CISCA. Later Ahmann went to work with the Chicago Department of Welfare and in 1957 became a field representative for the Catholic Interracial Conference.[18]

Internal changes in the Chicago CIC followed on the union of councils. In early 1959 a special committee consisting of Jerome Kerwin, Gordon Zahn, Cantwell, Robert Faulhaber, Clifford Campbell, and executive director Lloyd Davis met to devise long-range plans in the wake of changing national conditions.[19] True to the civil rights mood of the nations, the shift was

on from education to direct action as the best way to secure the rights of blacks. Gordon Zahn articulated this forcefully in a memo:

> I am not a little concerned about what I view as the present dominant note of CIC operations. In recent years we have moved from modest, but rather direct action programs to more elaborate and, in my opinion, over-organized—"power elite" public relations programs. I personally feel that too much energy is being expended upon such "publicity impact" affairs as big-name benefits which seem to produce little more than enough funds to finance the staff needed to organize the next big-name benefit.

Zahn did not favor "turning our attention to problems of metropolitan planning," as some had urged, but called for long-range planning that would involve "risk-taking and boat-rocking action."[20] A major reorganization ensued, resulting in the resignation of Lloyd Davis and his replacement by Philadelphia social worker John A. McDermott in 1960.

McDermott was a product of the Specialized Catholic Action movements of the late fifties and a graduate of Catholic schools.[21] He, like Zahn, believed in direct action tactics which were becoming the trademark of the national civil rights movement. McDermott took over with a sure hand and moved first to strengthen contacts with archdiocesan officials. Soon after arriving, he urged Cantwell to "Arrange a visit of CIC leaders with Cardinal Meyer to give him a report and request renewal of his annual gift. Can we ask for $10,000 this year?"[22] McDermott also contacted other archdiocesan officials such as Cooke of Catholic Charities, McManus in education, and Burke in the chancery, in order to assure their support. But his prime goal was direct action and he articulated this in a response to complaints he received concerning CIC participation in a "wade-in" at Chicago's segregated Rainbow Beach:

> While it is true that CIC is probably basically an educational organization, I have never understood it to be exclusively educational. There need be no contradiction between direct action programs and educational programs. The important questions are: "is the program right and sound? Will it work? Will it advance or

set back our work?" In my judgement our "wade-in" program successfully met all of these tests.... The momentum of change in race relations is constantly increasing. In fact, in my opinion, it would be fair to say that today no race relations agency which restricts itself to purely educational efforts can long retain the respect of the Negro community.[23]

The CIC under McDermott would become an important medium for Chicago Catholics promoting civil rights issues. But there were others.

FRIENDSHIP HOUSE

Another feature of the interracialist approach was Bishop Sheil's Friendship House. Baroness Catherine DeHueck was responsible for the origins of the organization, when she founded a house for the poor in Toronto in 1931 and in 1938 extended her apostolate to the black poor by opening an interracial center called Friendship House in Harlem. Her success drew the attention of Sheil, who offered to sponsor the establishment of a similar establishment in Chicago. In 1942 DeHueck persuaded Ellen Tarry, a black worker on the *Amsterdam News*, and Ann Harrigan, a teacher at a high school in New York, to move to Chicago and establish the new house. Harrigan came first and was later joined by Tarry and DeHueck, who assisted in securing storefronts on the South Side for the new operation.[24]

By November 5, 1942, the feast of St. Martin De Porres, the new center was open. The primary work of Friendship House consisted in facilitating friendly contact between the two races in a city so segregated that blacks and whites had no place to meet. Attracting volunteer workers and the services of Daniel Cantwell as chaplain, the House opened an Adult Education Center which offered lectures and discussions on matters relating to interracial justice: the Mystical Body, housing, the poll tax, the lay apostolate, foreign language, and Negro history. The most popular program of the House was the organization of family home visits between the races. Friendship House enthusiasts felt face-to-face meetings between the races would break

down the fear between them. The interracial home visits were highly successful, lasting into the sixties. A Mother's Club was formed to assist in financial matters, and a children's day-care center was opened. The corps of idealistic young women who worked full-time in the center lived a quasi-religious life, attending Mass regularly and ending each day by praying together the office of Compline. Like the Catholic Interracial Council, Friendship House was always on the verge of economic collapse and Bishop Sheil, who had brought them there, could give very little on-going support, but, miraculously, the House always seemed to find the needed funds at the appropriate moment. Eventually, as their programs grew, they were compelled to move their operation out of the Forty-third Street address to a permanent location on Indiana Street.

The House regularly reported on their activities to Cardinal Stritch, who characteristically mistrusted them as he did the CIC. He confided as much to Father Clifford, his theological advisor: "Confidentially, I am just a bit afraid of this group. They are unquestionably good people and have the best of intentions. I want to guide them and give them a clear mandate as regards to the Friendship House in Chicago."[25] Stritch need not have feared. Friendship House remained a small, struggling operation very much on the fringe of even the national civil rights movement. When Stritch departed Chicago in 1958, a new era of Catholic response to black issues began, spearheaded reluctantly at first but later with great force by Archbishop Albert G. Meyer.

THE MEYER AGENDA

Meyer did not come to Chicago with any kind of reputation for outspokenness on social issues. Indeed, in the bitter Kohler, Wisconsin, strike of the fifties, Meyer had been the soul of caution, refraining from public comment of any kind and choosing as his emissary to the tortured neogtiations between management and labor a priest who was sympathetic with the company. What little he did have to say on racial matters was found in a series of sermon outlines which he prepared while he was bishop of Superior between 1946 and 1953.

The year 1958 marked a turning point in Meyer's awareness of the racial situation. In that year he was associated with the annual statement of the Administrative Board of the National Catholic Welfare Conference drafted by Father John Cronin, assistant director of the Social Action Department of the NCWC. As a member of the Administrative Board, Meyer received an advance copy for consideration and there is no record that he offered any suggestions. But his name was affixed to the final draft and he subsequently used the text, especially the statement "The heart of the race question is moral and religious," as the springboard for later pronouncements. Matthew Ahmann wrote a note of thanks to Cronin for his role in drafting the document, observing: "Incidentally the statement has already had obvious constructive effects, in encouraging people to work with us, and other things. And it certainly is quotable."[26] The man who would quote it most readily was Albert G. Meyer.

MEYER SEIZES THE ISSUE

Meyer's first months at the head of the Chicago archdiocese were difficult. The tragic fire at Our Lady of the Angels had consumed much of his attention and the intricacies of mastering the enormous administrative structure of Chicago were nearly overwhelming. But racial issues were on the "front-burner" from the outset. In his first Lenten pastoral, in 1959, Meyer wrote:

> I would like to call special attention to the Statement issued by the Bishops of the United States on the occasion of their annual meeting in November of 1958 on the subject of racial justice and the Christian conscience.... I would like to emphasize the teaching of this statement, and to urge all of you to study it carefully and prayerfully, so that you may fully understand and realize in the practical conduct of your lives that "the heart of the race question is moral and religious. It concerns the rights of man and our attitude toward our fellow man...." The holy season of Lent is surely a most opportune time not only to reflect on these and similar profound truths but also to work for these truths with quiet and persevering courage....[27]

Soon after publishing the pastoral, Meyer was approached by Father Theodore Hesburgh, C.S.C., president of the University of Notre Dame and member of the Presidential Commission on Civil Rights. The Commission had been empaneled in 1957 and traveled around the country seeking testimony from parties concerned about the race issue. In February 1959 Cardinal Francis Spellman of New York had testified, and Hesburgh inquired whether Meyer would be willing to do the same. Meyer demurred, claiming that he did not have enough experience with local conditions to speak authoritatively. Hesburgh then pressed for a statement drafted by Egan and delivered in Meyer's name.[28] Meyer consented and, with the help of Nicholas von Hoffmann, Egan drafted the statement which Meyer carefully edited. Egan delivered the statement before Father Hesburgh and former Governor John S. Battle of Virginia on May 6, 1959, and took aim at the evils of racism. He went on to single out Chicago's most egregious instance of racial discrimination: residential segregation. Egan called for additional housing for blacks and for community organizations which would "ensure that Negroes do gain access to our communities, but not to the degree that we merely extend the boundaries of the racial ghetto."[29]

The reaction of the news media was positive. The Chicago *Defender* quoted Meyer's condemnation of residential segregation approvingly: "the restrictions against the most capable and self-reliant portions of the Negro population which call the loudest for remedy and which must be rectified most speedily."[30] The Jesuit weekly, *America*, wrote: "His calm and courageous statement offers the best hope that the job can be done. Catholics who have long looked to the bold and imaginative social Catholicism of the Midwest metropolis as a symbol of the American Church's special vitality will hail it, too, as shining proof that the mantle of leadership which slipped from his beloved predecessor in death has indeed fallen on resolute shoulders."[31] Meyer, however, was not altogether pleased with the publicity he received. The day before Egan delivered his address, Saul Alinsky had given a blunt speech urging the establishment of racial quotas of blacks in white neighborhoods.[32] This suggestion upset both ends of the spectrum:

whites who wanted to keep blacks out altogether, and blacks and their white supporters who felt blacks should be free to move wherever they desired. In the ensuing publicity, Alinsky's remarks were so intertwined with Meyer's as to make it appear that Meyer was requesting the quotas. Egan was also upset with the reporting and later noted that Meyer never referred to the Civil Rights Commission talk again. But he did not backtrack or publicly deny the statements. Indeed, he may have even been secretly pleased with the publicity. Father William Graney, assistant editor of the *New World*, wrote to Cantwell:

> From what I hear, he [Meyer] has received a large number of complaints about his statement. He refers to them as his "love letters." I think it was significant that the Archbishop was willing to make such a forthright statement so early in his career as Archbishop of Chicago. It seems to indicate his thinking and a course of action he might be willing to take in the future.[33]

Graney was on target. That the statement had been given at all represented a major break from the quiet policy of Cardinal Stritch. But it would take two racial incidents to move Meyer beyond mere words to positive action: Deerfield and Catholic high schools.

SUBURBAN INTEGRATION: AN UNCERTAIN START

In 1959 Meyer was still unsteady on racial issues. Cantwell and his coworkers were extremely happy with Meyer's interest in their work and his willingness to tackle difficult issues. But they may have been disconcerted over Meyer's reaction to the first challenge of his term, the integration of Deerfield, a suburb some twenty miles north of Chicago.

Until this time there had been concern only for black migration to cities and the movement of blacks into areas adjoining the black belt. There had been some efforts to integrate suburbs directly in the path of black growth, such as Oak Park, Berwyn, and Cicero to the west of the city, but in the sixties, black migration to areas such as Deerfield, Skokie, and Niles, not directly contiguous with the black belt, set off a new wave of white alarm. Morris Milgram, a Philadelphia developer and the head

of Modern Community Developers (MCD), a firm dedicated to building "open occupancy housing," contributed to this concern.

MCD's Illinois subsidiary, "Progress," found available land in the suburb of Deerfield and purchased fifteen acres known as Floral Park in April 1959. Two months later, Progress picked up another seven acres and named the site Pear Tree. MCD proposed to build thirty-nine houses on the first site and twelve on the second, and received speedy approval from the Deerfield Village Board of Trustees. Sewers, water lines, and model homes began to sprout in Floral Park. But by November, things began to change when a Deerfield minister named Jack Parker informed his vestrymen that ten or twelve of the Progress homes would be sold to blacks.

The news sped rapidly from the church to the village fathers. On November 13 Deerfield's building commissioner began looking for and finding code violations in the sample houses at Floral Park. On November 17 the Deerfield Park Board further slowed the project when they decided that the community desperately needed parks (even though a referendum the previous August had rejected such a "need"). On top of it all, an independent group called the Deerfield Citizen's Association began to call for an "overall land program," which on its face was a reasonable land management program, but was taken by some as a subterfuge to keep blacks out of the suburb. On November 18 an acrimonious meeting was held between community residents and Morris Milgram, at which MCD's plans were condemned as "totalitarian." As these events unfolded, Cantwell wrote to Meyer:

> Last week, while you were in Washington, a housing development was announced which I think I should bring to your attention. Morris Milgram ... has announced that he is going to build a racially integrated subdivision within the village limits of Deerfield, Illinois. The development will consist of 51 homes of high quality ranging in value from $30,000 to $35,000.... The announcement of this project for Deerfield has spirited some overt opposition and a much larger amount of anxiety....

Cantwell was particularly distressed by the refusal of Father John J. O'Mara, the pastor of Deerfield's only Catholic

church, to support efforts of the other religious leaders of the community who called for acceptance of the integrated housing development.[34] He asked Meyer:

> I call this to your attention in the hope that you might think it good to drop a short note to the pastor of the parish of Deerfield encouraging him to see this as an opportunity to carry out the program you enunciated in your statement before the President's Committee on Civil Rights.... If this project in Deerfield succeeds, as I surely hope it will, it will stand as a splendid example to the other outlying areas in Chicago and the metropolitan communities.[35]

Cantwell later spoke with Meyer about the O'Mara situation and the prelate urged Cantwell to reason with the pastor. But O'Mara would not budge and Cantwell reported to Meyer: "After talking with you, I tried to reach the pastor but he refused to see me. He took the position that he was pastor in Deerfield, and that when and if he wanted my help he would call·for it. He insisted that I should remember that he had jurisdiction."[36]

Meyer could have lowered the boom on O'Mara, but he chose not to. At that time he was preparing to go to Rome to receive the red hat of a cardinal, and the press of business and holidays curtailed normal activity. In the end, the brunt of Catholic support for integration in the Deerfield situation was carried by the North Shore chapter of the Catholic Interracial Council and an organization known as the Deerfield Citizens for Human Rights. Discussions were arranged and excerpts from Meyer's Civil Rights Commission testimony were sent to Deerfield Catholics. But O'Mara remained adamant and refused to contribute to these efforts toward community peace. Without the support of the parish, it was difficult for lay Catholics to make headway. This opposition along with other hitches caused Milgram to give up on the project.

In the midst of the controversy, Meyer received a letter from Mr. and Mrs. Anthony Sabato, a couple in Deerfield:

> Humbly we submit to you the sad plight of the Catholics of Deerfield. Although we constitute between twenty-five and thirty-five percent of the population of the town, and among us are many well-educated persons, we are letting "the agitator and

the racist" "seize the mantle of leadership"—in fact, many of our number have joined the ranks of the opposition, even in leadership positions.[37]

The Sabato letter, liberally quoting the passage from the 1958 statement, struck a responsive chord with Meyer. The image of the "mantle of leadership" resonated with his own sense that he had to do something about the festering racism in the Catholic community itself and in the community at large. His response in Deerfield would be atypical.

HIGH SCHOOL INTEGRATION

Deerfield was only one of the racial issues confronting Archbishop Meyer in 1959. The question of racial exclusion in the Catholic high schools of the South Side had also been a nagging problem since the days of Stritch. The desire of black Catholic children to get into such schools as Mercy High School for girls and Mount Carmel High School for boys had been complicated by the general dearth of high school facilities. Often school administrators cloaked a desire to exclude black applicants with the excuse that there simply were not enough seats. A typical example occurred at Mercy in 1957 when Mrs. James Lewis, a black Catholic, attempted to register her daughter Diane. She wrote to Stritch:

> I was told by Sister Jovita that I was not in the Mercy district and that I would have to be living south of Seventy-eighth Street.... My daughter and I were at Mercy at 10:30 in the morning of registration, only a half a [sic] hour after registration began. Many people came after us. Upon our arrival, we were informed by a student that this was not a public registration.... On August 16, 1957, I called Sister Mark inquiring again about Diane's registration for September. She informed me that there was no room for Diane. I asked if I could register her now for September 1958, this she refused.[38]

In 1958 there were only four Catholic high schools accepting blacks in any considerable number: St. Elizabeth, Hales, St. Malachy, and St. Philip Benizi. Other schools such as Cathedral High and De LaSalle accepted a few, but never in proportion to

the number living in their districts. Father Martin Farrell and other priests in the "negro apostolate" had long been familiar with these instances of racial exclusion but had never been able to get very far with Stritch. The cardinal complained that he knew firsthand about the crowded conditions in all Catholic high schools and did not want to complicate the problem by forcing black students on the religious who ran the schools. Inspired by Meyer's openness to racial integration, Farrell was emboldened to act.[39] Together with Father Timothy Sullivan, an assistant at all-black St. Anne's parish on Fifty-fifth and Wentworth and a member of the archdiocesan school board, he began to agitate for admission of blacks in four of the South Side Catholic high schools that excluded them: Mount Carmel, Aquinas, the Academy of Our Lady, and Mercy. Moreover, they pressed for additional black registrations in schools like St. Rita and De LaSalle, which already accepted them.

The goal of Farrell and Sullivan was to enroll twenty pupils per school and permanently end segregation and tokenism. This proposal caused a great imbroglio on the school board, where Farrell and Sullivan were vigorously challenged by the members of that body, and by Superintendent William McManus, to produce names and dates of refusal at the respective schools. The furor soon reached Archbishop Meyer, who called in Farrell and Sullivan to hear their story. Without hesitation, Meyer sympathized with Farrell's request and in March 1960 the archdiocesan school board formally ratified a policy of integration.[40] Meyer himself phoned reluctant principals and compelled action. Integration was achieved.

To insure the success of the policy, Farrell, Richards, and Sullivan scoured the Catholic grade schools for bright eighth graders and urged them to apply for seats in the local high schools. But one problem remained: whites avoided an integrated school by registering at several different schools and attending the one with the fewest blacks. McManus put a halt to this abuse by insisting that registration for all Catholic high schools occur on the same day and at the same hour throughout the archdiocese.[41] The school integration policy did what Farrell, Richards, and Sullivan hoped: it broke down the walls of segregation forever in the Catholic high schools of the black districts.

The only holdout to this policy of integration was Visitation. But that would soon end. Meyer waited until 1963 to cauterize the festering racism of Visitation. When racial disturbances broke out in the Englewood neighborhood in that year, Meyer compelled Monsignor Richard Wolfe to issue statements demanding an end to the violence.[42] Meyer further insisted that Wolfe allow blacks to attend Visitation High School. Monsignor Daniel Byrnes must have turned over in his grave.

MEYER SPEAKS OUT

By mid-1959 Meyer surely knew what he later expressed to a news reporter: the racial situation in Chicago was far more serious than it had been in Superior or Milwaukee and direct episcopal action was necessary. Meyer's chosen vehicle for his first public address on racial matters was the clergy conference. Since his days as seminary instructor and rector, Meyer had always placed great faith in the clergy conference as a means for clerical instruction and the dissemination of policy. In Superior and Milwaukee he had utilized these sessions effectively, and insisted that every priest attend.

In early 1960 Father Joseph Richards and Father Martin Farrell proposed the idea of having a clergy conference dedicated to a discussion of the racial issue. Trouble seemed to be brewing in the summer of 1960, as racially motivated incidents occurred in Park Forest and in Bessemer Park on the South Side.[43] Meyer agreed with the two priests' observation that Chicago's clergy needed more education on the race issue in order to break down fears and stereotypes and to help avoid panic when blacks moved into all-white neighborhoods. Tactfully, Meyer made the conference a joint effort of the convert makers and the interracialists.

Through Father Joseph Mangan, S.J., a seminary professor, Meyer asked Cantwell for input on the proposed conference. Cantwell resurrected an old plan he had concocted on the subject with Father John Hayes. He urged fresh ideas and approaches:

> The conference should not be just an opportunity for old war horses like myself to browbeat the priests of Chicago. It would be

better if old timers like myself step aside for younger men who would be more persuasive, more effective, and who would be listened to without the resistance habitually built up against us.

Above all, he insisted:

It is essential that the Cardinal should talk. His talk should be on the moral law and the mission of the Church.... In his talk there should be as little emphasis as possible, indeed if any, on the value of church property, etc.... His talk should be on the growth of the Mystical Body, its inner life, its catholic character. His appeal would be to our zeal and love, to going beyond justice toward charity and the thirst for souls, to winning Negroes not just accepting them.[44]

Meyer agreed to tackle the issue and asked Cantwell, McManus, and Egan to draw up a draft for his address to the priests. The conference met on September 20 and 21 in the huge auditorium of Resurrection parish on the West Side. It was a *tour de force* of organization and presentation. Richards led with a clear analysis of the growth and spread of the black population in the city. He was followed by Father Patrick Curran, who described the convert apostolate, and Father Rollins Lambert, Chicago's first black ordinand, on the attitude of the Negro toward the Church. But the high point of the meeting was Meyer's own strong but carefully worded address entitled "The Mantle of Leadership." In this statement Meyer offered the clearest delineation of archdiocesan racial policy of any archbishop of Chicago.[45] He exhorted his priests:

We must remove from the Church on the local scene any possible taint of racial discrimination or racial segregation from the whole community. We must do it, because the glory of Christ demands it. We must do it, if the motto taken from the Lord's Prayer and emblazoned on my coat-of-arms has true meaning: Thy Kingdom Come! We must do it, because only in the Church can human beings find their full stature. It is only in the Church that we find ours.

He then publicly enunciated specific policy statements:

Every Catholic child of the Negro race ... must have as free access to our schools as any other Catholic child on all levels of

our academic training, elementary and secondary, as well as the higher levels. The acceptance of Catholic children of the Negro race is based on the same policy which guides the acceptance of other Catholic children, whether in the schools of territorial or non-territorial parishes. In other words, pastors of territorial parishes as well as pastors of non-territorial parishes will accept these children—the pastors of territorial parishes for all Catholic children whose parents are domiciled within the parish boundaries and pastors of non-territorial parishes in the same manner in which de facto they accept Catholic children who otherwise do not qualify because of special language or national background which serves as the basis of the non-territorial parish.[46]

Meyer also included high schools, fraternal, and parish organizations, and hospitals in this injunction to equality. In conclusion he noted dryly: "If it should be necessary for a pastor to have a further explanation of these points, I shall always be happy to discuss particular cases with him."[47] The proceedings of the conference made big news. Screaming headlines of the *Chicago Daily News* announced: "INTEGRATION ORDERED BY CARDINAL MEYER."[48] Later, they won additional media attention when the speeches appeared in a sizeable booklet in early 1961. The clergy conference of September 1960 was a dream come true for the interracialist forces in Chicago.

SUBURBAN INTEGRATION AGAIN

It did not take long for the effects of Meyer's September 1960 dictum to be felt when suburban integration was attempted in Skokie, a largely Jewish community to the north of the city. Two black Catholic professionals, Mr. and Mrs. David Jones, purchased a home in Skokie in early 1961. Fear began to percolate through that suburb, as it had earlier in nearby Deerfield. But this time results were better, undoubtedly because of Meyer's strong words. The CIC moved quickly into the situation in order to dispel fear and tensions by publishing a fact sheet on the Joneses and contacting city and local church officials in the Skokie area.[49] Moreover, local Catholic priests like Father Arthur Sauer of St. Peter's parish in Skokie contributed to rather than obstructed a good settlement. Sauer had been a

charter member of Skokie's Human Relations Commission and quickly took a bold stand in defense of the Joneses from his pulpit in February 1961:

> Two weeks ago, a highly educated and cultured Negro family, a young man and his wife, with no children, moved to Skokie and into St. Joan of Arc's Parish. He and she are both college graduates. They are practicing Catholics. Culturally and socially, this family is equal to anyone here and even surpasses many of us in this respect.... I will say but a few words at this time: Let us, as Christians, be Christians and not let fear, hysteria, ugliness and all that is beneath the dignity of a human being come out of us.... We will not be another Deerfield, nor another Little Rock! Our Archbishop, Cardinal Meyer, has ordered us to act as true and good citizens, as true Catholics. We have a moral obligation to accept the races of the world ... otherwise we will have another New Orleans where many so-called "Catholics" have given a black eye to our Church.[50]

John McDermott, who had been encouraging Sauer all along, strongly praised the pastor and urged the *New World* to print the story of Sauer's involvement in the defusing of tensions in Skokie.[51] The Joneses were permitted to settle in peace. Skokie would not be another Little Rock nor would it be another Deerfield.

RAINBOW BEACH

McDermott himself went on the front lines of activism in the desegregation of Rainbow Beach, a public bathing facility between Seventy-fifth and Seventy-ninth Streets, along Lake Michigan. Around the time of the Trumbull Park riots, the beach had become an all-white refuge on the increasingly black South Side. Throughout the fifties a series of ugly incidents had occurred, targeting blacks who wished to use the beach. As the beaches north of Rainbow Beach were integrated, many white bathers determined to make Rainbow Beach the site of a "last stand" against integration. However, as the area west of the beach became more heavily black, segregation at Rainbow Beach was a dead letter.

Direct action techniques, adapted from the civil rights movement in the South, began on Saturday, June 24, 1961, when a group of fifteen blacks from the local branch of the National Association for the Advancement of Colored People visited the beach and then left without incident after about an hour and a half. When they returned on July 2, a crowd formed around the black bathers and forced them to leave. The following weekend of July 8 and 9, the NAACP pledged to return for a "wade-in" and the prospect of a major showdown loomed. The CIC convened a meeting of city religious leaders and sent a telegram to Police Superintendent O. W. Wilson urging him to protect the rights "of every Chicago citizen to use the public beaches without interference or intimidation." They also arranged to have a delegation of priests, ministers, and rabbis come to the beach to help calm tensions.

As the day of the "wade-in" approached, the Congress of Racial Equality, the Woodlawn Organization, and a group called PACE (Positive Action for Civil Equality) organized groups of blacks to go to the beach. A strong police contingent was in place and about twelve to fifteen Protestant ministers, seminary students, and Catholic clergy, including Monsignor John Egan and Fathers William Hogan, James Mollohan, Daniel Mallette, Gerard Weber, Claretian Patrick McPolin, and George Cullen, were present.[52] The "wade-in" took place without incident. These combined efforts secured peace, and on July 15 McDermott organized a wade-in of Catholic youth from South Side parishes, many of them leaders of YCS groups. Although a brief episode of violence occurred the next day between the police and white gangs, segregation's back had been broken at Rainbow Beach.

CLERICAL AND RELIGIOUS ACTIVISM

Rainbow Beach demonstrated another feature of the new civil rights enthusiasm, the public militancy of priests and sisters. Catholic priests and sisters, in full garb, often demonstrated and marched. Among the first to demonstrate publicly was Father Martin Farrell in his association with the Woodlawn Organization. When Meyer called Farrell in to ask him why he

had done such a thing, Farrell replied that he thought he should be with his people. Meyer gave him his blessing for further protest activities.[53] Another memorable incident was the CIC's picketing of the segregated Illinois Catholic Women's Club, which met at Lewis Towers on Michigan Avenue. As a rule priests were free to participate in these public demonstrations and did so, wearing their Roman collars. The 1963 March on Washington also saw significant participation by lay, clerical, and religious Catholics from Chicago. Matthew Ahmann wrote to Meyer: "It looks as though there will be a fairly large Catholic participation in the August 28 demonstration in Washington. It is my hope that a large number of priests will be scattered throughout the march."[54] With the coordinated effort of the CIC and Friendship House, more than 250 Chicagoans participated in the historic march, including several Chicago priests: George Clements, Anthony Vader, and Daniel Mallette.[55] A year later Monsignor John Egan, recovering from a serious heart attack, heeded Martin Luther King's call to march to Selma, Alabama. Clerical participation was banned only once, when serious violence threatened Martin Luther King's march through Cicero, Illinois.

All through 1964 the tempo of civil rights activity increased throughout the Chicago archdiocese. In March 1964 Cantwell asked for permission to join a group of Catholic priests in other dioceses to "make [ourselves] available in troubled situations where priestly witness for justice would be helpful and where local ordinaries would permit it."[56] Because public activity on the part of his priests in the jurisdiction of another bishop might arouse ill-will, Meyer withheld approval. But he did continue to allow activism of a similar sort in the archdiocese. When the Chicago Real Estate Board again proposed a referendum on open occupancy legislation, the Chicago Conference on Religion and Race (CCRR) openly denounced the move as a "despicable instrument to extend the dual housing market which forces negroes to live in a ghetto."[57] Meyer himself entered the lists of those against the proposed referendum and sent to all the clergy the statement of the CCRR on the proposed referendum, suggesting "that the enclosed Statement will prove helpful in discussing this question with men and women of your various

parish organizations."[58] When S. T. Sutton, chairman of the Property Owners Coordinating Committee, attacked the efforts of the Chicago Conference on Religion and Race as "a self-appointed coterie of priests, preachers and rabbis," the executive board of the CCRR, consisting of Monsignor Robert J. Hagarty, Dr. Robert L. Bond, and Rabbi Benzion C. Kaganoff, rebutted Sutton's "self-appointed" slam and once again urged their congregations "to refrain from signing petitions calling for a referendum on open-occupancy legislation."[59] The efforts of the Catholic and ecumenical communities contributed to the defeat of the referendum.

AN INTERRACIAL CONFERENCE

The idea of holding an interreligious conference on racial issues had first surfaced in the board meetings of the NCCIJ in August 1960. Soon afterward Matthew Ahmann, the father of the idea, presented it to John McDermott, and the two began making plans for a great gathering in Chicago to celebrate the one hundredth anniversary of the Emancipation Proclamation. In July 1961 Ahmann and McDermott prevailed on Cantwell to present the idea to Meyer:

> It seems to us that it would be a good idea if we could arrange a meeting across religious lines of churchmen involved in human relations problems around the country.... Nothing of this kind has ever been done and it seems to us that it would have good effects for the Church. Moreover, a great deal of good would come here at home and other parts of the world if religious people were to raise a united voice for human rights and against racial discrimination and segregation.[60]

The trio of Ahmann, Cantwell, and McDermott submitted a lengthy memorandum to Meyer summarizing the reasons for such a meeting and met with the cardinal on August 17, 1961. Meyer was receptive to the proposal and to the suggestion that the conference be held in Chicago. He submitted the memorandum to Archbishop William E. Cousins of Milwaukee, episcopal chairman of the Social Action Department (SAD) of the National

Catholic Welfare Conference (with whom the NCCIJ was affiliated), and to Archbishop Patrick A. O'Boyle of Washington, a former chairman of the SAD.[61]

O'Boyle responded within a few days, heartily endorsing the project, "in view of the national interest in the rights of the Negro at the time."[62] Cousins responded a month later: "From all that I could determine by inquiry with the Social Action Office and from those engaged in the general field of Social Welfare, the calling of such a meeting would be as timely now as it could ever be."[63] Moreover, SAD pledged to be a cosponsor of the event, as did the Department of Racial and Cultural Relations of the National Council of Churches and the Social Action Commission of the Synagogue Council of America. Meyer gave his approval to the project and appointed the Chicago branch of the Catholic Interracial Conference to oversee the preparations for the conference, scheduled for January 14 to 17, 1963.

By the end of May the meeting had formally been titled "National Conference on Religion and Race" and formal invitations went out, including one to President John F. Kennedy. Four topic areas were to be covered with regard to racial policies: the inner life of the local church and synagogue; the church and the synagogue in its institutional management; the role of the religious leader; and church and synagogue in relation to community.[64] Meyer's role in the Religion and Race Conference was not only to act as host but to deliver one of the major addresses. In late 1962 the demands of the newly opened Vatican Council prevented him from giving full-time attention to the task and so he called on Father John LaFarge to draft the main text for him. LaFarge completed the work and sent it to Cantwell, who shipped it to the cardinal in Rome. Meyer wrote to LaFarge:

> When Msgr. Cantwell forwarded these notes to me in Rome, I was so occupied with the work of the Council that I had little time to study them. I brought them home with me, and it was soon Christmas, besides the volume of work awaiting my arrival. The net result was that I could not work on the talk until only recently after Christmas. It was then that I realized how great your help was. I want to assure you that I am using the greater portion of your notes, having added and subtracted something of

my own and having the whole then "polished" by several others, including Msgr. Cantwell.[65]

The conference opened on January 14, 1963, in Chicago's Edgewater Beach Hotel. The talks given at the plenary sessions were the conference highlights, but the main work was done in thirty-two work groups composed of religious leaders from around the country. Here they dealt with the practical implementation of the ideas expressed in the talks. Historical-minded reporters compared the stellar array of religious leaders meeting in early 1963 with the participants at the World Congress of Religion which met in the city sixty years earlier.[66] Among the 657 delegates present in Chicago were leading figures of Protestant and Jewish communities, including J. Irwin Miller, president of the National Conference of Churches; Rabbi Julius Mark, president of the Synagogue Council of America; Dr. Abraham Heschel, who presented one of the talks; R. Sargent Shriver, former president of the CIC and now director of the Peace Corps; and Dr. Martin Luther King, Jr., who also spoke at the gathering. The presence of King gave the meeting an air of drama. King would deliver his famous "I have a dream" speech eight months later on the steps of the Lincoln Memorial. That Meyer and King should appear together in pictures was ironic because as recently as 1960 Meyer had vetoed the civil rights leader as a speaker at a Catholic Interracial Council function.[67] But by 1963 his attitude toward King had changed and he gave an address that must have warmed the civil rights leader's heart.

Meyer's speech was delivered on the first night of the conference during its plenary session:

> The unresolved race question is indeed a pathological infection in our social and political economy. It is also an obstacle to a right conscience before God. Our whole future as a nation and as a religious people may be determined by what we do about the race problem in the next few years.[68]

The conference concluded with a measured but inspiring address by Martin Luther King, Jr., and "An Appeal to the Conscience of the American People." In late January 1963, Meyer

appeared on Chicago's TV talk show host Irv Kupcinet's program and spelled out specific ways to fight racial discrimination, urging active participation in community and neighborhood organizations, joining in interracial activities, employing Negro workers, reading Negro publications, and getting to know blacks personally.[69] As a by-product of the convocation, a permanent secretariat for a National Council on Religion and Race was formed, and a Chicago branch was opened with Meyer's approval and financial support of $10,000.[70] In March 1963, Galen R. Weaver, of the United Church of Christ, was appointed executive director of the committee. The proceedings of the historic meeting were soon edited by Ahmann and published in a paperback format under the title *Race: Challenge to Religion.*[71]

AN INCREASED TEMPO

Before the 1963 conference and afterwards, Meyer continued his campaign for racial justice in the city. He commissioned Egan to report to him on efforts to educate priests for the work of the Negro apostolate. In a lengthy report Egan urged the appointment of a full-time "consultant for the Negro Parish Apostolate."[72] Meyer did not follow through on this suggestion, but did mandate a series of three sermons on the racial issue to be delivered in every parish in the archdiocese. He wrote to the priests:

> As regards the application of Christian principles to modern situations, we have among the most serious issues of the present day, the race question. Consequently, several sermons of this series will deal with this timely matter. Thus we shall also fulfill a promise made on the occasion of our Clergy Conference on this topic, calling for simultaneous sermons on this subject in all the parishes of the Archdiocese. Under no circumstances should these sermons be omitted in any parish of the Archdiocese.[73]

Press reaction to Meyer's dictum came from the *Chicago Daily News* religion writer, Dave Meade, who reported favorably on the substance of the three sermon outlines.[74] A black newspaper, the *New Crusader*, observed, "Maybe all churches of all

denominations could profit by following the cardinal's lead."[75] Only the *Defender* had some critical words: "A social malady of the virulence of race prejudice cannot be eradicated with mild prescriptions.... It is too bad that the [church] leadership had to wait until the Federal Courts came to grips with discrimination before asserting itself on the issue of racial equality. The church should have led the way."[76]

But if the editorial staff of the *Defender* did not feel the sermons were enough, their timing was perfect for another case of racial integration in Niles, a Chicago suburb. On December 29, 1961, the first black family, Mr. and Mrs. John Viera, moved into the village of Niles. Since the family was Catholic, Father John J. Flanagan, pastor of St. John de Brebeuf parish, paid them a personal visit. Two days later the sermon series on racial justice began, and Flanagan and his assistants, Francis C. Waldron and Leon Wagner, preached on the theme at all the Masses and urged the acceptance of the family into the parish. When some minor incidents marred the general peace surrounding the Vieras' move in, Flanagan quickly sought the help of the Catholic Interracial Council in containing potential difficulties and Meyer was also brought in on the matter. With the cardinal's support, Flanagan and the Rev. Robert W. Gish of Niles Community Presbyterian Church drafted a statement in the name of all the clergy in Niles urging "pride in our community as one of enlightenment and respect for the ideals of our country which pledges liberty and justice for all."[77]

On January 9, 1962, Flanagan attended a meeting of the village board with Gish and other clergymen to "shame into silence" those who came to criticize the board for not taking action against the black family. The critical moment came when Flanagan and his associates showed up at a property-owners meeting on January 16, a meeting he had been warned not to attend. When a motion was offered asking Flanagan to leave, it was defeated two to one.[78] On January 28, Flanagan wrote a letter to his parishioners, one of the first of its kind by a priest of the Archdiocese of Chicago in addressing the race problem. He concluded:

> So far, we have avoided the tragic mistakes of a Cicero or a Deerfield. We seem to be well on our way to meeting this challenge

intelligently and in a true Christian spirit.... I have been criticized for visiting Mr. and Mrs. Viera. This has shown "favoritism and preference," some have said. On the contrary this was a simple act of Christian courtesy for which I have no apology. If this family is good enough to be welcomed into the Church of Christ, surely they are good enough to be welcomed into our parish.[79]

Meyer carefully monitored the Niles situation through phone calls to Flanagan and received regular reports from McDermott and the Catholic Interracial Council.[80] His strong support for Flanagan translated his words in behalf of racial justice into positive action.

CLERICAL EDUCATION

No less daunting than confronting Catholic suburbanites was the task of continuing education for priests in the work of interracial justice. This was ably handled by Father Anthony Vader. Vader had been among the first priests to go into black convert work, in the footsteps of Farrell and Richards. In 1957 Stritch had given him permission to take classes in sociology at the University of Chicago, and in 1962 he had completed a master's thesis on racial segregation in the Chicago archdiocese. In the spring of 1964 Vader organized a study week in race relations for the priests of the archdiocese on the campus of the college seminary at Niles.

Sponsored by Meyer, who spoke on the first day, the seminar attracted 155 priests from 83 parishes and had an impressive array of speakers, including Dr. Daniel Thompson, a black sociologist from Howard University who spoke on the "Negro Religious Mentality," and Cyril Tyson, who discussed "The Negro Family: Structure, Stability and Authority in the Home." A recently ordained black Chicago priest, Father Kenneth Brigham, an assistant at Our Lady of Solace parish, shared his experiences as well.[81] On the third and fourth days of the seminar, group discussion by priests in predominantly black parishes took place, coupled with talks by Father Leo Mahon, now a missionary in Panama, and Father Bernard Cooke, S.J., from Marquette University, who discussed liturgical and scriptural issues related to the Church's work with blacks. Three colloquiums of

priests met to discuss the role of the Church in the civil rights movement, how to proclaim the message of Christ to the neighborhood, and how to celebrate a meaningful liturgy. A parish group discussed work with blacks in parishes. Each group made its recommendations, which included more diligent efforts to evangelize and catechize blacks, the creation of an experimental parish "by combining small, fumbling parishes without potential," and the formation of teams of priests to minister from one central location, "e.g., The Catholic Church of Englewood."[82] It also called for personal clerical participation in direct action movements. The recommendations of the study week represented some of the most advanced thinking of the Chicago clergy already under the spell of Vatican II.

ECUMENICAL ENDEAVORS

Heightened sensitivity to the racial issue also dovetailed with the convocation of Vatican II and the ecumenical prospects offered by the council. Working together with other denominations on matters of joint ethical concern no longer seemed to have the taint of *"communicatio in sacris,"* which both Stritch and Meyer had avoided so strenuously in their earlier years. This ecumenical spirit washed over the interracial movement. In late 1963 Cantwell informed Meyer that he had selected Dr. Eugene Carson Blake, Stated Clerk of the United Presbyterian Churches in America, to be the speaker at the annual Catholic Interracial Council dinner in 1964. Meyer had become more engaged in ecumenical endeavors, accepting one of several civil rights awards from the Second Methodist Conference on Human Relations during a banquet at the Conrad Hilton in August 1963. In receiving the honor Meyer related an anecdote from his experiences at Vatican II:

> Our gathering here this evening reminds me of the report which Bishop Corson, one of the three Methodist Observers at the Second Vatican Council, gave on his audience with the late Pope John XXIII: "He's very expressive, just the kind you love to be with. Whenever he wanted to say something to me he would pat me on the arm. And really, I had all I could do to keep from patting him

back." I am confident that this is also the spirit of our gathering here this evening, even though the "patting" is only metaphorical. I am also reminded of a similar report given by Reverend Leslie Davidson, president of the British Methodist Conference of his audience with Pope John. He said that he spent a half hour with the Pope and that Pope John said to him: "Let's forget those sad centuries when men met only to quarrel. Let's meet to love one another."[83]

Later that year, Meyer was the recipient of a similar award from the Chicago Human Relations Commission.

Meyer's activism in behalf of civil rights was significant, considering the extent to which he was preoccupied with the Vatican Council. In July 1963 he appeared at a special meeting of the National Catholic Interracial Council, convened in the wake of President Kennedy's submission of a civil rights bill to Congress in June. The meeting was held to consider ways and means to support civil rights efforts through concerted local interreligious work and involvement in direct action techniques. Meyer reiterated the thrust of his remarks in January: that all action had to revolve around correct principles. "Right actions" he insisted, "must stem from right principles.... Right principles of action derive from truth, justice, charity and freedom."[84] In anticipation of the March on Washington in August 1963, Meyer issued copies of the U.S. bishops' letter on racial harmony to all his clergy and requested the priests to "make the text of this letter the subject of your sermon next Sunday, August 25."[85]

Meyer's insistence in 1960 that archdiocesan institutions end racial segregation was also monitored carefully in the wake of the Conference on Religion and Race. In 1963 Edward Marciniak, now on the city Human Relations Commission, sent a lengthy memo to Meyer urging more work to secure black vocations to the priesthood. He attached an evaluation of the state of interracial relations within the Church, evaluating officially certified Catholic offices, agencies, and organizations for the number of blacks present in them or for the outreach to them. The report was disconcerting: virtually every one of the groups listed, from the chancery through the fraternal organizations, had few, if any, black employees or participants.[86] On April 9, 1964, exactly

one year before his death, Meyer issued a directive calling for fair employment practices in Church-related institutions. He mandated that since the archdiocese was "committed to fair employment, [it] must insist that pastors employ qualified applicants regardless of race. Preference on the basis of race is forbidden." He concluded:

> Confident that you will understand the necessity of these regulations, I now ask that you go beyond them, by making a zealous effort to include, as far as possible, both white and Negro lay teachers in the faculty of your parish school. A racially integrated faculty will teach our children lasting lessons on the virtues of racial justice and love. To give schoolchildren good example is a paramount duty incumbent upon all educators, and especially upon Catholic educators.[87]

His letter was passed on to the Department of Public Aid director, Raymond Hilliard, who wrote: "Your personal leadership means a very great deal to me in my official position because if the war against racial injustice is won in Chicago, automatically the war against poverty will also be won, because it has long been evident that if we attack one, we are also attacking the other."[88] Meyer's intense interest in the civil rights question led him to contribute to the Leadership Conference on Civil Rights in order to finance their lobbying for the Civil Rights Bill of 1964.[89]

ST. PHILIP NERI

Meyer was deeply preoccupied with Vatican II when he dealt with the last serious difficulty of racial segregation during his tenure in the archdiocese, St. Philip Neri School. St. Philip was one of the wealthiest parishes of the South Shore, and its pastor, Monsignor Vincent Moran, had been a powerful influence in archdiocesan circles and on the Archdiocesan Conservation Council. Moran had refused to admit black pupils to the advanced grades of St. Philip Neri School in late 1964, in the hopes of securing a more phased-in integration. When Mrs. Gloria Lewis complained that her eighth-grade son, Tommie, a convert to Catholicism, was denied entrance into the school, the

priests of Holy Angels Church wrote a lengthy letter to Meyer, protesting Moran's decision: "The number of Negro Catholic youngsters being refused admittance to St. Philip Neri School is causing hardship in families, scandal in the Southside Negro Catholic community and pastoral concern among the clergy of five or six parishes."[90]

Moran had informed a trio of priests, James Mollohan, Anthony Vader, and George Clements, that he personally approved all new admissions to the school and would not accept even Catholic children into the school "unless at least one parent is Catholic." Since the Lewises were not Catholic, Moran felt justified in excluding the child. However, after the three priests spoke with Moran, they found that a number of black Catholic parents had been told there was no room in upper grades of the school.[91] Meyer immediately called Moran to hear his side of the story, but he wrote to him:

> In the specific problem which prompted my phone call, I realize that there are aspects of the same which are not fully clear to me. I understand that it is one thing to lay down a clear policy, as I did in the Clergy Conference of several years ago, and another thing to apply it to the facts of a specific case or cases. Looking back, however, over the past several years, and even more at the present state of this problem in general, I am convinced that it is the only policy which we can accept and be consistent with our own teaching.[92]

Meyer departed for his last session of Vatican II, and the controversy raged on. When he returned, he found on his desk a lengthy report from McDermott detailing the complaints of those who had attempted to register their children in the upper grades of the school. At Meyer's urging, Moran capitulated in early February 1965. CIC president Robert J. Cronin wrote to Meyer:

> This morning the upper grades of St. Philip Neri Grammar School were integrated. The parishioners involved in the problem wish to thank you for your important help in bringing this about. For myself, it has been a heart rending and soul searching experience—being at odds with people within the Church.... I

begin, through this involvement, to see in a small way your own difficult role in Rome as the Church seeks to redefine its expression of the will of God.[93]

Meyer's "difficult role in Rome" was the part he played in Vatican II, the climax of his career, the climax of the age of confidence.

10

The Twilight of an Era

After the death of Stritch in May 1958, a summer-long interregnum ended for the Archdiocese of Chicago on September 24, 1958. While Archbishop Albert Meyer was attending an episcopal consecration of a classmate in Wilmington, Delaware, the apostolic delegate announced his succession to the see of Chicago. Why had Meyer been chosen for the post?

Unsubstantiated claims attest that the original choice had been Dubuque's Archbishop Leo Binz, but the intercession of Pius XII's powerful housekeeper, Madre Pasqualina Lenhart, had swayed the ailing pontiff to Meyer. But, in all likelihood, Meyer's real advocate was probably his old scripture professor from the Propaganda, Cardinal Ernesto Ruffini of Palermo, a member of the powerful Consistorial Congregation. Indeed, Ruffini later bragged that it was he who had pushed Meyer's candidacy for the post.[1]

Meyer's installation was set for November 15, the feast of St. Albert the Great. As we have already seen, his accession meant new policies in critical areas of administration, urban affairs, and interracial relations. But events in Chicago itself were soon overshadowed by other occurrences in Rome. Ten days before his departure from Milwaukee, Meyer had watched the coronation ceremonies for a new pope, the former Cardinal Roncalli of Venice, who had taken the name John XXIII. Meyer was in office a little more than two months when the pontiff made the earthshaking announcement of a council. Vatican II would in many ways affirm and institutionalize changes that

were already well established among some Chicago Catholics. In other respects, especially in the area of ecumenism and priestly life, it would plow new ground. In any case, Chicagoans closely followed the ebb and flow of conciliar events, not only because of their own interests but because their leader, Cardinal Meyer, would be one of the movers and shakers of Vatican II. Indeed, Meyer would become so wrapped up with the work of the council that the affairs of the Chicago archdiocese would be in a state of suspended animation for the duration of the conciliar period.

VATICAN II

While still in the process of taking possession of his churches in Rome, John XXIII announced to a group of stunned cardinals in January 1959:

> Venerable brothers and our beloved sons! We announce to you, indeed trembling a little with emotion, but at the same time with a humble resolution of intention, the name and proposal of a two-fold celebration: a diocesan synod for the city, and an ecumenical council for the Universal Church.[2]

Initially, skepticism and indifference reigned in the wake of the announcement. Veteran Roman bureaucrats remembered similar plans by Pope Pius XI in the late twenties. Moreover, in his later years Pius XII was also prone to overblown statements and the bureaucracy had learned to discount such papal rhetoric as flights of fancy. This pope's call seemed no different. However, as it became clear that the pontiff really intended to bring the Council together, official reaction solidified. The chief opposition to the council came primarily, but not exclusively, from the Roman Curia, which attempted to slow down the various stages of the preparation. Reaction among the various episcopates of the world varied: the French seemed indifferent while Italian cardinals like Ruffini wrote the Holy Father, enthusiastically backing his plans for a council. American bishops appeared at once confused and indifferent. Largely insulated from the theological and liturgical ferment that existed on the continent since the end of the war, many American prelates had

no idea of the need for a council. Meyer's early reactions seemed to be in this vein. After he was created a cardinal in 1959, he managed some limited participation in the preparations for the great event. But he had a diocese to manage and initially did not have a sense of the major issues soon to be vigorously debated on the floor of St. Peter's Basilica. By 1962 this would change, as Meyer grew increasingly more interested and engaged in the affairs of the council.

PREPARING FOR THE COUNCIL

Meyer's intellectual preparation for Vatican II occurred in Chicago between 1959 and 1962. Although many American bishops had neither time nor inclination to study, Meyer had never given up his scholarly interest in Scripture and dogmatic theology. He had been faintly aware of the changes in scriptural studies that had been gradually emerging since Pius XII's encyclical *Divino Afflante Spiritu*. In Chicago, the presence of Loyola University, a major research institution, and the work of Cantwell and Barta in the Adult Education Centers brought these ideas front and center.

Loyola University had been one of the first Catholic institutions in Chicago to incorporate the insights of historical critical methodology in the exegesis of Scripture and had held a major symposium on the topic for interested priests in 1959. In the wake of the symposium, a good deal of unease ensued, which Meyer described to his old Biblicum classmate Monsignor William Newton:

> You will recall that when we spoke about the present trends in scripture when we met in Rome, we both expressed concern about the direction in which these trends were taking us. When I returned from Rome, I discovered that many of my priests, especially the older ones, were greatly disturbed as a result of a Scriptural Symposium held at Loyola University for priests.

Meyer noted that they were concerned about "the application to the New Testament of the Literary Forms discernible in Old Testament History." Then, quoting an article from *Theological Studies* of December 1959 by Father David M. Stanley, S.J.,

Meyer pinpointed the reason for the discomfort of the older priests and his own as well:

> There are undoubtedly some who feel, even though perhaps they do not express their fears too openly, that the old ghost of Modernism, which Pius X was thought to have laid [to rest] within the household of the faith, has staged a reappearance, this time as a poltergeist.[3]

However, the questions raised at the Loyola symposium, like the problems of Chicago he learned from Egan and others, did not stimulate fear or defensiveness in Meyer but, rather, made him intensely curious to learn more.

This newly roused curiosity coincided with the plans of Cantwell to arrange a two-week summer session in Scripture for priests to be held at the Maryknoll seminary in nearby Glen Ellyn. Meyer gave his approval to the project, scheduled for the first two weeks in July of 1960, and Cantwell assembled a top-notch staff of speakers, including Carmelite Roland Murphy, Jesuits John L. McKenzie and George Glanzmann, and Passionist Barnabas Mary Ahern. Nearly 250 priests registered for the sessions. Meyer himself agreed to give a major address on July 8, in order to allay the fears of the priests that the Loyola symposium had first stirred. To this end he sought advice and counsel from his former mentor, Cardinal Augustine Bea, S.J. Bea willingly provided a complete text that answered his questions on the emerging historical-critical method of biblical exegesis.

Meyer was so taken with Bea's address that he delivered it verbatim to the assembled priests—almost as though it had come from heaven. The text solidly endorsed the historical-critical school of exegesis as fully consonant with the mind of the Holy Father.[4] "We are in a state of transition in biblical studies," Meyer told the priests. "The certainties that have resulted from research in the correlated subjects [history and archaeology] have made it imperative that we set aside some views that had become 'traditional.' The uncertainties that remain warn us further change may be necessary."[5] The conveners of the conference were ecstatic at Meyer's repetition and affirmation of Bea's words. One of the organizers, Maryknoll priest John F. McConnell, wrote:

Your Eminence's visit and conference did something for the Institute that nothing else could have done. Your words and the words of Cardinal Bea read by you gave the priests the reassurance that Catholic priests generally, I think, can derive only from authority. No matter how great their respect for scholarship and holiness, they are instinctively wary until they hear a word from someone who has a right to speak to them in the name of the Church.[6]

McConnell's letter underscored the key to Meyer's own intellectual transition on the crucial scriptural question: higher Church authority had mandated it. It was now his task, as an obedient churchman, to understand and internalize what higher ecclesiastical authority had mandated.

Meyer was quick to realize the implications of the new approach to Scripture for dogmatic theology. In a letter to Cardinal Bea, Meyer reported on the discussion stirred in the archdiocese:

Articles appearing in priestly periodicals [relating to new methods of exegesis] or in popular pamphlets on biblical subjects, continue to cause much comment. This seems to be chiefly so, because they champion viewpoints which are so very new to most priests, and seemingly, contrary to what they were taught in the seminary. In particular the use of the Scriptures in the field of Apologetics has raised a number of questions.[7]

Even though concerns continued to be raised about the implications of the new methods, Meyer did not back away from the methodology.[8] Instead he set to work revising Bea's address for publication in pamphlet form and convened a clergy conference in February 1961 devoted to the new Catholic approach to the interpretation of Scripture. Papers were delivered by Ahern and Jesuits Bernard Cooke and Francis Filas. In his concluding remarks Meyer urged, "we must give scholars time and freedom to make their advances, mindful that we cannot solve all problems now." But, he insisted:

Prudence, great prudence is required: both for the research scholar, so that he may not lightly expose himself to perils; and for the popularizer, lest he rashly run into print. The same is true

of the priest in the ministry in his preaching and catechizing, as well as the teacher in the school.[9]

However, his call for prudence was not an attempt to turn back the clock. Meyer realized that the issues raised by the new scriptural methods would need a thorough airing at the council and wrote to Bea: "I gather, however, that the ferment in this field is quite general, and of course not confined either to our country or to any one country. Undoubtedly, the forthcoming Council will deal with this general subject and I deem it necessary that it so do."[10]

On February 2, 1962, Pope John announced the council would open on October 11, 1962, the Feast of the Maternity of Mary. Meyer ordered prayers in all Chicago's churches for the success of the meetings and made his own preparations to travel to Rome. Selection of *periti*, or advisors to the council fathers, was to be made. Any number of Chicago priests would have been delighted and capable of advising Meyer at the council, but symbolically he chose instead two trusted Scripture scholars, Passionist Barnabas Mary Ahern and Jesuit Francis McCool. Ahern had met Meyer when the latter was the archbishop of Milwaukee and they renewed their acquaintance at the Glen Ellyn symposium. Ahern was a native of Chicago. A pious, erudite, and ascetical man, he had been the hit of the symposium. Ahern would render yeoman service in the formulation of critical conciliar documents and would himself be the teacher of the bishops in new scriptural methodology. A second theological advisor of Meyer's, Scripture scholar Francis McCool, S.J., was on the faculty of the Pontifical Bibilical Institute. McCool had been introduced to Meyer by Bishop Ernest Primeau, who knew the Jesuit as the confessor to the members of the archdiocesan-owned residence in Rome known as the Chicago House.

Meyer was clearly enthusiastic about the deliberations of the council. His last speech before his departure was to the Archdiocesan Council of Catholic Men, whom he told: "The Council will be the most important religious event of our lives."[11] On September 14 he departed for the council with Cletus O'Donnell aboard a passenger liner which docked first in Palermo, where he was able to visit his old professor, Cardinal

Ruffini. He then set out for Rome and took up residence at the Chicago House on Via Sardegna. From that moment on, the Chicago House would be a veritable beehive of activity. Formal and informal dinners, discussions of conciliar business and politics, feast day and birthday parties, all became opportunities for discussing conciliar issues, lessons in biblical criticism, and dabbling in Roman politics.

THE OPENING OF THE COUNCIL

On October 11, 1962, Pope John XXIII solemnly convoked the Second Vatican Council. A total of 2,450 council fathers were in attendance at the opening session along with observers from various Protestant denominations and the Orthodox churches. Just before taking part in ceremonies opening the council, Meyer wrote back to his people:

> The Holy Father has already expressed his hopes that the Council will accomplish a deep and pervading renewal of your life in Christ and with Christ. He has expressed his hopes that this renewal will be an inspiration to others so that the words of Christ can be fulfilled: "And I, if I be lifted up, will draw all things to Me."[12]

In his opening address, the pope set the tone for the council:

> The salient point of this council is not therefore, a discussion of one article or another of the fundamental doctrine of the Church which had been repeatedly taught by the Fathers and by ancient and modern theologians, and which is presumed to be well known and familiar to all.... For this a council is not necessary, but for the renewed, serene and tranquil adherence to the teaching of the Church in its entirety and preciseness as it still shines forth in the acts of the Council of Trent and the First Vatican Council ... the whole world expects a step forward toward a doctrinal penetration and formation of conscience in the faithful and perfect conformity to the authentic doctrine which however should be studied and expounded through the methods of research and through the literary forms of modern thought. The substance of the ancient doctrine of the Deposit of Faith is one

thing, and the way in which it is presented is another.... The Spouse of Christ prefers to make use of the medicine of mercy rather than of severity. She considers that she meets the needs of the present day by demonstrating the validity of her teaching rather than by condemnation.[13]

Albert Gregory Meyer, always attuned to the flow of papal utterance, spent the rest of his days as a council father integrating the insights of this opening address into his work at the council.

In a letter to Monsignor George Casey, Meyer gave some fascinating insights into the day-to-day workings of that first session of the council:

Yesterday, some rumors started floating around the coffee shop that there was a strong movement afoot to ask the Holy Father to change the date of the next session.... Again it is only a rumor.... The coffee shop will probably go down in history as one of the more important phases of the Council! As you have probably heard, it does not interfere with the continuation of the discussion during the morning, but is running continuously with the Council Fathers taking time out as they see fit (or as nature requires!) Some make a regular habit of it, others are rarely seen down there. I have been a rather regular customer of late.[14]

The first session had begun with an enormous dispute over the procedure of selecting committees to consider the prepared schemata of the council. What emerged, within minutes, was a clear split between progressives and conservatives that would last through the entire four sessions of Vatican II. Critical disagreements over the nature of revelation demanded further study and the bishops were able to accomplish relatively little in those opening months. Meyer had stepped out of the shadows in the first weeks of the session and firmly aligned himself with the council's progressive wing. But in the end the first session of the council had been nothing more than a shakedown cruise for many of the American bishops. If they came befuddled about the need for such a convocation of the world's bishops, they left convinced that serious and deep issues would have to be resolved.

Meyer found the whole experience exhilarating and told a reporter: "I don't think any Council Father could go back home the same. In a sense I found the Council to be better than the best retreat I ever made."[15] Meyer was clearly pleased with what was happening. He returned to Chicago on December 9 and was besieged by local media for his impressions of the first session. He cited his enhanced appreciation of the universality of the Church, the presence of Protestant observers, the quality and richness of the liturgical life. But, with an increased perception of his new political role, he refrained from making specific statements and comments. Nonetheless, he indicated that the key accomplishment of the first session was the "gradual crystallization of the objectives of the council in the minds of the Council Fathers." He singled out the opening address of Pope John: "I would like to mention that in retrospect every bishop will constantly look back to that address and study it in the light of his experience of these past weeks. I think it is the key to understanding the Council. I think it is the Pope's own keynote."[16]

Meyer was not alone in this estimation of the spiritual power of the pope. Bishop John Mark Gannon of Erie, Pennsylvania, wrote to Meyer after the beginning of the new year:

> The man in the Council who captured me body and soul was John XXIII. I listened to him on three occasions and when I closed my eyes I could hear the Holy Ghost speaking. I returned home with the thought that the Holy Ghost was trying to reach us poor ignorant mortals on earth through John and the spell is still with me.[17]

INTERSESSION I: 1963

The hiatus between the first and second sessions of Vatican II was filled with activity. Conciliar progressives had clearly captured the initiative at the council and sought to keep it by carefully watching for any evidence of procedural sabotage on the part of the Curia. Meyer kept Chicagoans abreast of the issues, and the *New World* kept up a steady diet of articles about the council and the council fathers, and provided incisive commentary and reporting by assistant editor Father William Graney.[18]

During the intersession period, conciliar politics spilled over into the public forum at the Catholic University. At the insistence of Apostolic Delegate Egidio Vagnozzi, Catholic University Rector Monsignor William McDonald had banned a university sponsored Lenten lecture series by leading theologians John Courtney Murray, S.J., Godfrey Diekmann, O.S.B., Gustave Weigel, S.J., and Swiss theologian Hans Küng. All of them, except for Murray, had been *periti* at Vatican II, and associated with the liberal cause. When pressed for reasons for this obvious violation of academic freedom, McDonald lamely explained that since many issues these theologians intended to discuss were still before the council, it would not be wise to give a forum to one particular point of view on the campus of the Catholic University.[19]

This decision created a fire storm of opposition in academic and ecclesiastical circles. Cardinal Ritter of St. Louis sent Meyer a copy of his letter to McDonald:

> As a member of the Board of Trustees of the Catholic University I was greatly displeased to learn of the University's decision to bar four priests, prominent in their fields of theological endeavor, from addressing the students. As a member of the American hierarchy, responsible for the University I deeply regret the deleterious effects such a short-sighted decision will have on our Catholic University's reputation. Personally I am indignant that such an incident could take place in any Catholic institution of higher learning in our country.[20]

Meyer shared Ritter's indignation and wrote to the St. Louis archbishop:

> I believe your letter expresses the thought of many of us, and I must confess that I had been prompted to write a similar one. It was my thought, however, that possibly Monsignor McDonald was simply in the unenviable position of having to take blame for a decision that was not his.... I am afraid, like yourself, that the prestige of the University has been seriously damaged.[21]

Meyer showed his sympathy for the theologians by permitting a sympathetic editorial in the *New World* by Father William Graney.[22] Moreover, when Küng visited Chicago to address

Cantwell's John A. Ryan Forum on the topic, "Freedom in the Church," Meyer met briefly with the Swiss theologian.[23] When Küng spoke at the massive McCormick place, he drew a crowd of 5,000—one of the largest audiences for a theological lecture in Chicago's history. In the heavily charged atmosphere of conciliar politics this affirmation of the right of free discussion could hardly have been missed by curial conservatives. Chicago Catholic leaders such as Cantwell were once again heartened by Meyer.

Looming over all this debate was the final illness and death of Pope John XXIII in June of 1963. Meyer returned to Rome for the papal obsequies and remained for the brief conclave that elected John's successor, Cardinal Giovanni Battista Montini— Pope Paul VI. Meyer returned from the papal conclave and coronation in time to host a meeting of 149 bishops at Chicago's Conrad Hilton Hotel to discuss the issues of the second session. The much-harassed Ahern presented information on his labors on the document on revelation, while Meyer summarized the discussions on religious liberty that had been brewing since the close of the first session.

SESSION II

The second session of the council, with its reflection on the meaning of Church, brought forth a consideration of the role of Catholicism in relationship to other Christian denominations. This concern produced the Decree on Ecumenism. Meyer informed O'Donnell, who remained in Chicago to administer the diocese after the death of Casey:

> It has been announced that we shall discuss De Oecumenismo, next. As you know, a fourth chapter had been added to this schema, dealing with the Jews. A fifth chapter will also be added on religious liberty. It had difficult sailing in the theological commission, to which it had to be sent for review at the request of the Holy Father, before being presented to the Council Fathers. This far, we do not have the printed copy of the final text.[24]

Meyer's interest in ecumenism was perhaps the biggest surprise of the council. In his early years as bishop he had

avoided even the semblance of *communicatio in sacris*, regularly forbidding Catholic participation in the YMCA and attendance even at the blandly nondenominational baccalaureate services that public high schools tacked on to their commencement ceremonies. Yet, once he became archbishop of Chicago his feelings began to change. Catholics and non-Catholics, he observed, could and did come together for fruitful cooperation in confronting serious urban problems.

A preliminary decree was prepared by the Secretariate for Christian Unity and the Oriental and Theological Commissions in the summer of 1963. But the last two chapters of the text on the Jews and the topic of religious liberty hit rough waters. Meyer wrote O'Donnell:

> The first three chapters, which we received in the regular schema last summer, were voted for acceptance for further discussion in detail, but my strong plea to have the same happen NOW for chapters four and five did not succeed. I understand that there were strong objections from different segments, on the basis that these chapters had not been received in sufficient time for enough study. Hence the vote to accept them as the basis of detailed discussion was not proposed, and it seems unlikely that it will be proposed before the end of this session. I am still hoping, but I doubt it very much.[25]

The council ended on a sad note for Meyer and the American bishops when news arrived of the death of President Kennedy. Yet, despite the gloom of the Kennedy assassination and the concern over the slow pace of conciliar deliberation, Meyer returned to Chicago in early December and briefed the priests on events in Rome and wrote to the people: "I certainly do not subscribe to the judgement of those journalists who have expressed disappointment with the work of the Council, or have even spoken of 'shattered hopes.'"[26]

INTERSESSION II: 1964

This intersession would be the busiest for Meyer. He threw caution to the winds and began implementing the letter and spirit of the council in Chicago. His first initiative was in the

arena of ecumenism. Even before the council, Meyer recognized the need for a practical alliance with other religious bodies in the city in pursuit of racial justice and allied urban problems. The high-water mark of ecumenism, during Meyer's years in Chicago, came when he co-hosted the 1963 Conference on Religion and Race. In the fall of that same year he took to the council floor to underscore his belief that "All should respect the religious sincerity of others and not regard differences of religious belief and practice as excuses for violating the moral obligation to treat all fellow citizens with respect, justice and charity."[27] He used the opportunity of his annual Lenten pastoral in 1964 to discuss the implications of the council's deliberations on ecumenism. "Although the Council has not concluded these discussions [on ecumenism], I have considered it fitting to place before you in this pastoral letter some general considerations on the subject.... In this way we feel we are sharing in the spirit of the Council itself."[28]

The day the lengthy pastoral was issued, Meyer spoke before a group of two hundred Protestant ministers gathered at Chicago Theological Seminary, summarizing the teaching of the pastoral.[29] As Meyer prayed with the ministers, begging pardon "for our controversies ... narrow mindedness or exaggerations ... for our intransigence and our harsh judgements," perhaps he or others there remembered, only ten years earlier, Stritch's injunction against Catholic participation in the Evanston meeting of the early fifties. Times had indeed changed.[30]

The promulgation of the Constitution on the Liturgy also gave Meyer the opportunity to implement the will of the council. On the way home from Rome in 1963 he appointed auxiliary bishop Aloysius Wycislo to head an Archdiocesan Liturgical Commission. Working closely with Monsignor Eugene Mulcahey, pastor of St. Jerome's parish, Wycislo assembled a blue-ribbon panel of fourteen priests, religious, and laypersons to form the commission. They met with Meyer on April 7, 1964, and began to lay plans for educating priests and lay people in spirit of the new liturgy.[31] In May, annual clergy conferences were dedicated to instruction in the new liturgy, with presentations by Jesuit Bernard Cooke, theologian Gerard Sloyan, Killgallon, and lay members of the liturgical commission, Joseph Evans and

William Quinn.[32] On the eve of his departure for Rome, Meyer promulgated an approved vernacular ritual, allowing the use of English in the administration of the sacraments and sacramentals, effective on September 14, with the vernacular Mass to begin on November 29.[33] Enthusiasm for the new liturgy built around the diocese as frequent articles in the *New World* gave instructions about the nature and spirit of the changes. To Reynold Hillenbrand these must have been heady days.

RELIGIOUS LIBERTY

As he returned to Rome for the third session of the council, the issue of religious liberty was uppermost in Meyer's mind. Originally, schematae on religious liberty and the Jews had been attached to a decree on ecumenism proposed during the second session. Meyer had worked diligently through the summer of 1964 for the passage of this document. He met with one of the leading voices for a document on religious liberty, Father John Courtney Murray, whom he had first encountered at a dinner in 1963 arranged by Bishop Ernest Primeau and Monsignor John S. Quinn. After Pope John had issued *Pacem in Terris* in 1963, the cause of religious liberty had picked up steam and Meyer became a leading proponent of some sort of declaration. Indeed, he deemed conciliar action on this issue essential to the credibility of ecumenical relations in the United States. As he had told O'Donnell when the second session of the council ended:

> At first glance, it may not seem important when this vote [on the Decree on Ecumenism to which chapters on the Jews and Religious Liberty had been attached] is taken up, but psychologically I think it is, because of the publicity which these chapters have already received. This will look like a delaying action, if we do not accept them now as a basis of discussion.... If it is not accepted now who knows what may happen to it in the interim.[34]

But the proposed statement did not sit well with some forces in the council. The politics of committees, composed of liberals and conservatives, were chipping away at the heart of the text. McCool, in Rome, alerted Meyer to the action in a letter dated January 21, 1964:

I have just heard that Fr. John [Courtney] Murray is in the hospital with a slight heart attack. I hope sincerely that he gets over it.... Because of his health I did not tell Fr. Murray when writing him of the rumor here which is rather preoccupying. That is that most of the emendations on the chapters on religious liberty and the Jews are hostile to the doctrine contained in those documents. Roman rumor is an old story, but this may well be true. Those who favor a document are inclined to let it go at that whereas its adversaries tend to be more active. We all hope that before January 31st many more comments favoring the document come in to Archbishop Felici. It can mean so much.[35]

Meyer did not waste any time picking up on McCool's exhortation to action. Just the day before his own archdiocesan pastoral on ecumenism was issued, Meyer wrote a lengthy letter to Pope Paul in behalf of religious liberty:

Various rumors have reached me that those opposed to these chapters have written strong objections to them. Therefore do I hasten to write to Your Holiness, confident that Your Holiness will understand.... I am confident that if these two chapters are accepted ... they will do much to promote the cause of religious unity.... Your Holiness, I am convinced that all Ecumenists—Protestants and Catholics alike—who have been engaged in the ecumenical movement, and who have an understanding of the mind of our separated brothers—are convinced that the question of religious liberty is THE NUMBER ONE AND MORE IMPORTANT QUESTION in the whole schema on Ecumenism. It is the number one question which underlies all of the various tensions that exist between Catholics and Protestants in the United States. The same would be true of the chapter on the Jews for our relations with them.... If the Bishops of the United States have to return home from a third session of the Council without these two chapters, the cause of the Catholic Church in the United States, I am afraid, will suffer greatly.[36]

Following up on the letter, Meyer publicly lobbied for the passage of a document on religious liberty. To a group of Protestant ministers he quoted a passage from Pope John XXIII's *Pacem in Terris* which read: "Every human being has the right to honor God according to the dictates of an upright conscience and the

right to profess his religion, privately or publicly."[37] Meyer's public statements and those of other progressive cardinals resulted in the salvation of the sections on religious liberty and the Jews by having them detached from the schema on ecumenism into free-standing documents at a meeting of theologians in Arricia, Italy, in February 1964.

While this made it easier to shepherd the work on ecumenism through the process of deliberation, it hardly stilled the controversy over the two new documents. The document on the Jews and other non-Christians certainly created its share of headaches. In a letter to Meyer in April 1964, Father McCool informed him that the document had been reworked by the Central Coordinating Committee and that the new text excluded a specific exoneration of the Jews from the traditional charge of deicide. Since this had been explicit in the first draft of the document, McCool observed: "the fact that the contents of the former statement were already generally known may cause some heart-burning among the Jews in America when the changes are made known."[38] On June 14, when the changes were formally approved, McCool again wrote Meyer: "Every reference to *deicida, Gens deicida* has been removed. Naturally there will be sharp disappointment in Jewish circles."[39] True to McCool's predictions, Jewish leaders were distressed. Meyer himself was contacted, via Monsignor Cantwell, by Rabbi Marc Tanenbaum, chairman of the Interreligious Affairs Department of the American Jewish Committee and by members of the Chicago Jewish community.[40] He was also visited by Rabbi Abraham Heschel, who vigorously urged him to insist on a restoration of the original exoneration. The two men talked long into the night, and although he complained privately to O'Donnell about the pressure, he addressed the council later that month to call for the restoration of the references.[41]

But Meyer was heavily involved in the document on religious liberty. When the reworked document was sent to the council fathers and reintroduced to the council on September 23, 1964, by Bishop Emile DeSmedt of Bruges, Meyer rose on that same day to speak in its behalf. He sensed the unanimity among the American and many European bishops on the need for a

document on religious liberty but knew full well that considerable resistance emanated from the Curia and the hierarchies of Spain and Latin America, who feared that such a decree would lead to religious indifferentism. They spoke strongly against the document and it once again passed through a series of revisions and reexaminations, causing confusion among the bishops as to just what stage the text was in at any given time. Eventually the document was sent back to committee with the intention of refining its language and some of its provisions, and resubmitting it as soon as possible for deliberation at the end of the third session. These delays created anxiety in Meyer and many American bishops who were eager to signal to the world that the Church was serious about ecumenism.

Parliamentary subterfuges to sidetrack deliberations occurred soon after the decision to refer the matter to committee. Archbishop Pericle Felici informed Cardinal Bea that the jurisdiction over the document was to be shifted from Bea's liberal Secretariate for Christian Unity to a mixed commission made up of liberals and conservatives.[42] When the members of the Secretariate caught their breath over this attempt to short-circuit the document, they leaked word to the council fathers and a hastily summoned meeting of seventeen cardinals, including Meyer, met at the residence of Dutch Cardinal Bernard Alfrink. The seventeen drafted a petition to the pope, dated October 11, 1964 (the anniversary of the opening of the council two years earlier), protesting the decision. This protest, called the *Non sine magno dolore* letter, compelled the pope, who may not have known of Felici's effort, to rescind the order and restore jurisdiction over the document to Cardinal Bea.

The danger to the substance of the document passed and the work of revision moved ahead. Meyer pressed publicly for the passage of the Declaration on Religious Liberty in a much-publicized address before Rome's Pro Deo University, given at a symposium on Pope Paul VI's encyclical *Ecclesiam Suam*. In words aimed at the critics of the declaration, who feared it would canonize an American-style church-state separation, Meyer sought to reassure them by explaining the meaning of the first amendment to the U.S. Constitution:

To be sure, it meant that there was to be in our country a separation between church and state, but not the kind of malevolent, anti-religious separation, which, at that time and for many generations thereafter, was the pattern in parts of Europe and which had so many baneful consequences. The kind of separation between Church and state envisioned by our founding fathers and provided for in the first amendment to the Constitution presupposed that religion is supremely important—so important and so sacred that the state must be prohibited from interfering in any way with its free exercise.[43]

As precious moments ticked away the declaration went through the arduous process of revision. With each passing week Meyer grew more pessimistic, writing to a friend on November 16 that it did not look likely a vote would be taken.[44] But the very next day the schema was finished and resubmitted to the floor. When the debate recommenced, with the promise that a vote would be taken, tension began to mount. Meyer, who now sat with the Council of Presidents, was working at his place on the morning of November 19 when lightning struck.

In the course of a discussion on a minor issue, the presiding cardinal, Eugene Tisserant, rose and informed the bishops that the council presidents had determined that since some of the council fathers felt they had insufficient time to consider the new text on religious liberty, voting would be postponed until the next session. The brief wave of applause that greeted the announcement was soon replaced by a roar of displeasure from the bishops. Meyer was stunned. Had he been missed in the poll of the council presidents? Certainly Tisserant had not asked him. He strode from his place to Tisserant and asked what this meant. He received no answer but that it had been done. Visibly angered, but not consumed with rage as later press reports and apocryphal retellings of this event have suggested, Meyer came down from the presidential dais and joined a knot of like-minded progressives including Ritter, Frings, and Leger.[45]

Meanwhile, bishops were scampering out of their places in the aula, signing a petition drafted hastily by Bishop Francis Reh, rector of the North American College, using typewriters of Archbishop Felici's secretariate, which opposed the declaration.[46] Beginning with the Latin words, *Instanter, Instantius,*

Instantissimus, "Urgently, more urgently, most urgently, we petition that a vote on the Decree on Religious Liberty be permitted before the end of this session." Several copies of the petition circulated around the council floor, gathering an indeterminate number of signatures. Before long these petitions were thrust in Meyer's lap and he agreed to present them to the pope in company with Cardinals Leger and Ritter. Cardinal Leger recalled of the meeting:

> The Pope received us and the Cardinal [Meyer] explained the situation with respect, yet with a certain vehemence. His attitude revealed a real passion to see the schema "de libertate religiosa" approved as early as possible. The pope's response was dictated with discretion. He recommended patience and the schema was sent back to the next session.[47]

In the aftermath of the incident, Meyer was shaken and melancholic.[48] The formal close of the third session of the council took place on November 21, 1964, and ended all hope for sending the kind of signal to the world that Meyer and the progressives sincerely wanted. He flew home in early December and, shortly after his arrival, spoke with reporters, openly telling of his disappointment that the council was denied the opportunity to vote on a statement proclaiming the right of religious freedom.[49] Despite the setback, John Courtney Murray, Meyer, and others continued to work on the declaration, revising and rewriting the text in preparation for the next session of Vatican II. True to his word, Pope Paul VI placed consideration of the text at the top of the agenda and it was finally promulgated in December 1965. Although the events of "Black Thursday" disappointed and dejected Meyer and other proponents of the declaration, the final document that emerged was probably better and stronger than the draft of the previous year.

In early December of 1964 Meyer met with his priests at Resurrection parish to inform them of developments at the council. When he walked into the huge auditorium filled with his clergy, he was greeted by five full minutes of cheers and ovations. For a man who so loved the priesthood and priests, this was one of the peak moments of a life and career that would soon be over.

RETURN TO CHICAGO

Meyer and his entourage were tired when they arrived home after the third session. Meyer had occasionally written home about a stiffness in his neck and headaches around his right ear, but he attributed it to the stress and intensity of the conciliar sessions. After meeting with the clergy at Resurrection parish, Meyer tackled the huge backlog of work that awaited him since September. But after the Christmas crunch, those close to him began to notice differences. His longtime spiritual director/confessor, Monsignor William Groessel of Milwaukee, visited him on New Year's Day, 1965, and remarked to a friend: "He wasn't his old self anymore."[50] Later that month, Meyer alarmed the house detective at his residence when the bathrobe-clad cardinal was discovered wandering around the house in the middle of the night, insisting he smelled gas. O'Donnell was immediately summoned and after a quick check for gas leaks put Meyer back to bed. He noticed, however, that Meyer was having a difficult time keeping his balance and focusing his normally intent eyes. Later that morning, O'Donnell placed a call to Dr. John Kiley, a neurologist at Loyola's Stritch School of Medicine, and described the problem. Kiley insisted Meyer be taken immediately to nearby Mercy Hospital where he and Dr. George O'Brien would check him. Meyer angrily submitted to the ambulance ride and was kept in the hospital four days. He was released with the public statement that he had suffered gall bladder problems.

On his return, Meyer's ability to focus or work on anything grew steadily worse. He was compelled to delegate more and more administrative duties to O'Donnell and shocked educational chief Monsignor William McManus by asking him to draw up a speech for him because he claimed he could not do it on his own. Realizing that his health was deteriorating, he finally agreed to submit to a series of tests. The day before he went into the hospital he wrote to Ahern:

> Since my strength is coming back only gradually I must confess that I am not exactly looking forward with anticipation to the next session of the Council, although I will do my best to prepare

for it. The most attractive part of it for me will be the opportunity to meet again with you and Father McCool since I owe so very much to both of you for the great help you extended to me.[51]

Sensitive to the criticisms leveled against the archdiocese over the medical treatment of Cardinal Stritch, O'Donnell requested opinions from leading specialists, including a cardiologist who had worked with former President Dwight Eisenhower. The tests revealed a malignant tumor on Meyer's brain about one inch from his right ear—the very ear Meyer had complained about during the council. Once the decision for surgery was made, Meyer accepted the news calmly and began to make methodical preparations for the operation and its aftermath. Groessel was brought down from Milwaukee to live in the room adjoining Meyer's at Mercy Hospital and prepare him spiritually for the ordeal. Meyer then turned almost matter-of-factly to funeral preparations. Much to O'Donnell's discomfort, he insisted that the auxiliary preside at his funeral (not Apostolic Delegate Egidio Vagnozzi, whom Meyer disliked), and that Archbishop William Cousins, his successor in Milwaukee, preach the funeral sermon. On February 28 the surgery was performed.

As those were the days before delicate lasers and more advanced cancer therapies, the surgeons were unable to remove the malignancy. Meyer lingered for the whole of March and the first weeks of April. Infrequent periods of lucidity allowed him to receive a few of the steady stream of visitors that came to his bedside. Finally on April 9, 1965, Albert Meyer passed away at the age of sixty-two and was laid to rest in the peaceful cemetery at Mundelein. On his tombstone the words from Pius XI's encyclical on priesthood were inscribed as a final instruction to the future priests of Chicago: "Prepare yourself with all seriousness for the great task to which God calls you."

+ + +

From April until August, Meyer's chief aide, Bishop Cletus F. O'Donnell, directed the affairs of the archdiocese. As Sheil before him, O'Donnell had hopes that his faithful service would merit him the Chicago see and cardinal's hat. But the needs of

Chicago seemed to be driven more by the rapidly growing racial tensions stimulated by the civil rights movement and rising black militancy. On June 16, 1965, John Patrick Cody, the archbishop of New Orleans, who won himself a reputation as a friend of civil rights when he masterminded the public excommunication of the notorious racist Leander Perez and some associates, was appointed to succeed Meyer.

Cody came to Chicago that August with as much support as any newcomer could have expected and took the diocese out of the state of suspended animation necessitated by Meyer's presence at the council. He pressed ahead with a torrent of overdue reforms: strong support for the new liturgy, improved clerical salaries, genuine archdiocesan insurance, upgraded school salaries and standards. Moreover he dealt firmly with some long overdue personnel issues when he imposed an administrator on the aging Bishop Bernard J. Sheil and he removed Monsignor Malachy Foley as rector of the seminary, tasks for which Meyer had neither the time nor the stomach.

But Cody's style of administration brought more problems than plaudits. Cody was clearly not in the "permissive" mode of his two predecessors and immediately began to centralize power into his own hands and act without consultation. Longtime favorites, such as Egan and Cantwell, were removed from positions of authority and sent out to parishes, while the offices and movements they had established withered. Indeed, one year after Cody's accession to office, journalist John Leo openly criticized the new archbishop on the pages of *Commonweal*:

> He has managed to convey the idea that nothing of value happened in the Archdiocese until he arrived. He is mistrustful of his priests, often giving them two full-time jobs to make sure they're not goofing off. Initiative is being discouraged, and the chancery bureaucracy is on the point of becoming paralyzed.[52]

By early 1966 Cody's tactics and the general ferment associated with the postconciliar era led more than four hundred Chicago priests to form what *Time* magazine called "the closest thing yet to a priests union," the Association of Chicago Priests (ACP). While this organization would never match the high expectations of its founders, its rise marked the capstone of the

permissive policies of Stritch and the progressive mood of the Meyer era in the Chicago Catholic community. Cody successfully undercut the ACP and grew increasingly more defensive and authoritarian. These policies only added to the disarray and division in the Chicago Church of the postconciliar years and provided a sharp departure from the ebullient confidence of the previous generation. Typical of other Catholic communities, Chicago Catholics became embroiled in debates on birth control and clerical life. Even the liturgical movement lost its vital connection with social action, and disgruntled pioneers such as Hillenbrand pulled away from old friends like Pat and Patty Crowley and scorned the slapdash liturgical reforms promulgated without sensitivity to beauty or engagement with the world. Indeed, an epoch had passed.

It is hazardous to guess what Chicago Catholicism would have been like if Albert Meyer had lived to the mandatory retirement age of seventy-five and retired in 1978. However, it certainly can be noted that Meyer lacked Cody's love for centralization and he managed to allow his subordinates adequate freedom to do their jobs. Meyer did make phone calls to recalictrant pastors and school principals to insist on racial justice, but one could hardly imagine him phoning to check on the faculties of a priest visiting Chicago from another diocese as Cody did. Moreover, he would have had the astute O'Donnell at his side, at least for a time, to steer him through the rocky shoals of ecclesiastical politics. O'Donnell's upward ascent was cut short by his transfer to the predominantly rural Madison, Wisconsin, diocese in 1967. This was no doubt done with Cody's blessing, who wanted no remnants of the old regime as a gathering point for clerical dissatisfaction. Finally, Albert Meyer was a much brighter and more naturally inquisitive man than his successor. His first response to new problems would have been to dig for more information on which to base wise decisions. Cody tended to act unilaterally and at times based on bad information.

Yet, even Meyer would have found the postconciliar years difficult. "What have we released from Rome?"[53] he is reported to have said in the declining days of the third session of the council. Although he, like most other bishops, was caught up in the euphoria generated by the council sessions, he also noticed

the cracks of division, the extreme polarization of positions, and perhaps (even though he would never have admitted it publicly) the indecisiveness of Pope Paul VI, which caused the reform movement to sputter and stop.

Above all, Meyer would have mourned the loss of confidence—that sure knowledge that the Church, with all her spots and wrinkles, still represented the last best hope of mankind. The confidence bred of neo-scholasticism and papal direction was the lodestar of the lives of Stritch, Meyer, and their contemporaries. It was this mood of confidence, in everything from Church doctrine to social justice, that stands in even bolder relief in the years since its passing.

Abbreviations

AAC	Archives of the Archdiocese of Chicago
AAM	Archives of the Archdiocese of Milwaukee
AAD	Archives of the Archdiocese of Detroit
ADT	Archives of the Diocese of Toledo
AACin	Archives of the Archdiocese of Cincinnati
ADN	Archives of the Diocese of Nashville
ACUA	Archives of the Catholic University of America
AUND	Archives of the University of Notre Dame
ANCWC	Archives of the National Catholic Welfare Conference
CBNA	Chicago Branch National Archives
CHS	Chicago Historical Society
FDRL	Franklin D. Roosevelt Library
HSTL	Harry S Truman Library
UICA	University of Illinois Chicago Archives

Notes

INTRODUCTION

1. Albert G. Meyer to Stritch, August 3, 1953, Box 2828, Stritch Papers, Archives of the Archdiocese of Chicago (hereafter AAC).

2. "The Biggest U.S. Archdiocese," *Life*, December 26, 1955, pp. 62–69.

3. Stritch to Dan Herr, February 28, 1958, Stritch Papers, AAC.

4. Telegram, Dell'Acqua to Stritch, February 5, 1958, Stritch Papers, AAC.

5. Dell'Acqua to Stritch, January 17, 1958, Stritch Papers, AAC.

6. Stritch to Angelo Dell'Acqua, February 5, 1958, Stritch Papers, AAC.

7. Dell'Acqua to Stritch, February 13, 1958, Stritch Papers, AAC.

8. Stritch to Dell'Acqua, February 24, 1958, Stritch Papers, AAC.

9. Press Release, NCWC Press Department Papers, Archives of the Catholic University of America (hereafter ACUA).

10. Interview with Bishop Cletus F. O'Donnell, May 3, 1984, and Monsignor James Hardiman, June 28, 1988.

11. This is alluded to in John Cooney's controversial biography of Spellman, *The American Pope: The Life and Times of Francis Cardinal Spellman* (New York: Times Books, 1984), pp. 245, 248–256.

12. Pietro Fumasoni-Biondi to Stritch, July 8, 1957, Chancery Files, Stritch Papers, AAC.

13. Stritch to Spellman, March 6, 1958, Stritch Papers, AAC.

14. Dan Ryan to Ernest Primeau, March 8, 1958, Stritch Papers, AAC.

15. Stritch to Edward A. Tamm, March 10, 1958, Stritch Papers, AAC.

16. *Congressional Record*, March 19, 1958, pp. 4195–4196.

17. Stritch to J. Gerald Kealey, March 4, 1958, Stritch Papers, AAC.

18. Hardiman interview.

19. Joseph Emmenegger to Meyer, April 28, 1958, Meyer Papers, AAC.

20. Office Memorandum from SAC (Special Agent in Charge) Auerbach to Mr. Hoover, April 28, 1958, FBI Office Files, 94-4-1411-18. At the request of Judge Tamm and Monsignor Fitzgerald, Hoover took a personal interest in Stritch's case and expedited these matters.

1. "THIS IS CHICAGO"

1. "Chicago Roars Great Ovation to Archbishop," *Chicago Tribune*, March 7, 1940.

2. Ibid.

3. Quoted in an undated clipping from *Nashville Register* in Stritch Papers, Archives of the Archdiocese of Chicago (hereafter AAC).

4. Marie Cecilia Buehrle, *The Cardinal Stritch Story* (Milwaukee: Bruce Publishing Co., 1959), p. 14.

5. "Concluding Address" in *Proceedings of First National Catholic Social Action Conference*, May 14, 1938, Milwaukee, Wisconsin, p. 400.

6. Muench Diary, Muench Papers, Archives of the Catholic University of America (hereafter ACUA), p. 67.

7. "Mirrors of Toledo: Bishop Stritch, " *Toledo News-Bee*, January 21, 1922, Clipping File, Toledo City Library.

8. For additional information on Stritch's years in Milwaukee, see the author's "Samuel Stritch and Milwaukee Catholicism, 1930–1940," *Milwaukee History* 13 (Autumn 1990): 70–91.

9. The memoir of one of his personal secretaries, Monsignor John D. Fitzgerald, gives an excellent description of Stritch agonizing over a problem priest. Copy of the "John Fitzgerald Memoir" given by Thomas Stritch to the author.

10. Muench Diary, p. 19, Muench Papers, ACUA.

11. Ibid., p. 63, Muench Papers, ACUA.

12. Ibid., p. 45, Muench Papers, ACUA.

13. The two best sources for this development are Charles Shanabruch's *Chicago's Catholics: The Evolution of an American Identity* (Notre Dame, Ind.: University of Notre Dame Press, 1981) and Edward R. Kantowicz, *Corporation Sole: Cardinal Mundelein and Chicago Catholicism* (Notre Dame, Ind.: University of Notre Dame Press, 1983). Harry Koenig has edited four volumes on the history of the parishes and institutions of the Archdiocese of Chicago. See *History of the Parishes*, 2 vols. (Catholic Bishop of Chicago, 1980) and *History of the Institutions*, 2 vols. (Catholic Bishop of Chicago, 1980).

14. "Civic Booster Lost in Death of Cardinal Mundelein," October 3, 1939, *Chicago Tribune*.

15. Eileen M. McMahon, "What Parish Are You from?" (Ph.D. diss., Loyola University, 1989), p. 344.

16. For a description of this dimension of Catholic life at large in the Midwest, with some good examples from Chicago, see Stephen J. Shaw's essay, "The Cities and the Plains, A Home for God's People: A History of the Catholic Parish in the Midwest" in Jay P. Dolan, ed., *The American Catholic Parish: A History from 1850 to the Present*, vol. 2 (New York: Paulist Press, 1987), pp. 327–354.

17. Roger L. Treat, *Bishop Sheil and the CYO* (New York: Julian Messner Inc., 1951).

18. The best discussion of student life at St. Viator's is provided by John Tracy Ellis's delightful memoir, *Faith and Learning: A Church Historian's Story* (Lanham, Md.: University Press of America, 1989), pp. 3–10.

19. The no-hitter story is repeated in two articles in *Time* magazine, "Meat and a Bishop," July 24, 1939; "The Bishop's 25th," May 11, 1953. Robert Burns, an employee of the Sheil School, inspected the score books of the game and found the evidence that the so-called no-hitter had never happened. Interview with Robert Burns, January 4, 1988.

20. Edward A. Kantowicz, *Corporation Sole*, p. 180.

21. See ibid., pp. 152–153. Monsignor John S. Quinn, Sheil's successor at St. Andrew's parish, related the story about the appointment of Sheil. Interview with Monsignor Quinn, March 2, 1984.

22. Born in 1905, Campbell was a Chicago native, and the son of a successful woolen manufacturer. He was graduated from Augustinian-run St. Rita's High School and College on the South Side and later completed law studies at Loyola University, receiving his bachelor's degree in 1926; was admitted to the Illinois Bar in 1927; received his L.L.M. in 1928. He formed a partnership with fellow attorney William O. Burns.

23. For instance of this see correspondence in the Campbell papers dealing with rental agents, especially one Philip Peck regarding the Congress Street building, Campbell Papers, in Chicago Branch of National Archives (hereafter CBNA).

24. Martin Carrabine, S.J., to Campbell, November 9, 1937, Campbell Papers, RG 200, Box 2, November-December 1937, CBNA.

25. For Agnes Meyer's role in Sheil's career see Sanford Horwitt's life of Saul Alinsky, *Let Them Call Me Rebel* (New York: Alfred Knopf, 1989), pp. 179–180, 195–196.

26. Campbell to Aubrey Williams, November 26, 1937, Campbell Papers, RG 200, National Youth Administration, November–December 1937, CBNA.

27. "Exit Mr. Cummings," *Time*, November 28, 1938.

28. Campbell to Corcoran, November 13, 1937, Campbell Papers, RG 200, Box 2, NYA, November-December 1937, CBNA.

29. Roosevelt to Sheil, February 10, 1938, Presidential Personal File (hereafter PPF), 5177, Franklin D. Roosevelt Library (hereafter FDRL).

30. Franklin D. Roosevelt to Bernard J. Sheil, January 25, 1938, PPF, 5177, FDRL.`

31. "Mundelein Denies Views of Coughlin Represent Church," *New York Times*, December 12, 1938.

32. Memo, PPF, 5177, FDRL.

33. Sheil to Harry D. Wohl, February 23, 1939, Campbell Papers, RG 200, Box 1, "Attack During Newspaper Strike, 1939," CBNA.

34. Corcoran to Missy LeHand, July 24, 1939, PPF, 5177, FDRL.

35. Roosevelt to Honorable Frank Knox, October 4, 1939, Presidential Secretary File (hereafter PSF), "K," FDRL.

36. Harold Ickes, *The Lowering Clouds: The Secret Diary of Harold L. Ickes*, vol. 3 (New York: Simon and Schuster, 1955), pp. 63–64.

37. This memo is in the bound version of the Myron Taylor Correspondence, FDRL.

38. George Q. Flynn, *Roosevelt and Romanism* (Westport, Conn.: Greenwood Press, 1976), p. 117.

39. Hillenbrand to Uncle Henry, February 9 [no year], Hillenbrand Papers, Archives of the University of Notre Dame (hereafter AUND).

40. Hillenbrand to Parents, September 17, Hillenbrand Papers, AUND.

41. Ibid.

42. Hillenbrand to George [Hillenbrand], October 7, Hillenbrand Papers, AUND.

43. Hillenbrand Diary, Epiphany 1929, Hillenbrand Papers, AUND.

44. Hillenbrand Diary, February 22, 1929, Hillenbrand Papers, AUND.

45. Robert McClory, "Hillenbrand: U.S. Moses," *National Catholic Reporter*, September 7, 1979.

46. Hillenbrand Diary, February 29, 1929, Hillenbrand Papers, AUND.

47. "De Modo in quo Deo Justificatos Inhabitat," a copy of this is in the Feehan Library at St. Mary of the Lake Seminary. Robert Tuzik provides a concise discussion of the subject matter of Hillenbrand's dissertation in his dissertation "The Contribution of Msgr. Reynold

Hillenbrand (1905–1976) to the Liturgical Movement in the United States: Influences and Development" (Ph.D. diss., University of Notre Dame, 1989), pp. 28–29.

48. See Joseph J. Bluett, "Current Theology: The Mystical Body of Christ 1890–1940," *Theological Studies* 3 (June 1942): 261–262.

49. Letter of Monsignor Stanislaus Piwowar to author, October 23, 1987.

50. Letter of Monsignor George Higgins to author, October 29, 1982.

51. Roger Biles, *Big City Boss in Depression and War: Mayor Edward J. Kelly of Chicago* (DeKalb: Northern Illinois University Press, 1984), pp. 21–22.

52. Interview with Monsignor Daniel Cantwell, December 14, 1983.

53. "Homily Preached at the Eucharist Celebrating the Life and Passing of Monsignor Reynold Hillenbrand, Pastor Emeritus, Sacred Heart Church, Hubbard Woods, Ill. Monsignor Daniel M. Cantwell Pastor, St. Clotilde Church, Chicago, May 25, 1979." Author has copy.

54. Virgil Michel, "The Basis of Social Regeneration," *Orate Fratres* 9 (1935): 545.

55. The classic work on Virgil Michel is still Paul Marx's *Virgil Michel and the Liturgical Movement* (Collegeville, Minn.: Liturgical Press, 1957). More recently, R. W. Franklin and Robert L. Spaeth have written *Virgil Michel: American Catholic* (Collegeville, Minn.: Liturgical Press, 1988).

56. *Philosopher's Chronicle*, 1937–1938 [no pagination], Feehan Library, St. Mary of the Lake Seminary.

57. Hillenbrand to Haas, January 21, 1938, quoted in Dennis Robb, "Specialized Catholic Action in the United States, 1936–1949: Ideology, Leadership, and Organization" (Ph.D. diss., University of Minnesota, 1972), p. 52.

58. *Summer School of Catholic Action for the Clergy Conducted at St. Francis Seminary, St. Francis, Wisconsin, July 5–30, 1937*, 4 vols., Salzmann Library, St. Francis Seminary, Milwaukee, Wisconsin.

59. "Cathedral Sermons on Labor Arouse Widespread Interest," *New World*, April 1, 1938.

60. "Noted Speakers on Economics at the Cathedral," *New World*, March 18, 1938.

61. Barbara Warne Newell, *Chicago and the Labor Movement* (Urbana: University of Illinois Press, 1961).

62. "Eleven Catholic Labor Schools Open Sessions" *New World*, November 1, 1940.

63. John M. Hayes, "Work of the Priest," *Proceedings of Summer School of Social Action for Priests* (Mundelein, Ill.: St. Mary of the Lake Seminary, 1938), vol. 4, p. 499.

64. Rev. Donald J. Kanaly, "The J.O.C.," in ibid., p. 424.

65. Letter of Monsignor Donald Kanaly to author, October 6, 1985.

66. Christopher J. Kauffmann, *Faith and Fraternalism: The History of the Knights of Columbus, 1882–1982* (New York: Harper and Row, 1982), p. 336.

67. John M. Huels, O.S.M., "Popular Appeal of the Sorrowful Mother Novena" (Rome: Edizioni Marianum, 1976).

2. CHICAGO IN WAR AND COLD WAR

1. "Enthronement Address of Archbishop Stritch at Cathedral Thursday," *New World*, March 15, 1940.

2. See James C. Schneider, *Should America Go to War? The Debate over Foreign Policy in Chicago, 1939–1941* (Chapel Hill: University of North Carolina Press, 1989).

3. Edward Kantowicz, *Corporation Sole: Cardinal Mundelein and Chicago Catholicism* (Notre Dame, Ind.: University of Notre Dame Press, 1983), p. 234.

4. Harold Ickes, *The Lowering Clouds: The Secret Diary of Harold Ickes*, vol. 3 (New York: Simon and Schuster, 1955): 110.

5. This was a comment Roosevelt made to Myron Taylor, quoted in Gerald Fogarty, S.J., *The Vatican and the American Hierarchy from 1870 to 1865* (Wilmington, Del.: Michael Glazier, 1985), p. 263.

6. See my "Samuel Stritch and Milwaukee Catholicism, 1930–1940," *Milwaukee History* 13 (Autumn 1990): 70–91.

7. "No Official Stand on Neutrality Statement," *Catholic Herald Citizen*, September 23, 1939.

8. Spellman to Roosevelt, February 5, 1940, PSF, FDRL.

9. Ibid.

10. Stritch to Spellman, January 20, 1940, PSF, FDRL.

11. Ibid.

12. Roosevelt to Spellman, February 13, 1940, PSF, FDRL.

13. Dan Herr, "Samuel Cardinal Stritch: Prince Among Men," *Sign*, January 1957, pp. 11–15; 75–77.

14. Stritch to Bishop John B. Morris, Box 2941, Chancery Files, Stritch Papers, AAC.

15. Stritch to Earl Southard, December 4, 1940, Box 2941, Chancery Files, Stritch Papers, AAC.

16. Stritch to Monsignor William F. Cahill [no date], Box 2941, Chancery Files, Stritch Papers, AAC.

17. George Casey to Thomas J. Coffey, O.M.I., September 8, 1941, Box 2941, Chancery Files, Stritch Papers, AAC.

18. Stritch to John B. Morris, December 3, 1941, Chancery Files, Stritch Papers, AAC.

19. Stritch to Archbishop John J. Cantwell, August 30, 1941, Chancery Files, Stritch Papers, AAC.

20. Stritch to McNicholas, October 28, 1942, Box 2942, Chancery Files, Stritch Papers, AAC.

21. Stritch to John F. Noll, April 20, 1942, Box 2949, Chancery Files, Stritch Papers, AAC.

22. "War Message Text," Box 2945, Chancery Files, Stritch Papers, AAC.

23. Harold M. Mayer and Richard C. Wade, *Chicago: Growth of a Metropolis* (Chicago: University of Chicago Press, 1969), pp. 368–370.

24. "Hey Soldier! Fall in at the C.Y.O. Saturdays—On the House," *New World*, March 28, 1941.

25. "Open New NCCS Center in Chicago," *New World*, August 29, 1941.

26. Stritch to M. J. Ready, July 30, 1941, Chancery Files, Stritch Papers, AAC.

27. "USO Sign Goes Up on NCCS Club," *New World*, May 8, 1942.

28. This protest was made in the context of a general protest to the president and Secretary of War Henry Stimson by the Administrative Board of the NCWC. Archbishop Edward Mooney of Detroit, the chairman that year, had written the letters to Stimson and Secretary of the Navy Frank Knox but had received negative replies. In the September 1943 meeting of the board the suggestion was made that Stritch "make a personal suggestion to the Secretary of the Navy, Mr. Knox, that he withdraw the objectionable statements in his letter...." This correspondence and suggestion are found in the minutes of the September 28, 1943, meeting of the Administrative Board, National Catholic Welfare Conference Papers.

29. "St. Peter Canisius" in Harry S. Koenig, *A History of the Parishes of the Archdiocese of Chicago*, vol. 1 (Chicago: Catholic Bishop of Chicago, 1980), p. 776.

30. "Survey of Catholic War Activities in the Archdiocese of Chicago," 1943, Box 2953, Chancery Files, Stritch Papers, AAC.

31. "Chicago Catholic Women Join Plan for Defense Activities," *New World*, April 11, 1941; "Polish Relief Organizations Busy in 130 Chicago Units," *New World*, April 10, 1942.

32. "Chicagoans Attend First Field Mass at Camp Forrest on Easter Sunday," *New World*, April 18, 1941.

33. "St. Camillus" in Koenig, *A History of the Parishes of the Archdiocese of Chicago*, vol. 1, p. 164. This Mass was popular until the sixties.

34. John M. Huels, *The Saturday Night Novena* (Rome: Edizione Marianum, 1976).

35. "Survey of Catholic War Activities," Stritch Papers, AAC.

36. See Reports of the Superintendent, 1942–1944, Education Department, AAC.

37. Stritch to Harry C. Rynard, December 2, 1942, Chancery Files, Stritch Papers, AAC.

38. At the November 1939 meeting that had elected Stritch chairman of the Administrative Board of the National Catholic Welfare Conference, the bishops had adopted a resolution seeking to preserve the exempt status of priests, seminarians, and religious in the event that national preparedness required enactment of a conscription law. The expected bill (known as the Burke-Wadsworth Bill) was introduced after the fall of France in June 1940, with separate versions introduced in the House and the Senate. It immediately renewed isolationist fears that this was one more administration ploy to bring the United States into war. The bishops were drawn into the debate not only because of their divided opinions on the Roosevelt preparedness policies, but also, as the Legal Affairs Department of the NCWC pointed out, because the new legislation lacked the exemptions for seminarians and male religious that had been part of the 1917 conscription act. The possibility that seminarians and religious brothers could be drafted led Stritch to convene a special meeting of the Administrative Board at the Drake Hotel in Chicago on July 4.

Although many bishops and a number of Catholic editors urged outright opposition to the bill, Stritch urged the Administrative Board to completely sidestep the issue of whether to have conscription or not, insisting on complete neutrality in this issue. If there was to be a conscription law, they wanted certain exemptions. The board drafted a position paper to Secretary of War Henry Stimson requesting the exemptions of seminarians and religious brothers, and for the remainder of the summer Stritch sent letters to all bishops urging them to press their congressmen and senators to vote for the proposed exemptions. Stritch himself wrote to President Roosevelt in the name of the bishops: "Any consideration of national defense provisions includes a strengthening of those spiritual forces, without which liberty cannot

be sustained.... We beg that in the consideration of the measures necessary for national defense, there be no thought of weakening the agencies of religion." Beginning almost immediately after the July 4 meeting, Monsignor Michael Ready, the secretary of the NCWC, served as the bishops' chief lobbyist in pressing the exemptions on important senators and congressmen.

In late August, Roosevelt finally replied to Stritch's letter of mid-July. In a response drafted by Stimson, the president accepted exemptions for priests and divinity students but seemed unwilling to bend on the issue of religious brothers. Ultimately, the coordinated letter-writing campaign paid off. Roosevelt and Stimson's reservations notwithstanding, Congressman John McCormack proposed an amendment that provided the necessary exemptions for seminarians, priests, and brothers. In the Senate, Edwin C. Johnston of Colorado introduced an amendment to the bill which exempted priests and students preparing for the ministry. By September the reconciled version was passed and signed by Roosevelt. Although brothers were not formally included in the legislation, a rule of the Selective Service System in 1941 formally designated them as Ministers of Religion, thereby exempting them.

39. Edward Burke to Donald M. Carroll, March 18, 1943, Chancery Files, Stritch Papers, AAC.

40. Donald F. Kelly to Stritch, June 25, 1943, Chancery Files, Stritch Papers, AAC.

41. Stritch to Donald Kelly, June 29, 1942, Chancery Files, Stritch Papers, AAC.

42. Francis A. West to Stritch, July 7, 1944, Chancery Files, Stritch Papers, AAC.

43. Joseph M. Lynch to Stritch (no date), Chancery Files, Stritch Papers, AAC.

44. Stritch to Edward M. Flannery, August 3, 1943, Chancery Files, Stritch Papers, AAC.

45. Bernard E. Burns to Stritch, August 2, 1944, Chancery Files, Stritch Papers, AAC.

46. Stritch to Lawrence Keating, July 18, 1942, Chancery Files, Stritch Papers, AAC.

47. Albert J. Buckley to Stritch, January 8, 1943, Chancery Files, Stritch Papers, AAC.

48. Bernard E. Burns to Stritch, August 2, 1944, Chancery Files, Stritch Papers, AAC.

49. Arthur E. Douaire to Stritch, February 12, 1945, Box 2967, Chancery Files, Stritch Papers, AAC.

50. Bernard E. Burns to Stritch, August 2, 1944, Chancery Files, Stritch Papers, AAC.

51. Edward R. Kantowicz, "Polish Chicago: Survival Through Solidarity" in Peter d'A. Jones and Melvin G. Holli, *The Ethnic Frontier* (Grand Rapids: Eerdmans, 1977), pp. 180–209.

52. Earl Boyea, "The National Catholic Welfare Conference: An Experience in Episcopal Leadership, 1935–1945" (Ph.D. diss., The Catholic University of America, 1987), pp. 376–381.

53. Stritch to Howard Carroll, December 17, 1945, Box 2967, Chancery Files, Stritch Papers, AAC.

54. Stritch to E. Dzierwa, March 24, 1941, Box 2942, Chancery Files, Stritch Papers, AAC.

55. Interview with Bishop Aloysius Wycislo, July 14, 1988.

56. "Essentials of a Good Peace," Statement of the Administrative Board of the NCWC, November 11, 1943, in Raphael M. Huber, ed., *Our Bishops Speak* (Milwaukee: Bruce Publishing, 1952), p. 116.

57. "Papal Peace Guide," *New World*, June 18, 1943.

58. Ready to Stritch, October 27, 1943, Box 2956, Chancery Files, Stritch Papers, AAC.

59. Guido Gonella, *A World to Reconstruct: Pius XII on Peace and Reconstruction* (Milwaukee: Bruce Publishing Co., 1944), trans. T. Lincoln Bouscaren, S.J., p. v.

60. Perhaps the single most important instance of this was Truman's warmth toward former President Herbert Hoover and his appointment of the once scorned Republican to a committee to study the organization of the executive branch.

61. Stritch to Harry S Truman, PPF, Harry S Truman Library (hereafter HSTL).

62. "John Fitzgerald Memoir."

63. Truman to Sheil, April 19, 1954, Post Presidential File, HSTL.

64. "Gael E. Sullivan Is Dead at 51; Started Helicopter Mail Service," *New York Times*, October 28, 1956.

65. Gael Sullivan to Stritch, January 6, 1943, Box 2958, Chancery Files, AAC. Stritch to Sullivan, January 15, 1943, ibid.

66. Stritch to J. Edgar Hoover, December 13, 1937, Document 94-4-1411-1, Section 1, Serial 1-38, Subject File, Federal Bureau of Investigation Records,

67. Stritch to Tamm, December 27, 1945, Chancery Files, Stritch Papers, Box 2968, AAC. Tamm was unable to prevent the closure of the hospital. Cf. Tamm to Hunt, January 4, 1946, (copy) Chancery Files, Box 2968, Stritch Papers, AAC.

68. Tamm to Stritch, January 4, 1946, Chancery Files, Box 2968, Stritch Papers, AAC.

69. Tamm to Stritch, July 12, 1946, Chancery Files, Box 2968, Stritch Papers, AAC.

70. Stritch to McNicholas, no date 1947, McNicholas to Stritch, November 6, 1947, McNicholas Papers, Archives of the Archdiocese of Cincinnati [hereafter AACin].

71. Tamm to Stritch, February 3, 1948, Chancery Files, Box 2968, Stritch Papers, AAC.

72. Tamm to Stritch, June 21, 1948, Chancery Files, Box 2968, Stritch Papers, AAC.

73. Memorandum for Mr. Tolson, Mr. Nichols, March 16, 1951, Document 94-1-1085-16, FBI Files.

74. Stritch to Alter, April 9, 1946, Alter Papers, Archives of the Diocese of Toledo (hereafter ADT).

75. Stritch to Casey, March 27, 1946, Box 2971, Chancery Files, Stritch Papers, AAC.

76. Casey to Edward J. Kelly, March 29, 1946, Box 2971, Chancery Files, Stritch Papers, AAC.

77. Truman to Stritch April 25, 1946, Box 2975, Chancery Files, AAC. Stritch to Truman, May 10, 1946, Box 2975, Chancery Files, AAC. At this meeting with Truman, Stritch also discussed the plight of Polish Refugees at a camp in Guanajuato, Mexico. He won Truman's assurances here that American funds would continue to flow to the Mexican camp despite the cessation of hostilities. See Truman to Stritch, April 30, 1946, Box 2975, Chancery Files, AAC.

78. "Biographical No. 126, Samuel Cardinal Stritch," NCWC News Service Files, March 3, 1958, Archives of the Catholic University of America (hereafter ACUA).

79. O'Grady played an important role in Chicago affairs during these years. For a complete biography see Thomas Tifft's "Toward a More Humane Social Policy: The Work and Influence of Monsignor John O'Grady" (Ph.D. diss., Catholic University of America, 1979).

80. Stritch to O'Grady, October 10, 1952, Chancery Files, Stritch Papers, AAC.

81. Stritch to Spellman, May 6, 1953, Chancery Files, Stritch Papers, AAC.

82. Stritch to Thomas L. Noa, December 2, 1949, Chancery Files, Box 2994, Stritch Papers, AAC.

83. Stritch to Ready, January 16, 1937, Ready Papers, Archives of the NCWC.

84. "Confidential Questionnaire on Communism" [no date], Chancery Files, Box 2996, Stritch Papers, AAC.

85. Higgins to Mooney, May 12, 1953, Mooney Papers, Archives of the Archdiocese of Detroit.

86. Stritch to Alter, July 16, 1945, Alter Papers, ADT.

87. Thomas Stritch to author.

88. "Hinsdale Pastor Announces Weekly Prayers for Peace," *New World*, December 29, 1950.

89. "Readers of The New World Rise to Attack, Defend Father Gillis," *New World*, July 17, 1953.

3. RIDING THE WHIRLWIND

1. "Broadcast for V-E Day," Box 2967, Chancery Files, Stritch Papers, AAC.

2. *Annals*, Dominican Sisters of Visitation Convent, Chicago, Archives of the Dominican Sisters of Sinsinawa Mound.

3. Stritch to Mother Mary Samuel, O.P., October 31, 1945, Box 2966, Chancery Files, Stritch Papers, AAC.

4. "Report on Archdiocesan Debt Structure," Chancery Files, Stritch Papers, AAC.

5. Interview with Monsignor James Hardiman, June 28, 1988.

6. Stritch to McNicholas, March 11, 1944, Archives of the Archdiocese of Cincinnati (hereafter AACin).

7. George Casey to Sister M. Gerald, O.P., January 9, 1943, Box 2954, Chancery Files, Stritch Papers, AAC.

8. Muench Diary, p. 76, Muench Papers, ACUA.

9. Memo, Casey to Stritch [undated but in 1943 file], Box 2953, Chancery Files, Stritch Papers, AAC.

10. For facts on parish formation in the earliest years of Chicago Catholicism see Charles Shanabruch, *Chicago's Catholics: The Evolution of an American Identity* (Notre Dame, Ind.: University of Notre Dame Press, 1981). Cardinal Mundelein was also a parish founder; see Kantowicz, *Corporation Sole*.

11. Stritch to Edward Saunders, October 15, 1952, Chancery Files, Stritch Papers, AAC.

12. *Residential Construction and Related Data*, Office of Housing and Redevelopment, 1954, copy in Chancery Files, Stritch Papers, AAC.

13. Much of this will be covered in chapters 6 and 7. And see Arnold Hirsch, *Making the Second Ghetto* (New York: Cambridge University Press, 1983), for a thorough treatment of the process of racial succession.

14. Interview with Harold Mayer, April 10, 1989.

15. Kenneth Jackson, *Crabgrass Frontier: The Suburbanization of the United States* (New York: Oxford University Press, 1984), pp. 190–219.

16. "St. George, Tinley Park," in Harry S. Koenig, *History of the Parishes of the Archdiocese of Chicago* (Chicago: Catholic Bishop, 1980), vol. 2, pp. 1559–1563.

17. By 1946, Catholic families were moving to the southwestern boundaries of the city, resulting in the establishment of St. Helena of the Cross in Fernwood and St. Thomas More in the Wrightwood neighborhood. Of the formation of St. Thomas More, the parish historian wrote a line that was often repeated in describing the formation of new parishes in this period: "single family dwellings were constructed on the prairies west of Western Avenue ... the majority of the newcomers had moved out of older neighborhoods on the south side of the city." A mix and match congery of parishes reflected the changing population patterns of the south and southwestern sides of the city. On the fringes, new parishes like St. Daniel the Prophet (Archer and Nashville), St. Mary, Star of the Sea (south of Fifty-ninth St. and west of Pulaski Road), and St. John Fisher (South Washtenaw). The northwest quadrant of St. John Fisher jutted into the rapidly expanding suburb of Evergreen Park, where St. Bernadette Parish would open. In nearby Chicago Ridge, Father William Gentleman, a former assistant to Bishop Sheil, assumed the direction of the Mission of Our Lady of the Ridge in 1948 after its elevation to parochial status. The same occurred in nearby Hazel Crest when the expansion of the Catholic population made St. Anne's Mission a parish in its own right in 1949.

18. Koenig, "St. Irenaeus," in *History of the Parishes*, vol. 2, pp. 1464–1468.

19. Michael Ebner, *Creating Chicago's Northshore* (Chicago: University of Chicago Press, 1988) is the best text to consult in studying this region.

20. Samuel Cardinal Stritch, *The Church and Neighborhood Conservation*, pamphlet, copy in Stritch Papers, AAC.

21. The graphs at the end of this chapter chart at five-year intervals the growth of Catholic life in Chicago in several vital areas.

22. Andrew Greeley, "The Catholic Suburbanite," *Sign* 37 (February 1958): 30–32.

23. Andrew Greeley, *The Church in the Suburbs* (New York: Sheed and Ward, 1959), p. 189.

24. Neil P. Hurley, "The Church in Suburbia," *America* 98 (November 16, 1957): 194–199.

25. Paul Brindel, "A Pox on Suburbia," *Voice of St. Jude* 22 (April 1957): 6–10.

26. Gibson Winter, "The Church in Suburban Captivity," *Christian Century* 72 (September 28, 1955): 1110–1112. He elaborated further

on these themes in his book *The Suburban Captivity of the Churches* (Garden City, N.Y.: Doubleday, 1961).

27. "Archdiocesan Conservation Council Report, 1962," Meyer Papers, AAC.

28. "Million More Catholics Here by 1985," *New World*, October 19, 1962.

29. Stritch to Rev. Austin G. Schmidt, S.J., August 5, 1942, Box 2951, Chancery File, Stritch Papers, AAC.

30. Stritch to Rev. Joseph D. Connerton, November 14, 1953, Chancery Files, Stritch Papers, AAC.

31. Stritch to Cicognani, September 12, 1953, Stritch Papers, AAC.

32. Increasingly under the control of conservative cardinals like Alfredo Ottaviani, the Roman Curia had begun to crack down in inter-creedal cooperation of any kind and had issued a strong warning against such activity in August 1953 in the wake of the "scandal" of Catholic observers at the World Council of Churches Conference on Faith and Order at Lund, Sweden, in 1952.

33. Stritch to Rev. R. C. Hartnett, S.J., June 5, 1954, Stritch Papers, AAC.

34. Pastoral Letter of His Eminence Samuel Cardinal Stritch, Archbishop of Chicago, Feast of Saints Peter and Paul (copy in Stritch Papers, AAC).

35. Francis J. Connell to Stritch, July 5, 1954, Stritch Papers, AAC.

36. "The Gulf," *Christian Century* 71 (July 21, 1954): 869–871.

37. Stritch to Sister Mary of the Passion, August 13, 1954, Stritch, Papers, AAC.

38. Stritch to Rev. Charles Boyer, S.J., August 31, 1954, Stritch Papers, AAC.

39. Stritch to McNicholas, March 11, 1944, McNicholas Papers, AACin.

40. James Sanders, *The Education of an Urban Minority* (New York: Oxford University Press, 1977), p. 189.

41. Ibid., p. 190.

42. The most comprehensive study of Catholic high schools in Chicago during this period is George Fornero's doctoral dissertation, "The Expansion and Decline of Enrollment and Facilities of Secondary Schools in the Archdiocese of Chicago, 1955–1980: A Historical Study" (Ed.D. diss., Loyola University, 1990).

43. Stritch to Henry Althoff, August 14, 1944, Box 2826, Chancery File, Stritch Papers, AAC.

44. Stritch to Rev. Edward Brueggeman, S.J., December 7, 1954, Box 2833, Stritch Papers, AAC.

45. Stritch to Henry Althoff, August 14, 1944, Box 2826, Stritch Papers, AAC.

46. Ibid.

47. Stritch to Robert F. Trisco, April 12, 1955, Stritch Papers, AAC.

48. Stritch was instrumental in pushing a released time provision through the Illinois legislature.

49. Alice O'Rourke, O.P., *Let Us Set Out: Sinsinawa Dominicans, 1949–1985* (Sinsinawa: Sisters of St. Dominic, 1986), p. 30.

50. "Choose Chicago Heights for Regional High School," *New World*, July 29, 1949. Stritch to "Dearly Beloved in Christ," September 7, 1949, Box 2990, Stritch Papers, AAC.

51. "Marian Catholic High School, Chicago Heights" in Harry S. Koenig, ed., *Caritas Christi Urget Nos: A History of the Offices, Agencies, and Institutions of the Archdiocese of Chicago*, vol. 1 (Chicago: Catholic Bishop of Chicago, 1981), pp. 510–514.

52. "Suggestions for Financing of Proposed Catholic High Schools," memorandum [no date], Chancery Files, Stritch Papers, AAC.

53. One example was Monsignor Francis Lavin of St. James, who could only contribute $2,000. Stritch wrote him "I know full well the difficulties which you face and I want you to know I don't expect the unreasonable or impossible." Stritch to Lavin, March 25, 1958, Stritch Papers, AAC. Other pastors of suburban areas having young families and heavy mortgages could not make the assessment as well.

54. Interview with Bishop William E. McManus, October 28, 1988.

55. McManus to Stritch, January 3, 1944, Box 2961, Chancery Files, Stritch Papers, AAC.

56. McManus to Stritch, October 1, 1945, Box 2966, Chancery Files, Stritch Papers, AAC.

57. Typical of McManus's outspoken behavior was an incident at a 1952 press conference for Catholic college presidents. During the course of the dialogue he impulsively interjected his opinion that Senator Joseph McCarthy was a menace to higher education. This rebuke of McCarthy won him instant headlines and grumblings from bishops who supported the Wisconsin Catholic Senator. McManus later claimed that he escaped censure because Stritch felt the same way about McCarthy. McManus interview.

58. Stritch also coordinated Catholic opposition to the Barden Bill, a federal education bill introduced in Congress in 1948 which apportioned aid in proportion to the total number of pupils in a

district. What made the bill controversial and offensive to Catholics was a provision to count Catholic schoolchildren in calculating the total amount of aid to be given to states, but then to exclude them from any of the benefits, due to the separation of church and state. For many years the bishops of the United States had opposed federal aid to education for fear of establishing too much governmental control over what they deemed a parental right. In the forties the Education Department of the NCWC modified its rigid opposition in view of the fact that many school districts in poorer areas of the nation had an insufficient tax base to sustain a decent elementary and secondary school system. The Catholic position, argued vigorously by Father McManus of the Education Department of the NCWC as well as the conference's Legal Department, insisted that, if federal aid were to be given, it should be given on a per-child basis irrespective of the school attended. This would have made it possible for Catholic schoolchildren to share in the benefits that they were being counted for. In Chicago, Stritch mounted a campaign against the Barden Bill through the *New World* and personal intercession with local congressmen and senators. See "Federal Aid to Education," Statement by Rev. William E. McManus, Assistant Director, Department of Education, National Catholic Welfare Conference before Subcommittee on Education of the Senate Committee on Labor and Public Welfare, April 25, 1947. Copy in the Mooney Papers, Archives of the Archdiocese of Detroit. Stritch to Rev. Edward V. Dailey, July 2, 1949, Chancery Files, Stritch Papers, AAC. One congressman who voted against the Barden Bill at Stritch's urging was Congressman Sidney Yates of the 9th Congressional District. See Stritch to Yates, July 21, 1949, Box 2996, Chancery Files, Stritch Papers, AAC.

The McCollum case, a complaint by an Illinois resident, Mrs. Vashti McCollum, protesting the use of public school facilities for released-time provisions. Although the principle of released-time had been upheld in the Everson case, some bishops were fearful that the McCollum matter might call its constitutionality into doubt and thereby cripple religious education programs. Stritch and archdiocesan attorneys as well as the legal and education departments of the NCWC worked hard to prevent just such an occurrence and were successful. Although released-time programs at public schools were banned, the principle of released time was not abandoned. This was further upheld in the 1952 Zorach case. For Stritch's role in coordinating the McCollom defense see Alter to Stritch, February 14, 1947, Alter Papers, ADT; Stritch to Alter, February 22, 1947, Alter Papers, ADT.

On these matters see also Harold A. Buetow, *Of Singular Benefit: The Story of U.S. Catholic Education* (New York: Macmillian, 1970), pp. 267–276.

59. Stritch to McManus, April 16, 1957, Stritch Papers, AAC.

60. The following material is taken from my doctoral dissertation, "Meyer of Milwaukee: The Life and Times of a Midwestern Archbishop" (University of Notre Dame, 1985).

61. McManus to author.

62. This was St. Rosalie parish in Harwood Heights. A school was eventually built.

63. "Children and Nuns Victims in Chicago as Flames Race through Grammar School," *New York Times*, December 2, 1958.

64. "Archbishop's Statement," *New World*, December 5, 1958.

65. This was related to me by Monsignor Jack Egan, who was in residence at Our Lady of the Angels rectory at the time of the fire and was a participant in the funeral ceremonies.

66. Meyer to "Reverend and dear Father," January 23, 1959, Meyer Papers, AAC. "Installation of Sprinklers to Be Finished in August," *New World*, April 28, 1961.

67. My efforts to interview the priests who worked at the parish during this tragic episode were unsuccessful. One of them wrote that he had no desire to relive the memories which were among the most painful of his life. Unsubstantiated rumors still circulate that the person who started the fire has confessed, but no names have been mentioned and the official materials in the Archives of the Archdiocese of Chicago are closed to researchers.

68. McManus interview.

69. Kantowicz, *Corporation Sole*, pp. 159–161.

70. Interview with Bishop Cletus F. O'Donnell, September 6, 1983.

71. Interview with Rev. Francis McElligott, December 10, 1983.

72. Sheil's defenders insist that the press first referred to him as "senior auxiliary." However, Sheil never publicly disavowed the use of the term.

73. This was related to me by Casey's closest clerical friend, Monsignor Donald Masterson. Interview with Masterson, September 6, 1983.

74. The reality of divided loyalties among the priests was confirmed by virtually everyone who had close contact with Casey and Burke. For example, John Egan and William Quinn were known as "Burke Men" while Cletus O'Donnell and Donald Masterson were clearly beholden to Casey.

75. Interview with Monsignor John S. Quinn, March 2, 1984; Interview with Bishop Cletus F. O'Donnell.

76. Burke to Meyer, December 26, 1960, Meyer Papers, AAC.

77. "Six Pastors Appointed; Msgr. Edward M. Burke to St. Bartholomew's," *New World*, October 20, 1961.

78. Klupar's report is a validation of James O'Toole's observation that the administrative reforms of consolidating bishops, such as William Henry O'Connell in Boston, were never as thoroughgoing and efficient as once supposed. In Chicago, it was clear by the Meyer era that the reforms of Cardinal Mundelein, the prince of consolidating bishops, were seriously out of date. See James M. O'Toole, "The Role of Bishops in American Catholic History: Myth and Reality in the Case of Cardinal William O'Connell," *Catholic Historical Review* 72 (October 1991): 595–615.

79. Meyer to William G. Simpson, January 2, 1964, Meyer Papers, AAC.

80. Memorandum of William G. Simpson to Meyer, May 8, 1964, Meyer Papers, AAC.

81. *Minutes of Meeting with Stein, Roe and Farnham*, September 30, 1963, Meyer Papers, AAC.

82. Bishop Cletus O'Donnell to author.

83. O'Donnell to Meyer, October 9, 1963, Meyer Papers, AAC.

4. BISHOP SHEIL AND CHICAGO CATHOLICISM

1. Edward Kantowicz, *Corporation Sole: Cardinal Mundelein and Chicago Catholicism* (Notre Dame, Ind.: University of Notre Dame Press, 1983), p. 173.

2. Stritch to Cicognani, November 23, 1940, Box 2831, Chancery Files, Stritch Papers, AAC.

3. Sheil to Stritch, February 19, 1941, Box 2945, Chancery Files, Stritch Papers, AAC.

4. Stritch to Sheil, February 26, 1941, Box 2945, Chancery Files, Stritch Papers, AAC.

5. Campbell to John O'Grady, June 16, 1936, O'Grady Papers, ACUA.

6. Stritch to Ready, December 18, 1939, Ready Papers, ANCWC.

7. Stritch's role in blocking the promotion of Sheil was revealed in a letter to Cardinal Meyer from a Vatican official when Sheil arranged to have himself created an honorary archbishop. In noting Sheil's request, the official stated: "The Secretariate of State is aware of the remarks submitted by your eminent predecessor when there was a question of appointing Bishop Sheil to a residential See. The present instance, however, is one of a merely honorary title which would not

carry with it any additional authority or jurisdiction...." See Achille Lupi to Meyer, April 22, 1959, Meyer Papers, AAC.

8. Memorandum of Ralph C. Leo, 1942, George Drury Papers, in possession of the author.

9. Concern for democratic ideology was a popular theme in the World War II period. See Philip Gleason, "Americans All: World War II and the Shaping of American Ideology," *Review of Politics* 43 (October 1981): 483–518.

10. "Name New CYO Education Director," *New World*, October 17, 1941.

11. Taped interviews with George Drury, December 1987–January 1988.

12. Catherine De Hueck, "Educational Department Catholic Youth Organization Plan of the New Organization," manuscript copy in papers of Florence Weinfurter, in possession of the author.

13. Drury interview.

14. "Rev. James A. Magner Gives Forum Talk," *New World*, March 22, 1940.

15. "Dr. Adler Speaker at Mercy Forum," *New World*, February 16, 1940.

16. An example of this comparison to labor schools is found in "Teaching the Workers," *Commonweal* 37 (February 26, 1943): 478.

17. "Sheil School Opens Doors," *New World*, January 22, 1943.

18. Ibid.

19. "Benet Library Founder Observes 80th Birthday," *New World*, March 25, 1949.

20. Announcement of Courses, First Term 1943–1944, Sheil School of Social Studies, Drury Papers, in possession of author.

21. Mary Elizabeth Carroll, "Bishop Sheil: Prophet without Honor," *Harpers* 211 (November 1955): 45–51.

22. "Education for Democracy," Address of His Excellency, The Most Reverend Bernard J. Sheil, D.D., Founder, Director, C.Y.O. to the Sheil School Forum, November 19, 1943, Sheil Papers, AAC.

23. *Bulletin*, Sheil School of Social Studies, First Term 1943–1944, Drury Papers.

24. "Open Church Art Course," *New World*, July 9, 1943.

25. "Action the Epiphany of Being" [undated talk], Drury Papers.

26. James O'Gara, "Chicago's 'Catholic Times Square,'" *America* 82 (January 28, 1950): 492–495.

27. "On Bishop Sheil," *Commonweal* 51 (March 3, 1950): 558.

28. "Church Must Battle for Negro Rights, Bishop Sheil tells Catholic Convention," clipping, *Chicago Sun*, September 29, 1942,

Cantwell Papers, Box 28, Folder 28-9, Chicago Historical Society (hereafter CHS).

29. "To the Negro," *Time*, February 22, 1943, clipping, Cantwell Papers, Box 28, Folder 28-9, CHS.

30. "Bishop Sheil's Speech," *Chicago Defender*, 1942, clipping, Cantwell Papers, Box 28, Folder 28-9, CHS.

31. "Jim Crowism and the Catholic Church," *Chicago Defender*, March 1943, clipping, Cantwell Papers, Box 28, Folder 28–9, CHS.

32. Interview with Dora Somerville, March 15, 1989.

33. "Restrictive Covenants vs Brotherhood," Address delivered by the Senior Auxiliary Bishop of Chicago on May 11, 1946, for the Chicago Council Against Racial Discrimination, *Catholic Mind* 44 (December 1946): 713–717.

34. He also pressed, without success, for an FEPC in Illinois, a position opposed by Cardinal Stritch.

35. "Jewish Gift to the Pope," Address by His Excellency, The Most Reverend Bernard J. Sheil, D.D., Auxiliary Bishop of Chicago on January 2, 1940, Sheil Papers, AAC. Interestingly enough, the group had raised $125,000 for the pontiff and had given it to Sheil. Sheil only conveyed $75,000 of this gift to the Holy See. What happened to the rest is unknown. See Stritch to Cicognani, May 5, 1942, Box 2946, Chancery Files, Stritch Papers, AAC.

36. "Address Delivered by the Most Reverend Bernard J. Sheil, D.D., Auxiliary Bishop of Chicago and Founder-Director of the Catholic Youth Organization before Meeting of Temple Sholom in the Standard Club, Chicago, Illinois, on October 21, 1942," Sheil Papers, AAC.

37. "Lawyers' Decalogue Society Gives Award to Bishop Sheil," *New World*, March 5, 1948.

38. "Sheil Receives B'nai B'rith Award," *New York Times*, July 13, 1951.

39. Campbell to Keeshin, December 28, 1956, Campbell Papers, RG 200, Box 9, Correspondence 1956, CBNA.

40. Among the programs Sheil inaugurated in this new phase of CYO activity included community recreation centers, counseling and guidance clinics, commercial skills training centers, seeing-eye dog schools and special programs for Japanese, Puerto Ricans, and blacks. By the time the CYO empire was dissolved in 1954, there were six departments employing ninety-five full-time staffers.

41. See Alden V. Brown, *The Grail* (Notre Dame, Ind.: University of Notre Dame Press, 1989).

42. Interview with Anna May Smith, October 15, 1989, Chicago, Illinois.

43. I am indebted to Father Mark Sorvillo for this insight.

44. George Drury to the author. Taped interview, September 1987.

45. Drury interview.

46. Haston once commented to Robert Burns, who plumped for a new program for the organization: "It may be fine Bob, but where am I going to find the goddamned money!" Interview with Robert Burns, former CYO staffer, January 4, 1988.

47. Burns interview.

48. Drury interview.

49. "Join the Union," May 15, 1946. A copy of this circular was given to me by Nina Polycn Moore.

50. Sheil to Cantwell, March 14, 1946, Cantwell Papers, Box 1, Folder 1-6, CHS.

51. Daniel Cantwell to Sheil, June 1, 1946, Cantwell Papers, Box 1, Folder 1-6, CHS.

52. Charles C. Smith to Cantwell, July 17, 1946, Cantwell Papers, Box 1, Folder 1-6, CHS.

53. Charles C. Smith to Daniel M. Cantwell, July 17, 1946, Cantwell Papers, Box 1, Folder 1-6, CHS.

54. Cantwell to Sheil, July 19, 1946, Cantwell Papers, Box 1, Folder 1-6, CHS.

55. Interview with Father Cornelius McGillicuddy, November 27, 1987.

56. Burns interview.

57. Ibid.

58. Nina Polcyn to George Drury, postcard [no date], Drury Papers.

59. Interview with Dr. Edward Gargan, January 4, 1988.

60. Burns interview.

61. "Why Bishop Sheil Left the CYO," *Chicago Daily News*, January 24, 1955.

62. Quinn interview.

63. Drury interview.

64. Anna May Smith interview.

65. Interview with Judge Abraham Lincoln Marovitz, June 21, 1989.

66. WFJL had problems paying for records from the K. O. Asher Wholesale Distribution Company. See K. O. Asher to George C. Casey, January 6, 1951, Box 3004, Chancery Files, Stritch Papers, AAC.

67. Stritch to Sheil, May 10, 1949, Box 2995, Chancery Files, Stritch Papers, AAC.

68. Stritch to Sheil, February 12, 1951, Box 3008, Chancery Files, Stritch Papers, AAC.

69. Quinn interview.

70. Drury interview.

71. J. Francis McIntyre to Sheil, October 18, 1945, copy in Box 2971, Chancery Files, Stritch Papers, AAC.

72. Sheil to McIntyre, October 22, 1945, copy in Box 2971, Chancery Files, Stritch Papers, AAC.

73. McIntryre to Stritch, January 19, 1946, Box 2971, Chancery Files, Stritch Papers, AAC.

74. McIntryre to Stritch, April 30, 1947, Box 2971, Chancery Files, Stritch Papers, AAC.

75. Stephen S. Jackson to McIntyre, April 28, 1947, Box 2971, Stritch Papers, AAC.

76. Stritch to Sheil, May 5, 1947, Box 2980, Chancery Files, Stritch Papers, AAC.

77. "Bishop Sheil Has Pneumonia," *New York Times*, November 9, 1951.

78. "Labor's Bishop," *Newsweek* 28, July 15, 1946.

79. F.W. Specht to Stritch, March 18, 1948, Box 2988, Chancery Files, Stritch Papers, AAC.

80. Stritch to William O'Connor, June 13, 1953, Box 2827, Chancery Files, Stritch Papers, AAC.

81. Sheil to John F. Noll, May 26, 1945, Campbell Papers, Box 6, April-June 1945, CBNA.`

82. "Condemning Communism Bishop Sheil Warns against 'Witch Hunts' in Address to Veterans," June 23, 1947, NCWC Press Department Files, ACUA.

83. "Misguided Liberals Should Rediscover Supernatural Springs of Democratic Idea, Bishop Bernard J. Sheil Warns," September 11, 1950, NCWC Press Department Files, ACUA.

84. Donald F. Crosby, S.J., *God, Church and Flag: Senator Joseph R. McCarthy and the Catholic Church, 1950–1957* (Chapel Hill: University of North Carolina Press, 1978), pp. 139–140.

85. "For Joe: 'Phooey!'" *Time*, April 19, 1954.

86. Crosby, pp. 165–167.

87. William J. Rogers to Stritch, September 8, 1954, Stritch Papers, AAC.

88. Horwitt, pp. 253–254.

89. Quinn interview; Burns interview.

90. "Report on Catholic Youth Organization September 16, 1954," Box 2831, Chancery Files, Stritch Papers, AAC.

91. Kelly to Stritch, Stritch Papers, Chancery Files, AAC.

92. Higgins to Cantwell, September 21, 1954, Catholic Council on Working Life Papers, Box 7, Folder July-October 1954, CHS.

93. Mary Elizabeth Carroll, "Bishop Sheil Prophet without Honor," *Harper's* 211 (November 1955): 45–51.

94. Drury interview.

95. Gargan interview.

5. HILLENBRAND AND HIS DISCIPLES

1. Michael Ducey, O.S.B., "The National Liturgical Weeks and American Benedictines," *American Benedictine Review* 6 (Summer 1955): 156–157. Ducey was a monk of St. Anselm's Monastery in Washington, D.C.

2. "Program of the Liturgical Week," *Orate Fratres* 14 (September 9, 1940): 516; *Proceedings of the National Liturgical Week Held at Holy Name Cathedral*, Chicago, October 21–25, 1940 (Newark: Benedictine Liturgical Conference, 1941), *passim*; "Liturgical Congress Opens Oct. 21," *New World*, October 18, 1940; "National Liturgical Week Successful," *New World*, November 1, 1940.

3. *Proceedings of Liturgical Week*, pp. 5–11.

4. "Liturgy School Opens Monday," *New World*, July 11, 1941; "Three Day Liturgical Meeting Opens at Cathedral Tuesday," *New World*, October 8, 1943.

5. William Edward Wiethoff, "Popular Rhetorical Strategy in the American Catholic Debate Over Vernacular Reform" (Ph.D. diss., University of Michigan, 1974), p. 36.

6. "St. Aloysius" in Harry S. Koenig, *History of the Parishes of the Archdiocese of Chicago*, vol. 1, p. 51.

7. Gerald Ellard, S.J., "Progress of the Dialogue Mass in Chicago," *Orate Fratres* 14 (November 26, 1939): 19–25.

8. Quoted in Dennis Robb, "Specialized Catholic Action in the United States, 1936–1949: Ideology, Leadership, and Organization" (Ph.D. diss., University of Minnesota, 1972), p. 138.

9. Hillenbrand to Lorraine Cunningham, October 26, 1942, Hillenbrand Papers, AUND.

10. Stritch to Hillenbrand, April 6, 1945, Hillenbrand Papers, AUND.

11. Stritch to John W. Schmid, September 16, 1946, Chancery Files, Stritch Papers, AAC.

12. John W. Schmid to Stritch, September 21, 1946, Chancery Files, Stritch Papers, AAC.

13. Stritch to Schmid, September 24, 1946, Chancery Files, Stritch Papers, AAC.

14. Monsignor Jack Egan recalls being in the cardinal's office just after Voss and Marhoefer had their audience with Stritch. Interview with Monsignor John Egan, January 28, 1988.

15. Daniel Cunningham to Hillenbrand, April 1, 1940, Box 2943, Chancery Files, Stritch Papers, AAC.

16. Hillenbrand to Deferrari, August 24, 1940, Box 2943, Chancery Files, Stritch Papers, AAC.

17. Former seminarian Robert Heywood wrote of this dictum in a letter to his friend Rollins Lambert. A copy of this letter is in the Cantwell Papers. Heywood to "Dear Rollins," March 11, 1944, Box 1, Folder 1-4, CHS.

18. Culhane to Stritch, August 31, 1943, Chancery Files, Stritch Papers, AAC.

19. Stenger to Stritch, October 26, 1943, Chancery Files, Stritch Papers, AAC.

20. Stritch to Mooney, June 30, 1941, Chancery Files, Stritch Papers, AAC.

21. Stritch to John J. Clifford, S.J., March 10, 1945, Box 2964, Chancery Files, Stritch Papers, AAC.

22. Ibid.

23. Edward M. Kerwin to Stritch, May 9, 1941, Box 2943, Chancery Files, Stritch Papers, AAC.

24. Stritch to Kerwin, May 10, 1941, Box 2943, Chancery Files, Stritch Papers, AAC.

25. Stritch to Kerwin, November 4, 1941, Box 2943, Chancery Files, Stritch Papers, AAC.`

26. Hillenbrand to Stritch, November 16, 1941, Box 2943, Chancery File, Stritch Papers, AAC.

27. Stritch to Hillenbrand, November 17, 1941, Box 2943, Chancery Files, Stritch Papers, AAC.

28. Hillenbrand to Cantwell, March 27, 1950, Cantwell Papers, Folder 1–8, Box 1, CHS.

29. Stritch to McNicholas, November 24, 1941, Chancery Files, Stritch Papers, AAC.

30. For information about the Montgomery Ward's situation see Frank M. Kleiler, "The World War II Battle of Montgomery Ward," Chicago History 5 (Spring 1976): 19–27.

31. "Sewell Avery vs. Uncle Sam," Work, May 1944.

32. Catholic Labor Alliance publicist Edward Marciniak alludes to this in a letter. Marciniak to "Dear Dick," May 15, 1954, Catholic

Conference on Working Life Papers, Box 6, Folder March-June 1954, CHS.

33. "Farewell Address, Feast of Our Lady of Snow," August 5, 1944, Cantwell Papers, Box 1, Folder 1-4, CHS.

34. Hayes to Cantwell, August 23, 1944, Box 1, Folder 1-4, Cantwell Papers, CHS.

35. George Higgins to Cantwell, August 16, 1944, Box 7, Folder 7-10, Cantwell Papers, CHS.

36. Hillenbrand to Cantwell, April 3, 1950, Cantwell Papers, Box 1, Folder 1-8, CHS.

37. Andrew M. Greeley, *Confessions of a Parish Priest* (New York: Simon and Schuster, 1986), p. 114.

38. Memo in Cantwell Papers, 1949, Box 1, Folder 1-8, CHS.

39. Hillenbrand to Stritch, April 18, 1952, Stritch Papers, AAC.

40. Hillenbrand to Patrick Crowley, December 17, 1959, Cantwell Papers, Box 4, Folder 4-3, CHS.

41. Cantwell to Hillenbrand, December 31, 1959. Cantwell Papers, Box 4, Folder 4-3, CHS.

42. Egan interview.

43. His obituary in the *Chicago Catholic* was banal for a man of Hillenbrand's accomplishments. See "Msgr. R. Hillenbrand Dies," *Chicago Catholic*, May 25, 1979. Egan arranged to have the *National Catholic Reporter* report more extensively on his mentor. See Pam Bauer, "Hillenbrand: 'Anticipated Vatican II,'" *National Catholic Reporter* June 1, 1979; see also Robert McClory, "Hillenbrand: U.S. Moses," ibid.

44. Dennis Geaney, O.S.A., "From the Editor's Notebook," *Upturn*, Association of Chicago Priests, June-July 1985, p. 9.

45. Burke to Stritch (no date), Box 2988, Chancery Files, Stritch Papers, AAC.

46. "Frs. Egan, Quinn Named to New Posts," *New World*, October 25, 1946.

47. For an anecdotal life of Egan see Margery Frisbie, *An Alley in Chicago: The Ministry of a City Priest* (Kansas City, Mo.: Sheed and Ward, 1991).

48. Conleth Overman, C.P., "Cana Adventure," *Catholic Mind* 45 (February 1947): 123–128.

49. The best description of the work of the Cana Conference is found in Jeffrey Burns, "American Catholics and the Family Crisis 1930–1962, The Ideological and Organizational Response," (Ph.D. diss., University of Notre Dame, 1982), pp. 217–261.

50. Egan to Stritch, June 10, 1950, Box 2998, Chancery File, Stritch Papers, AAC.

51. "Defines Cana as Force for Practical Religion," *New World*, July 8, 1949.

52. "Cana Conference Publishes Manual for Directors' Use," *New World*, June 9, 1950.

53. "Father Egan Tells Cana Conference Progress in Chicago; 1900 Couples Instructed in 10 Months," *New World*, August 29, 1947.

54. Stritch to Hillenbrand, December 12, 1952, Box 3012, Chancery File, Stritch Papers, AAC.

55. Burns, pp. 222–223.

56. Burns, pp. 279–286.

57. Indeed John Cogley complained about this metamorphosis in an article "The Religious Revival," *Commonweal* 65 (January 18, 1957): 407; Burns discusses the middle-class character of the movement on pp. 321–324.

58. Stritch to Rev. Edmund P. Joyce, C.S.C., February 28, 1958, Chancery Files, Box 2825, Stritch Papers, AAC.

59. See my own "Milwaukee Catholicism 1945–1950: Seed-Time for Change" in Steven M. Avella, ed., *Milwaukee Catholicism: Essays on Church and Community* (Milwaukee, 1991), pp. 151-171.

60. The CFM still exists and apparently is headquartered in Ames, Iowa, as of this writing.

61. See Mary Irene Zotti, *A Time of Awakening: The Young Christian Worker Story in the United States* (Chicago: Loyola University Press, 1991).

62. Interviews with Vincent Giese, December 15, 1988; George Drury, December 1987–January 1988; Martin Farrell, September 30, 1983, and Russell Barta, November 30, 1987.

63. "Daniel M. Cantwell: Priest for the Laity" in Tim Unsworth, *The Last Priests in America* (New York: Crossroad, 1991), pp. 42-47.

64. Cantwell to Washington Housing Association, March 1, 1956, Cantwell Papers, Box 3, Folder 3-2, CHS.

65. For a general treatment of Catholic participation in union organizing in the thirties, see Neil Betten, *Catholic Activism and the Industrial Worker* (Gainesville: University Presses of Florida, 1976).

66. See Douglas P. Seaton, *Catholics and Radicals: The Association of Catholic Trade Unionists and the American Labor Movement from Depression to Cold War* (Lewisburg, Pa.: Bucknell University Press, 1981)

67. Ibid., p. 152.

68. Edward Marciniak to "Dear Dick," May 15, 1954, Catholic Conference on Working Life Papers, Box 6, Folder March-June 1954, CHS.

69. Lucy Read to Harry Read, September 18, 1941, Harry Cyril Read Papers, Archives of the Catholic University of America (hereafter ACUA).

70. Roger Biles, *Big City Boss in Depression and War: Mayor Edward J. Kelly of Chicago* (DeKalb: Northern Illinois University Press, 1984), p. 118.

71. Quoted in Bob Senser, "A Guy's Job in Life," reprint from *Voice of St. Jude*, Box 5, Folder September-October 1953, Catholic Council on Working Life Papers, CHS.

72. Raymond John Maly, "The Catholic Labor Alliance: A Laboratory Test of Catholic Social Action" (M.A. thesis, University of Notre Dame, August 1950), p. 15.

73. Cantwell to Stritch, August 15, 1947, Cantwell Papers, Box 9, Stritch Folder, CHS.

74. Tim Unsworth, "On Chicago's Daniel Cantwell," *Commonweal* 116 (June 16, 1989): 365–367.

75. Maly, pp. 40–49.

76. Barta interview.

77. "21 East Superior," *Sign* 37 (July 1958): 51–53.

78. Minutes, CLA Meeting, February 4, 1947, Catholic Council on Working Life Papers (hereafter CCWL), Box 1, Folder, 1947, CHS.

79. Cantwell to Reverend O. M. Cloran, S.J., January 28, 1957, Box 3, Folder 3-3, Cantwell Papers, CHS.

80. Cantwell to Most Rev. James W. Gleeson, January 9, 1962, Cantwell Papers, Box 5, Folder 5-6, CHS.

81. Andrew Greeley describes these meetings in his autobiography, *Confessions of a Parish Priest*, pp. 159-161. Interview with Father Jake Killgallon, September 17, 1987.

82. Interview with Father Leo Mahon, July 15, 1989.

83. John LaFarge, "The Chicago Catechism," *America* 98 (June 28, 1958): 363.

84. Killgallon interview.

85. "The Inner Forum," *Commonweal* 34 (July 25, 1941): 333–334.

86. "A Brief History of Childerly read at the meeting of the Calvert Foundation of Chicago, 10 January 1946," Box 2977, Stritch Papers, AAC.

87. Memo, Cantwell to Mary Dolan, Lloyd Davis, Russ Barta, Ed Marciniak, October 5, 1958, Box 8, Folder 8-3, Cantwell Papers, CHS.

88. Daniel Cantwell to Bernard Dauenhauer, October 8, 1959, Cantwell Papers, Box 4, Folder 4-3, CHS.

6. CHICAGO CATHOLICISM AND URBAN ISSUES

1. See Devereux Bowly, *The Poor House: Subsidized Housing in Chicago* (Carbondale: Southern Illinois University Press, 1978), p. 18.

2. Ibid., pp. 28–47.

3. These were the Parklawn and Greendale housing projects. The latter was one of the New Deal's famed "Greenbelt Cities."

4. Stritch to Elizabeth Wood, August 11, 1942, Box 2951, Chancery Files, Stritch Papers, AAC.

5. Stritch to Mrs. Joseph Loftus, September 18, 1942, Box 2948, Chancery Files, Stritch Papers, AAC.

6. Daniel M. Cantwell, "Facts in Negro Segregation" (masters thesis, Catholic University of America, June 1942).

7. Ibid., p. 93(a).

8. U.S. Census Reports, 1890–1960. See also Nicholas Lemann, *The Promised Land: The Great Black Migration and How It Changed America* (New York: Alfred Knopf, 1991).

9. "Negro population is piling up within a very limited area" (1944?) Catholic Interracial Council Papers (hereafter CIC Papers), Box 1, Folder 1932–1945, Chicago Historical Society (hereafter CHS).

10. Arnold R. Hirsch, *Making the Second Ghetto: Race and Housing in Chicago* (New York: Cambridge University Press, 1983), p. 23.

11. Minutes of the Meeting of the Officers and Board of Directors of the Chicago National Public Housing Conference, Cantwell Papers, Box 17, Folder 17-4, CHS.

12. See Thomas W. Tifft, "Toward a More Human Social Policy: The Work and Influence of Monsignor John O'Grady" (Ph.D. diss., Catholic University of America, 1979), pp. 364–447. O'Grady would be a significant figure in the development of Chicago Catholicism's response to urban renewal and neighborhood conservation.

13. "Restrictive Covenants," *Work* (September 1943).

14. Quoted in "Negro Population is piling up within a very limited area" (1944?), CIC Papers, Box 1, Folder 1932–1945, CHS.

15. "Quilici Demands End to Restrictive Real Estate Pacts," clipping, March 6, 1945, Cantwell Papers, Box 17, Folder 17-5, CHS.

16. Robert C. Weaver to Robert R. Taylor, February 14, 1945 (copy), Cantwell Papers, Box 17, Folder 17-5, CHS.

17. Cantwell to Robert R. Taylor, March 20, 1945, Box 17, Folder 17-5, Cantwell Papers, CHS.

18. Taylor to Cantwell, April 6, 1945, Box 17, Folder 17-5, Cantwell Papers, CHS.

19. Hirsch, p. 30.

20. Shufro to Cantwell, September 7, 1944, Cantwell Papers, Box 17, Folder 17-4, CHS.

21. Milton Shufro to Cantwell, November 27, 1943, Cantwell Papers, Box 17, Folder 17-4, CHS.

22. "Restrictive Covenants," *Work* (September 1943); "An Open Letter to the Governor," *Work* (October 1946); "Chicago Has Its Own 'D.P.' Problem," *Work* (April 1947); "Is Skyscraper Housing the Answer?" *Work* (August 1948).

23. Edward J. Kelly to Cantwell, April 3, 1946, Box 9, Folder Stritch, Cantwell Papers, CHS.

24. Cantwell to Dwight H. Green, August 21, 1946, Cantwell Papers, Box 1, Folder 1-6, CHS.

25. Bowly, p. 77.

26. Cantwell to Edward J. Kelly, December 3, 1946, Box 17, Folder 17-6, Cantwell Papers, CHS.

27. Daniel Cantwell, "Riot Spirit in Chicago," *Commonweal* 54 (July 27, 1951): 375–377.

28. Hirsch, p. 101.

29. Ibid., p. 112.

30. Two Catholic hospitals, Mercy at 2537 Prairie Avenue and Lewis Maternity at 3001 S. Michigan, were the largest Catholic institutions in the area. St. Ignatius School, run by the Sisters of Mercy, was also in the area. St. James parish and St. John's parish also fell within the boundaries of the South Side Planning Board. The boundaries of the South Side Planning Board fluctuated. Initially their area began at Twelfth Street and extended south to Forty-seventh. It then went west to the railroad tracks of the Pennsylvania Line and east to Lake Michigan. Later when the University of Chicago began to take an interest in urban renewal, the northern boundary was dropped to Thirty-first Street and the southern boundary of the area was extended to Fifty-seventh Street.

31. Thomas J. Reed to Stritch, March 5, 1946, Chancery Files, Stritch Papers, AAC.

32. Reed was born in Chicago October 30, 1904, and was graduated from Presentation School. He attended the archdiocesan seminaries and was ordained in 1928 by Mundelein. After a first assignment at St. Ambrose parish on the South Side, he was assigned to work with the Chicago-based Church Extension Society and became a special aide to Bishop William O'Brien, director of Extension.

33. The rocky history of the Mercy and Loyola relationship is discussed in a fairly genteel fashion in Joy Clough, R.S.M., *In Service to*

Chicago: The History of Mercy Hospital, booklet (Mercy Hospital and Medical Center, 1979).

34. "Cardinal Stritch Gives Name to Medical School," *New World*, May 14, 1948.

35. "Loyola Fulfillment Fund Opens Drive for Medical, Dental School Buildings," *New World*, June 18, 1948.

36. Stritch to Reverend Sister Superior, October 4, 1945, Box 2968, Chancery Files, Stritch Papers, AAC.

37. "Huge Building Program Set by Mercy Hospital," *New World*, March 22, 1946.

38. "Doctors, Architects Lay Plans for Mercy Sisters' Hospital," *New World*, February 28, 1947; "New Mercy Hospital to Make City 'World Medical Capital,' Says Cardinal as Drive Opens," *New World*, July 18, 1947.

39. A copy of this report is in the Stritch Papers, AAC.

40. Hirsch, p. 127.

41. Reed to Stritch, February 3, 1949, Box 2995, Chancery Files, Stritch Papers, AAC.

42. Reed to Stritch, December 19, 1950, Box 3001, Chancery Files, Stritch Papers, AAC.

43. Stritch to Reed, November 29, 1950, Box 3001, Chancery Files, Stritch Papers, AAC.

44. Bowly, p. 65.

45. Cantwell to George J. Tourek, February 2, 1950, Cantwell Papers, Box 18, Folder 18-3, CHS.

46. "Statement," 1950, Cantwell Papers, Box 18, Folder 18-6, CHS.

47. Stritch to Muench, January 11, 1952, Box 3012, Chancery Files, Stritch Papers, AAC.

48. Stritch to Cantwell, March 9, 1950, Cantwell Papers, Box 9, Folder "Stritch," CHS.

49. Cantwell to Stritch, March 23, 1950, Cantwell Papers, Box 9, Folder "Stritch," CHS.

50. Hirsch, pp. 225–228.

51. The defeat of the seven sites did not deter Cantwell's advocacy of public housing and he spoke out forcefully for his positions. He was strongly opposed to those who tried to undermine public housing by submitting it to public referendums. In 1951 when bills were introduced in the Illinois Legislature to require popular referendums on public housing, Cantwell protested to Senator John Gorman: "[The referendum] ... is in the long run subversive of good government.... It removes responsibility for the general welfare from representatives who are constituted to guard the common good with impartial, cool

and deliberate judgement. Our government has never been a government by referendum, but a government by representatives. Government by referendum is essentially chaos." Cantwell to John J. Gorman, February 12, 1951, Cantwell Papers, Box 19, Folder 19-1, CHS.

In the following year the city council attempted to do away with rent control, and Cantwell, as head of the Housing Conference, sought Cardinal Stritch's permission to testify against the move. Stritch did not agree with Cantwell's opposition to the removal of rent control (considering it a "question of justice") but he gave permission for the priest to appear before the city council nonetheless.

In 1953 the state legislature considered the Larson Bill, a proposal that effectively eliminated the possibility of more low-rent public housing in the state by once again submitting it to the vote of localities for which it was proposed. This time Stritch seemed to concur with Cantwell's position and appeared to allow Cantwell to testify against the measure in his name. However, Cantwell's presumption of Stritch's approval was only the result of a typographical error. This gave the prelate another opportunity to warn Cantwell to be careful about his public statements: "Referring to my letter of March 12, 1953, I find that there was an unfortunate mistake in the letter in the last sentence. I intended to say to my typist 'and NOT as my representative in that organization.' I am sorry that this mistake was made and I think you will appreciate why I want to correct it.... I hold to my conviction that we do need some low rent public housing. Anybody may quote me on this point but not beyond this point." Stritch to Cantwell, March 23, 1953, Cantwell Papers, Folder "Stritch," CHS.

52. Gallery to Stritch, September 20, 1951, Box 3005, Chancery Files, Stritch Papers, AAC.

53. Gallery to Stritch, September 29, 1951, Box 3005, Chancery Files, Stritch Papers, AAC.

54. Stritch to Gallery, October 18, 1951, Box 3005, Chancery Files, Stritch Papers, AAC.

55. Copy of this memo is in Box 3005, Chancery Files, Stritch Papers, AAC.

56. O'Grady to Raymond M. Foley, October 18, 1951, Box 3007, Chancery File, Stritch Papers, AAC.

57. Letter of Monsignor John Egan to author, February 22, 1990.

58. Stritch to Cantwell, November 8, 1952, Cantwell Papers, Box 9, Folder "Stritch," CHS.

59. Interview with Father John Ireland Gallery, April 24, 1989.

60. Further information on Alinsky can be found in his own

Reveille For Radicals (New York: Random House, 1969) and in Sanford D. Horwitt, *Let Them Call Me Rebel* (New York: Alfred Knopf, 1989) and P. David Finks, *The Radical Vision of Saul Alinsky* (New York: Paulist Press, 1984). See also, Robert A. Slayton, *Back of the Yards: The Making of a Local Democracy* (Chicago: University of Chicago Press, 1986).

61. J. I. Gallery, "How to Build the Neighborhood of Tomorrow," *Work*, July 1952. See also a pamphlet on the West Kenwood Association in the Alinsky Papers, University of Illinois at Chicago Archives (hereafter UICA).

62. The documents of this transaction are in the St. Cecilia Parish File in AAC.

63. "St. Cecilia" in Harry S. Koenig, *A History of the Parishes of the Archdiocese of Chicago*, vol., 1, pp. 180–182.

64. "The Contribution of One Pastor," *Catholic Charities Review* 35 (October 1951): 215–216. See also "The Pastor and the Conservation of His Parish," memo in Box 3005, Chancery Files, Stritch Papers, AAC.

65. "Pastors Conference on Conservation," St. Cecilia's rectory, October 10, 1951, Box 3012, Chancery Files, Stritch Papers, AAC.

66. Ibid.

67. Reed to Stritch, October 31, 1952, Box 3015, Chancery Files, Stritch Papers, AAC.

68. Stritch to "Dear Reverend Father," November 19, 1952, Box 3015, Stritch Papers, AAC.

69. Samuel Cardinal Stritch, "Neighborhood Conservation," *Catholic Charities Review*, February 1953, pp. 33–35.

70. "St. Sabina," in Koenig, *A History of the Parishes*, vol. 2, pp. 858–862.

71. Julian H. Levi to Reed, April 30, 1953, Box 3007, Chancery Files, Stritch Papers, AAC.

72. Reed to Stritch, September 24, 1954, Box 3008, Chancery Files, Stritch Papers, AAC.

73. Interview with Father John Quinn Corcoran, October 14, 1988.

74. In a conversation with the author, Monsignor Daniel Cantwell tagged John Quinn Corcoran's efforts in Garfield Park as nothing more than a ruse to keep blacks out of the area. Cantwell to author.

75. A copy of this pamphlet is in Box 3008, Chancery Files, Stritch Papers, AAC.

76. Stritch to Reed, August 26, 1954, Box 2835, Chancery Files, Stritch Papers, AAC.

77. Gallery interview.

78. Stritch to Fitzgerald, September 30, 1955, Box 2837, Chancery Files, Stritch Papers, AAC.

79. Stritch to Kelly, January 15, 1954, Box 2832, Chancery File, Stritch Papers, AAC.

80. V. E. Gunlock to Edward J. Kelly, March 16, 1954, Box 2832, Chancery File, Stritch Papers, AAC.

81. "Holy Guardian Angels Church," in Koenig, *A History of the Parishes*, vol. 2, pp. 1650–1653.

82. Interview with Father Leo Coggins, July 10, 1989; see also "St. Charles Borromeo," in Koenig, *A History of the Parishes*, vol. 2, pp. 1640–1645.

83. "St. Jarlath Church," in Koenig, *A History of the Parishes*, vol. 2, pp. 1653–1656.

84. "Holy Trinity Church," in Koenig, *A History of the Parishes*, vol. 1, pp. 399–403.

85. "St. Philip Benizi Church," in Koenig, *A History of the Parishes*, vol. 2, pp. 1671–1674.

86. "Our Lady of the Gardens Church," in Koenig, *A History of the Parishes*, vol. 1, pp. 675–677.

87. Stritch to Reed, October 14, 1957, Chancery Files, Stritch Papers, AAC.

88. Interview with Father Martin Farrell, September 30, 1983.

89. O'Grady to Reed, April 4, 1957, copy in Box 2839, Chancery Files, Stritch Papers, AAC.

90. Memo: Mr. F. J. Lewis's objections to St. James project [no date], Box 2825, Chancery Files, Stritch Papers, AAC.

7. COMMUNITY ORGANIZING AND PROFESSIONAL CONCERNS

1. "Chicago Has Its Own 'D.P.' Problem," *Work*, April 1947.

2. For Lucey's efforts see Stephen A. Privett, "Robert E. Lucey: Evangelization and Catechesis among Hispanic Catholics" (Ph.D. diss., Catholic University of America, 1985), pp. 113–191; see also Saul E. Bronder, *Social Justice and Church Authority: The Public Life of Archbishop Robert E. Lucey* (Philadelphia: Temple University Press, 1982).

3. Stritch to Michael Ready, October 2, 1944, Chancery Files, Stritch Papers, AAC.

4. Ibid.

5. For a study of Mexicans in Chicago see Louise Ano Nuevo Kerr, "The Chicano Experience in Chicago: 1920–1970" (Ph.D. diss.,

University of Illinois, 1976). Mr. Thomas Kelliher, a graduate student at the University of Notre Dame, is at work on a dissertation on ministry to Hispanics in the Archdiocese of Chicago.

6. Stritch to Monsignor Thomas A. Meehan, December 16, 1955, Chancery Files, Stritch Papers, AAC.

7. Rev. Thomas Matin, C.M.F., to Stritch, December 24, 1948, Chancery Files, Stritch Papers, AAC.

8. "Memorandum Number Two to His Eminence Samuel Cardinal Stritch" from Saul D. Alinsky–Industrial Areas Foundation, June 24, 1955; copy in O'Grady Papers, ACUA.

9. Burke to Stritch, undated memo, Chancery Files, Stritch Papers, AAC.

10. Interview with Father Leo Mahon, July 15, 1989.

11. Mahon's papers and material relating to the Mission of San Miguelito are to be found in the Archives of the University of Notre Dame.

12. P. David Finks, *The Radical Vision of Saul Alinsky* (New York: Paulist Press, 1984), pp. 82–83.

13. Alinsky to Stritch, November 1, 1954, Box 2833, Chancery Files, Stritch Papers, AAC.

14. "Revised Application of the Industrial Areas Foundation," December 21, 1955, Alinsky Papers, UICA.

15. "Near North Side Resume," Alinsky Papers, UICA.

16. Confidential Memo: Egan to Stritch, March 26, 1958, Stritch Papers, AAC.

17. Ibid.

18. Additional information can be gained from reading Hirsch, pp. 135–170; also Julia Abrahamson, *A Neighborhood Finds Itself* (New York: Harper and Row, 1959) and Peter H. Rossi and Robert A. Dentler, *The Politics of Urban Renewal* (New York: Free Press, 1961).

19. Reed to Stritch, July 15, 1954, Chancery Files, Stritch Papers, AAC.

20. Reed to Stritch, July 28, 1954, Chancery Files, Stritch Papers, AAC.

21. Hirsch, pp. 165–166. An example of the aspirations of Catholic reformers for the city is found in Joseph B. Schuyler, S.J., "Urban Society and Soldiarism," *Social Justice Review* 44 (December 1951): 257–261.

22. "Shiny New Islands Don't Solve Housing," *New World*, April 18, 1958.

23. "Conserving Chicago's Neighborhoods," *New World*, May 2, 1958.

24. "Common Good Takes Precedence over the Rights of Individuals," *New World*, May 7, 1958.

25. Statement by the Cardinal's Conservation Committee on the Hyde Park–Kenwood Urban Renewal Plan issues by the Very Rev. Msgr. John J. Egan, Executive Director, June 11, 1958, Cantwell Papers, Box 20, Folder 20-4, CHS.

26. "Catholic Unit Denies Opposing Urban Renewal," *Chicago Sun Times*, July 12, 1958.

27. The accusation that the Church was a stumbling block to urban renewal was voiced even after the Hyde Park-Kenwood battle was over. In 1963 *Time* magazine published a scathing attack on the Catholic Church in Chicago for its "opposition" to Mayor Daley's urban renewal plans (*Time*, March 15, 1963). Monsignor George Higgins offered a forceful rebuttal in his syndicated column "The Yardstick." See "Time Ignored Facts in Hitting Church's Urban Renewal Role," *New World*, April 5, 1963.

28. Cantwell to Egan, May 26, 1958, Cantwell Papers, Box 20, Folder 20-2, CHS.

29. Ben W. Heineman to R. Sargent Shriver, June 12, 1958, Cantwell Papers, Box 20, Folder 20-4, CHS.

30. Cantwell to Shriver, June 19, 1958, Cantwell Papers, Box 20, Folder 20-4, CHS.

31. Memo: Marciniak to Cantwell and Egan, July 25, 1958, Cantwell Papers, Box 20, Folder 20-4, CHS.

32. Edward Burke to Cantwell, July 28, 1958, Box 20, Folder 20-4, CHS.

33. "Layman Rips Church Stand on Hyde Park," unidentified clipping, Cantwell Papers, Box 20, Folder 20-4, CHS.

34. "Archbishop in Middle of Housing Fight," clipping, Cantwell Papers, Box 20, Folder 20-4, CHS.

35. "New Archbishop," "Hyde Park-Kenwood," *Chicago Tribune*, September 25, 1958.

36. Egan, quoted in "Archdiocese Rejects Hyde Park–Kenwood Urban Renewal Plan," *New World*, Sept. 26, 1958.

37. Ibid.

38. Interview with Monsignor John Egan, October 19, 1981.

39. O'Grady to Meyer, October 3, 1958, Meyer Papers, AAC.

40. Francois Houtart, *Aspects sociologiques du catholicisme americain* (Paris: Collection de Sociologie Religieuse, 1957).

41. Copies of these talks and papers are in the Stritch Papers, AAC.

42. Stritch to Reed, August 24, 1955, Box 2877, Chancery Files, Stritch Papers, AAC.

43. Memo of Thomas J. Reed, March 20, 1959, Meyer Papers, AAC.

44. "Msgr. Egan Heads Expanded Council," clipping, *Hyde Park Herald*, May 20, 1959, Catholic Interracial Council Papers [hereafter CIC], Box 34, Folder 1959 News Clippings, CHS.

45. Interview with Michael Schiltz, April 18, 1988.

46. "A Study Program on Religion, Community Life and Chicago's Housing," CIC Papers, Box 37, Folder April 1960, CHS.

47. "Organization for the Southwest Community: An Evaluation—October 1965," Office of Urban Affairs Papers, Box 3295, AAC.

48. John A. McMahon, "Conservation at St. Sabina's," *Catholic Charities Review* 38 (January 1954): 11–13.

49. Eileen McMahon discusses the history of this organization at length in her, "What Parish Are You From? A Study of the Chicago Irish Parish Community and Race Relations" (Ph.D. diss., Loyola University of Chicago, 1989), pp. 256–283.

50. Egan to Meyer, January 5, 1959, Meyer Papers, AAC.

51. Finks, *The Radical Vision of Saul Alinsky*, p. 124.

52. Stanley A. Koven, "The Day the Chicago Racists Lost," *Catholic World* 191 (August 1960): 308–314.

53. Memo: To Saul D. Alinsky, From: Nicholas von Hoffman; Re: O.S.C., June 21, 1963, Alinsky Papers, UICA.

54. Egan to Meyer, April 17, 1964, Meyer Papers, AAC.

55. The failure of the OSC to achieve an integrated neighborhood is described in McMahon, pp. 292–332. However she does point out that the rate of neighborhood transition was considerably more well-paced because of the efforts of OSC.

56. Reed to Stritch, September 20, 1957, Box 2839, Chancery Files, Stritch Papers, AAC.

57. Meyer to Paul Marcinkus, May 25, 1960, Meyer Papers, AAC.

58. Interview with Father Anthony Janiak, September 3, 1987.

59. *New World*, April 25, 1958.

60. "West Woodlawn Residents Look Toward 'Bright Future," *New World*, July 4, 1958.

61. "Woodlawn Block Club Council," *New World*, August 8, 1958.

62. Egan interview.

63. "Church supports 'hate group,'" *Chicago Maroon*, March 3, 1961, clipping, Alinsky Papers, UICA.

64. "Laud 5 Woodlawn Pastors Who Quit Unit in U of C. Expansion Row," *Chicago Daily Defender*, April 25, 1961, clipping, Alinsky Papers, UICA.

65. Harold E. Fey, "Open or Closed Cities—A Reply to Replies," *Christian Century*, June 5, 1961.

8. THE CHALLENGE OF RACE:
STRITCH, the UNCERTAIN TRUMPET

1. Stritch to Richard O. Gerow, April 20, 1940, Chancery Files, Stritch Papers, AAC.

2. Stritch to Eckert, April 29, 1940, Box 2943, Chancery Files, Stritch Papers, AAC.

3. The best source for information about the Great Migration to Chicago is James R. Grossman's, *Land of Hope: Chicago, Black Southerners, and the Great Migration* (Chicago: University of Chicago Press, 1989); Nicholas Lemann has also come out with a work on the Great Migration which focuses specifically on Chicago. Because of Stritch's southern background, Lemann argues that Stritch was better prepared than most northern prelates to welcome blacks into northern urban centers and integrate them into urban life. In point of fact, as this chapter demonstrates, Stritch only supported integration in a lukewarm fashion. His primary interest in black Chicagoans was to convert them to Catholicism.

4. A good description of black life in prewar Chicago is to be found in Allan H. Spear, *Black Chicago: The Making of a Negro Ghetto, 1890–1920* (Chicago: University of Chicago Press, 1967).

5. Grossman, *Land of Hope*, pp. 173–174.

6. "St. Elizabeth Church," in Harry S. Koenig, *A History of the Parishes of the Archdiocese of Chicago* (Chicago: Catholic Bishop, 1980) vol. 1, pp. 245–252.

7. "St. Elizabeth High School Is Story of Home Mission," *New World*, March 30, 1951.

8. "St. Anselm Church" in Koenig, *History of the Parishes*, vol. 1, pp. 72–75.

9. "Corpus Christi Church" in Koenig, *History of the Parishes*, vol. 1, pp. 216–219.

10. "Holy Family Church" in Koenig, *History of the Parishes*, vol. 1, pp. 378–382.

11. Hillenbrand to John LaFarge, [no date] 1940, Chancery Files, Stritch Papers, AAC.

12. Joseph G. Richards, "Growth and Spread of the Negro Population" in *The Catholic Church and the Negro in the Archdiocese of Chicago*, Clergy Conference, September 21–20, 1960, p. 3.

13. Memo of Archbishop Stritch to Rev. Edmund Goebel [no date], Archives of the Archdiocese of Milwaukee.

14. Interview with Bishop Cletus F. O'Donnell, September 6, 1983.

15. Stritch to John Clifford, S.J., February 13, 1942, Box 2946, Chancery Files, Stritch Papers, AAC.

16. Dorothy Maydem to George Casey, March 27, 1942; Box 2948, Chancery Files, AAC.

17. George J. Casey to Dorothy Maydem, April 9, 1942, Box 2948, Chancery Files, Stritch Papers, AAC.

18. Arthur G. Falls to Stritch, December 26, 1941, Box 2943, Chancery Files, Stritch Papers, AAC.

19. Stritch to Falls, December 27, 1941, Box 2943, Chancery Files, Stritch Papers, AAC.

20. Stritch to Cicognani, August 5, 1941, Box 2875, Chancery Files, Stritch Papers, AAC.

21. "Visitation Parish" in Koenig, *History of the Parishes*, vol. 2, pp. 968–974.

22. Interview with Father Martin Farrell, September 30, 1983.

23. Farrell interview.

24. "Honor Paid to Beloved Pastor of Visitation," *New World*, September 26, 1952.

25. Arthur G. Falls to Stritch, December 12, 1949, Box 2996, Chancery Files, Stritch Papers, AAC.

26. Farrell interview.

27. Edward Marciniak to "Stuart," February 4, 1950, CIC Papers, Box 1, Folder 1950, CHS.

28. Sister Kenneth Kreuser to author, April 5, 1989.

29. Annals of the Dominican Sisters, December 1952, Dominican Archives, Sinsinawa, Wisconsin. Emphasis is my own.

30. This was the same Cayton who participated with St. Clair Drake in the sociological study *Black Metropolis* (New York: Harper, rev. 1982).

31. Special report given by Fathers Joseph Richards and Martin Farrell,"The Catholic Church and the Negro in the Archdiocese of Chicago," 1955, a mimeographed paper given to the author by Father Martin Farrell.

32. Spencer A. Wilson to Stritch, August 28, 1943, Chancery Files, Stritch Papers, AAC.

33. Stritch to Wilson, August 28, 1943, Chancery Files, Stritch Papers, AAC.

34. Christopher C. Wimbish to Stritch, January 5, 1944, Box 2963, Chancery Files, Stritch Papers, AAC.

35. Stritch to Morrison, July 3, 1943, Chancery Files, Stritch Papers, AAC.

36. Stritch to Ernestine Martin, July 2, 1943, Chancery Files, Stritch Papers, AAC.

37. Mother Samuel Coughlin to Stritch, August 6, 1944, GA 12, Box 6/42, Dominican Archives, Sinsinawa, Wisconsin.

38. Stritch to Sister Mary Samuel, O.P., August 17, 1944, GA 12 Box 6/43, Dominican Archives.

39. Stritch to Mother Mary Corona, O.S.F., May 30, 1946, Box 2969, Chancery Files, Stritch Papers, AAC.

40. Robert Heywood to Francis Quinn, January 7, 1946, Cantwell Papers, Box 29, Folder 29-1, CHS.

41. Stritch to Heywood, January 11, 1946, Cantwell Papers, Box 29, Folder 29-1, CHS.

42. Report on 8 A.M. Mass at St. Ambrose Church, Forty-seventh Street and Ellis Avenue, Sunday June 25, 1950. Mass said by Father Quinn—Sermon by Father Quinn, Box 2997, Chancery Files, Stritch Papers, AAC.

43. Martin M. McLaughlin to Stritch, July 6, 1950, Box 2997, Chancery Files, Stritch Papers, AAC.

44. Memo, Stritch to Casey (no date), Box 2997, Chancery Files, Stritch Papers, AAC.

45. F. J. Quinn to George Casey, July 10, 1950, Box 2997, Chancery Files, Stritch Papers, AAC.

46. Stritch to Quinn, September 15, 1950, Box 2997, Chancery Files, Stritch Papers, AAC.

47. Quinn to Stritch, October 10, 1950, Box 3001, Chancery Files, Stritch Papers, AAC.

48. Julianne Fernandez to Stritch, September 5, 1951, Box 3005, Chancery Files, Stritch Papers, AAC.

49. Stritch to Julianne Fernandez, September 11, 1951, Box 3005, Chancery Files, Stritch Papers, AAC.

50. Henry Matimore to Burke, December 29, 1956, Chancery Files, Stritch Papers, AAC.

51. Stritch to Rev. Henry Mattimore [sic], January 4, 1957, Chancery Files, Stritch Papers, AAC.

52. *Work*, November 1943.

53. Heywood to Quinn, January 7, 1946, Cantwell Papers, Box 29, Folder 29-1, CHS.

54. Arnold Hirsch, *Making the Second Ghetto* (New York: Cambridge University Press, 1983), p. 52.

55. Stritch's silence could certainly have been justified by the appeal of Commissioner Thomas Wright of the city Human Relations Commission for press restraint in reporting such incidents in order to avoid sensationalizing the incidents.

56. Memorandum on Airport Homes—60th and Karlov, Mayor's Commission on Human Relations, Cantwell Papers, Box 17, Folder 17-6, CHS.

57. Daniel M. Cantwell, "Riot Spirit in Chicago, *Commonweal* 54 (July 27, 1951), pp. 375–377.

58. Telegram, Falls to Stritch, December 6, 1946, Box 2970, Chancery Files, Stritch Papers, AAC.

59. Ruth Hughes to Stritch, December 11, 1946, Box 2971, Chancery Files, Stritch Papers, AAC.

60. Stritch to Rita Hughes, December 13, 1946, Box 2971, Chancery Files, Stritch Papers, AAC.

61. Pauline O'Connor to Edward Marciniak, August 15, 1944, Catholic Council on Working Life Papers (hereafter CCWLP), Box 1, Folder 1944, CHS.

62. Memo to Mayor Martin H. Kennelly from Augustine J. Bowe and Thomas H. Wright of Commission on Human Relations, October 29, 1948, Appendix I, Racial Violence in the Park Manor Community. Cantwell Papers, Box 18, Folder 18-3, CHS.

63. Conversation with Father Chawk, St. Columbanus, July 25, 1949, Cantwell Papers, Box 18, Folder 18-4, CHS.

64. Cantwell, "Riot Spirit," p. 376.

65. George Bressler to Stritch, December 20, 1949, Box 2990, Chancery Files, Stritch Papers, AAC.

66. Stritch to George Bressler, December 22, 1949, Box 2990, Chancery Files, Stritch Papers, AAC.

67. William Gremley, "The Scandal of Cicero," *America* 85 (August 25, 1951): 495–497.

68. "Examine Conscience on Cicero Race Riots" *New World*, August 3, 1951.

69. Memo from Bayard Rustin: Joint Committee of the American Friends Service Committee and the Catholic Interracial Council, Re: Immediate Plans for Dave McNamara's work in the Cicero-Berwyn Area, September 11, 1951. CIC, Box 2, Folder 1951, CHS.

70. Confidential Memorandum, To: File; From: D. McNamara; Subject: Catholic Priests in Cicero and Berwyn, October 12, 1951. CIC, Box 2, Folder 1951, CHS.

71. Cantwell to Stritch, December 20, 1954, Cantwell Papers, Box 9, Folder Stritch, CHS.

72. The Work of the Catholic Interracial Council of the Archdiocese of Chicago for the period January 1954 through June 1954, CIC Papers, Box 6, Folder 1954, CHS.

73. Homer A. Jack, "Test at Trumbull Park," *Christian Century* 73 (March 21, 1956): 366–368.

74. Marciniak to Editor of the Christian Century, April 18, 1956, Cantwell Papers, Box 20, Folder 20-3, CHS.

75. "The Cardinal Speaks Up," *Daily Defender*, June 14, 1956, clipping, Cantwell Papers, Box 29, Folder 29-7, CHS.

76. Stritch to Martin McNamara, April 19, 1957, Box 2838, Chancery Files, Stritch Papers, AAC.

77. James A. Griffin to Stritch, July 2, 1945, Box 2965, Chancery Files, Stritch Papers, AAC.

78. Stritch to Griffin, July 5, 1945, Box 2965, Chancery Files, Stritch Papers, AAC.

79. Gerald O'Hara to Francis Hyland, April 30, 1954. Copy in Stritch Personal Papers, AAC.

80. Stritch to Francis E. Hyland, May 6, 1954, Chancery Files, Stritch Papers, AAC.

81. Francis E. Hyland to Stritch, May 24, 1954, Chancery Files, Stritch Papers, AAC.

82. Stritch to Hyland, June 5, 1954, Chancery Files, Stritch Papers, AAC.

83. Stritch to Clair Driscoll, April 15, 1955, Chancery Files, Stritch Papers, AAC.

84. Stritch to Aloisius Muench, July 7, 1955, Box 2831, Chancery Files, Stritch Papers, AAC.

85. Office Memorandum from: SAC Auerbach to: Mr. Hoover, December 3, 1957, 94-4-1411-14 FBI Office Files.

86. Memo: Barrett to Stritch (no date), Box 2943, Chancery Files, Stritch Papers, AAC.

87. Maude Johnston to Stritch, March 23, 1944, Friendship House Papers, Box 1, Folder January-May, 1944, CHS.

88. Interview with Father Anthony Vader, February 25, 1989.

89. Sister Praxedes of Providence to Stritch, July 26, 1945, Box 2966, Chancery Files, Stritch Papers, AAC.

90. Stritch to Sister Praxedes of Providence, July 30, 1945, Box 2966, Chancery Files, Stritch Papers, AAC.

91. Memo of Monsignor George Casey (no date), Box 2943, Chancery Files, Stritch Papers, AAC.

92. Memo: Stritch to Monsignor John A. Barrett, December 30, 1948, Box 2987, Chancery Files, Stritch Papers, AAC.

93. Report on Discrimination in Catholic Hospitals, submitted by Chicago Friendship House, September 30, 1955. A copy of this report is in the Stritch Personal Papers, AAC.

94. Ibid., p. 3.

95. Inaugural Address, A. M. Mercer, M.D., President Cook County Physicians' Association, January 1950, Box 3000, Chancery Files, Stritch Papers, AAC.

96. Samuel Cardinal Stritch, "Interracial Justice in Hospitals," reprint from *Interracial Review*, November 1955, Cantwell Papers, Box 9, Folder 9-3, Stritch, CHS.

97. Cantwell to Stritch, October 25, 1955, Cantwell Papers, Box 9, Folder 9-3, CHS.

98. Reports of these visits are in the CIC Papers, Box 13, CHS.

99. Stritch to Joseph Hurley, October 26, 1943, Chancery Files, Stritch Papers, AAC.

100. Stritch to Msgr. T. V. Shannon, June 10, 1941, Chancery Files, Stritch Papers, AAC.

101. Stritch to Cicognani, June 6, 1946, Box 2969, Chancery Files, Stritch Papers, AAC.

102. Stritch to Cicognani, September 24, 1946, Box 2969, Chancery Files, Stritch Papers, AAC.

103. In the conversation, the need to deal with marriage problems among blacks was raised with "no thought at all of asking for any relaxation of the law or any special legislation, but only to make studies of what under the existing law of the Church is possible." Ibid.

104. The impetus for founding the CSS had come indirectly from Franklin D. Roosevelt, who had identified the South as "economic problem number one" in a speech in the late thirties. This had given rise to a number of private organizations which had as their intention the building of a greater South. In April 1939 the National Catholic Educational Association passed a resolution at their annual meeting mandating that the South be represented in the program of the Second National Catholic Social Action Congress scheduled for June of that year. At the Cleveland meeting the southerners were so enthusiastic that they called for the formation of a permanent standing committee to assist "the southern Bishops and priests in their endeavor to make more articulate the voice of the Catholic Church in the Southland." Stritch was one of the most enthusiastic backers of the move. In April 1940 the Catholic Conference of the South was formed and promptly applied to the Administrative Board of the National Catholic Welfare Conference for recognition. The organization's name was changed to "Catholic Committee of the South" and it was designed to be a board to coordinate discussion of regional issues.

105. Stritch to Cicognani, September 24, 1946, Box 2969, Chancery Files, Stritch Papers, AAC.

106. Interview with Father Rollins Lambert, February 11, 1989.

107. Interview with Father Kenneth Brigham, March 11, 1989.

108. Quoted in a a special report given to Stritch by Joseph Richards and Martin Farrell, "The Catholic Church and the Negro in the Archdiocese of Chicago," 1955, personal copy of author.

109. Stritch to Cicognani, June 6, 1946, Box 2969, Chancery Files, Stritch Papers, AAC.

110. Interview with Father Jake Killgallon, September 17, 1987.

111. This continues to be the position of Farrell and Richards's most active white disciple, Father Anthony Vader. See his "Mission to Black America," *Chicago Studies* 23 (August 1984): 169–181. Vader interview.

9. CHICAGO CATHOLICS IN THE CIVIL RIGHTS ERA

1. Cantwell to Father Bernard Dauenhauer, October 8, 1959, Cantwell Papers, Box 4, Folder 4-3, CHS.

2. "Race War—A Challenge," *Work*, July 1943.

3. The best discussion of the origins and development of the Catholic Interracial Council of New York is Martin Zielinski's, "'Doing the Truth': The Catholic Interracial Council of New York, 1945–1965" (Ph.D. diss., Catholic University of America, 1989).

4. Stritch to John LaFarge, S.J., December 22, 1943, Chancery Files, Stritch Papers, AAC.

5. "Race War—A Challenge," *Work*, July 1943.

6. Other members of this committee included activist Edward Marciniak; real estate agent J. Goodsell Jacobs; Eugene Murphy of the Bruce Publishing Company; Jerome Kerwin of the University of Chicago; George Clark, an accountant; Edward Tiedebohl, a lawyer; government employees Bryan Hammond and Cassius Foster; insurance executive Melvin McNairy; and Taft C. Raines, M.D. See "Report to His Excellency, the Most Reverend Samuel A. Stritch on a Proposed Catholic Interracial Council" (no date), Box 2966, Chancery Files, Stritch Papers, AAC.)

7. Morrison to Stritch, October 8, 1945, Box 2966, Chancery Files, Stritch Papers, AAC.

8. Constitution and By-laws of the Catholic Interracial Council of the Archdiocese of Chicago, Box 2969, Chancery Files, Stritch Papers, AAC.

9. "Report to His Excellency, the Most Reverend Samuel A. Stritch on a proposed Catholic Interracial Council," October 1945, Box 2966, AAC.

10. Stritch to Morrison, October 15, 1945, Box 2966, Chancery Files, Stritch Papers, AAC.

11. Cantwell also apologized for the fact that one of the founders, John McNairy, was not a practicing Catholic. Cantwell promised "to restore him to active Catholic life...." Cantwell to Stritch, October 15, 1946, Box 2969, Chancery Files, Stritch Papers, AAC.

12. Stritch to Cantwell, October 18, 1946, Chancery Files, Stritch Papers, Box 2969, AAC.

13. Stritch to Cantwell, December 11, 1946, Box 2969, Chancery Files, Stritch Papers, AAC.

14. Daniel M. Cantwell, "Race Relations—As Seen by a Catholic," *American Catholic Sociological Review* 7, no. 4 (December 1946): 242–258.

15. Daniel M. Cantwell, ed., *Catholics Speak on Race Relations* (Chicago: Fides Press, 1952).

16. Daniel M. Cantwell, "Catholics and Prejudice," *Voice of St. Jude*, 18 (July 1952): 6–8, 32.

17. Memo to Fr. Egan, Fr. Imbiorski, Russ Barta, Ed Marciniak; From: Fr. Cantwell, April 17, 1957, Cantwell Papers, Box 3, Folder 3-3, CHS.

18. "Ahmann Lauded for Role in Religion-Race Meeting," *New World*, January 25, 1963.

19. For the minutes of this first meeting see, Committee on Long-Range Study of the CIC, CIC Papers, Box 30, Folder April 1–21, 1959, CHS.

20. Gordon C. Zahn to Lloyd Davis, June 16, 1959, CIC Papers, Box 31, Folder June 1–16, 1959, CHS.

21. Interview with John McDermott, December 18, 1987.

22. McDermott to Cantwell, March 3, 1961, CIC Papers, Box 42, Folder March 1–15, 1961, CHS.

23. Report on Rainbow Beach, September 1, 1961, Meyer Papers, AAC.

24. For the full story of Friendship House see Mary Clinch, "Crossing the Color Line: The Story of Friendship House" (unpublished manuscript, no date) in Friendship House Papers, CHS. Interview with Betty Schneider, February 12, 1988.

25. Stritch to John J. Clifford, S.J., December 5, 1951, Box 3004, Chancery Files, Stritch Papers, AAC.

26. Matthew Ahmann to John Cronin, December 9, 1958, Social Action Department Papers, ACUA.

27. Excerpt from "The Holy Season of Lent," Lenten Pastoral Letter, 1959, Most Rev. Albert Gregory Meyer, Archbishop of Chicago, CIC Papers, Box 35, Folder [undated, 1959], CHS.

28. Interview with Monsignor John Egan, October 19, 1981.

29. The President's Commission on Civil Rights, Federal Building, Chicago, Illinois, May 6, 1959. Most Rev. Albert Gregory Meyer, D.D., S.S.L, Archbishop of Chicago. Copy in Meyer Papers, AAC.

30. "The Housing Inquiry," May 13, 1959, *Daily Defender*.

31. "Archbishop Meyer on Housing," *America*, May 23, 1959. Clipping in Meyer Papers, AAC.

32. Alinsky text in Cantwell Papers, CHS.

33. William F. Graney to Cantwell, May 26, 1959, Cantwell Papers, Box 4, Folder 4-1, CHS.

34. "5 Deerfield Ministers Ask Acceptance of Integrated Housing," *Chicago Sun-Times*, November 20, 1959.

35. Cantwell to Meyer, November 24, 1959, Cantwell Papers, Box 8, Folder 35 8-3, CHS.

36. Cantwell to Meyer, December 7, 1959, Cantwell Papers, Box 8, Folder 8-3, CHS.

37. Mr. & Mrs. Anthony G. Sabato to Meyer, December 26, 1959, Meyer Papers, AAC.

38. Mrs. James Lewis to Stritch, August 22, 1957, Chancery Files, Stritch Papers, AAC.

39. Interview with Father Martin Farrell, September 30, 1983.

40. "Catholic High Schools in Chicago to Integrate," March 19, 1960; "Girls' Schools Test Integration," unidentified clippings, Cantwell Papers, Box 8, Folder 8-2, CHS.

41. Interview with Bishop William E. McManus, November 1, 1981.

42. Farrell interview.

43. A Report on the Bessemer Park Disturbance July 25–August 18, 1960, CIC Papers, Box 38, Folder August-September 20, 1960, CHS.

44. Cantwell to Joseph Mangan, S.J., May 16, 1960, Cantwell Papers, Box 8, Folder Meyer-Clergy Conference 8–2, CHS.

45. A copy of this draft is in the Cantwell Papers, see Cantwell to Meyer, August 19, 1960, Cantwell Papers, Box 8, Folder 8-2, CHS.

46. "The Mantle of Leadership" by His Eminence Albert Cardinal Meyer, Archbishop of Chicago, in "The Catholic Church and the Negro in the Archdiocese of Chicago," Clergy Conference, September 20–21, Resurrection Auditorium. Privately published by the Archdiocese of Chicago.

47. Ibid.

48. Clipping in Cantwell Papers, dated Friday January 20, 1961, Cantwell Papers, Box 8, Folder 8-2, CHS. See also "Suburbs Face Integration," clipping from *Community Reporter* in Cantwell Papers, ibid.

49. Report on CIC Activity in Skokie, February 1961, CIC Papers, Box 42, Folder February 18–28, 1961, CHS.

50. Letter from Father Arthur Sauer, Administrator, St. Peter's Catholic Church, Skokie, Illinois, read at all Masses on Sunday,

February 12, 1961, CIC Papers, Box 41, Folder February 1–17, 1961, CHS.

51. McDermott to William F. Graney, February 21, 1961, CIC Papers, Box 42, Folder February 18–28, 1961, CHS. See also "Community Effort Curbs Panic over Integration," clipping from *New World* in CIC Papers, Box 42, Folder March 15–30, 1961, CHS.

52. "Three Faiths Close Ranks at the Wade-Ins," *Chicago Daily News*, August 5, 1961.

53. Farrell interview.

54. Ahmann to Meyer, August 21, 1963, Meyer Papers, AAC.

55. "Catholics Set Washington March Plans," *New World*, August 25, 1963.

56. Cantwell to Meyer, March 11, 1964, Cantwell Papers, Box 8, Folder 8-7, CHS.

57. "Clergymen Denounce 'Racial' Referendum," *New World*, March 6, 1964.

58. Meyer to "Reverend and Dear Father," March 20, 1964, Meyer Papers, AAC.

59. "Religion, Race Group Answers Attack of Property Owners Unit," *New World*, June 12, 1964.

60. Cantwell to Meyer, July 28, 1961, Cantwell Papers, Box 8, Folder 8-4, CHS.

61. Meyer to Cousins, August 17, 1961, and Meyer to Patrick A. O'Boyle, August 17, 1961, Meyer Papers, AAC.

62. O'Boyle to Meyer, August 21, 1961, Meyer Papers, AAC.

63. Cousins to Meyer, September 18, 1961, Meyer Papers, AAC.

64. Program Committee Summary, May 16, 1962, Meyer Papers, AAC.

65. Meyer to John LaFarge, S.J., January 8, 1963, Meyer Papers, AAC.

66. "1893's World Parliament of Religions Recalled," *New World*, January 25, 1963.

67. Meyer to Cantwell, November 7, 1960, Meyer Papers, AAC.

68. Meyer quoted in "Church Leaders Probe Race Issue," *New World*, January 18, 1963.

69. "Cardinal Meyer Suggests Ways to Fight Racial Discrimination," *New World*, January 25, 1963.

70. "Cardinal Meyer Gives $10,000 to Race Group," *New World*, March 15, 1963.

71. Matthew Ahmann, ed., *Race: Challenge to Religion* (Chicago: Henry Regnery Press, 1964).

72. Memo to His Eminence Albert Cardinal Meyer from Very Rev. Msgr. John J. Egan, October 19, 1961, Meyer Papers, AAC.

73. Meyer to "Dear Reverend Father," October 28, 1961, Cantwell Papers, Box 8, Folder 8-4, CHS.

74. "Priests Told to Preach on Racial Equality," *Chicago Daily News*, February 24, 1962.

75. "Love Ye One Another," *New Crusader*, March 3, 1962, clipping, Meyer Papers, AAC.

76. "Cardinal Meyer on Equality," *Daily Defender*, February 28, 1962, clipping in Meyer Papers, AAC.

77. See Flanagan Statement in CIC Papers.

78. "Niles Cited for Responsible Leadership in Racial Integration," *New World*, May 18, 1962.

79. Copy of this letter is in the Meyer Papers, AAC.

80. There were three of these reports, all found in the Meyer Papers, AAC.

81. "Chicago Priests Probe Problems of Negro," *New World*, April 17, 1964; "Parley on Negro Called 'Good Beginning,'" *New World*, April 24, 1964.

82. See recommendations of Niles Study Day, Meyer Papers, AAC.

83. Second Methodist Conference on Human Relations, August 28, 1963, Response to Award Citation, Meyer Papers, AAC.

84. "Address to National Catholic Interracial Council," July 27, 1963, Meyer Papers, AAC.

85. Meyer to "Dear Reverend Father," August 19, 1963, Meyer Papers, AAC.

86. Edward Marciniak to Meyer, February 5, 1963, Meyer Papers, AAC.

87. Meyer to "Dear Reverend Father," April 9, 1964, Meyer Papers, AAC.

88. Raymond M. Hilliard to Meyer, May 5, 1964, Meyer Papers, AAC.

89. Ahmann to Meyer, May 21, 1964, Meyer Papers, AAC.

90. Gerald P. Scanlon et al. to Meyer, September 2, 1964, Meyer Papers, AAC.

91. Ibid.

92. Meyer to Vincent Moran, September 4, 1964, Meyer Papers, AAC.

93. Robert J. Cronin to Meyer, February 8, 1965, Meyer Papers, AAC.

10. THE TWILIGHT OF AN ERA

1. Interview with Monsignor John S. Quinn, September 10, 1983.

2. *Council Daybook* (Washington, D.C.: Press Department, National Catholic Welfare Conference, 1963), vol. 1: 2.

3. Meyer to William Newton, May 9, 1960, Meyer Papers, AAC.

4. "Meyer's Address," CIC, Box 40, Folder 1960, undated, Chicago Historical Society.

5. Ibid.

6. John F. McConnell, M.M., to Meyer, July 19, 1960, Meyer Papers, AAC.

7. Meyer to Bea, November 19, 1960, Meyer Papers, AAC.

8. For an example of these criticisms see Francis Filas, S.J. to Meyer, July 23, 1960, Meyer Papers, AAC.

9. "Summary and Remarks," His Eminence Albert Cardinal Meyer, *The New Catholic Approach to the Interpretation of Sacred Scripture* (Archdiocese of Chicago, Clergy Conference February 23–24, 1961), p. 27, Meyer Papers, AAC.

10. Ibid.

11. Address, "Institute of Lay Action Archdiocesan Council of Catholic Men," September 9, 1962, Meyer Papers, AAC.

12. "Cardinal Sends Message," *New World*, October 12, 1962.

13. *Council Day Book*, 1:27.

14. Meyer to George Casey, November 25, 1962, Meyer Papers, AAC.

15. "Cardinal Returns from Rome, Gives His Views on Council," *New World*, December 14, 1962.

16. Ibid.

17. John Mark Gannon to Meyer, January 9, 1963, Meyer Papers, AAC.

18. Examples of this commentary include "Changes in Inter-Faith Attitudes," *New World*, April 5, 1963, and "Cardinal Alfrink: Church Should Sacrifice Non-Essential Elements," *New World*, July 5, 1963.

19. *Catholic Herald Citizen*, February 20, 1963.

20. Ritter to McDonald, February 19, 1963, copy in Meyer Papers, AAC.

21. Meyer to Ritter, February 27, 1963, Meyer Papers, AAC.

22. "On Catholic U. Controversy," *New World*, March 8, 1963.

23. Meyer to Cantwell, March 14, 1963, Meyer Papers, AAC.

24. Meyer to O'Donnell, November 14, 1963, Meyer Papers, AAC.

25. Meyer to O'Donnell, November 24, 1963, Meyer Papers, AAC.

26. "Significance of Council's Work Lauded," *New World*, December 20, 1963.

27. Vincent A. Yzermans, ed., *American Participation in the Second Vatican Council* (New York: Sheed and Ward, 1967), p. 307.

28. "Ecumenism," Pastoral Letter of Cardinal Albert G. Meyer, Lent 1964, Meyer Papers, AAC.

29. "Cardinal Meyer Speaks at Ministers' Gathering," *New World*, January 24, 1964; "Churchmen Praying," *America* 110 (February 8, 1964): 179.

30. Despite the publicity attendant on his letter and the meeting with the ministers, Meyer still held back from going "too far." When the suffragan episcopal bishop, James W. Montgomery, invited archdiocesan chancellor Francis Byrne to attend the installation of some cathedral canons and participate in the procession in ecclesiastical regalia, Meyer wrote back to Byrne: "The answer to this must be 'no' and the reason given must be that it is still too immature. Actually something like that will be allowed according to the new text on Ecumenism. Since this text, however has received only a tentative approbation, and has not been solemnly promulgated (or even actually voted on), I would prefer to have you refrain from going in robes, or 'participating in the service.'" Meyer to Byrne, October 16, 1964, Meyer Papers, AAC.

31. Minutes of the First Plenary Session of the Chicago Archdiocesan Liturgical Commission, April 7, 1964, Meyer Papers, AAC.

32. "Priests Will Examine, Discuss Vatican II Document on Liturgy," *New World*, May 15, 1964.

33. Meyer to "Dearly Beloved in Christ," September 9, 1964; see also Meyer to "Dear Reverend Father," September 9, 1964, Meyer Papers, AAC.

34. Meyer to O'Donnell, November 24, 1963, Meyer Papers, AAC.

35. McCool to Meyer, January 21, 1964, Meyer Papers, AAC.

36. Meyer to Pope Paul VI, January 24, 1964, Meyer Papers, AAC.

37. "Religious Liberty Statement Need Cited by Cardinal," Press Release, January 24, 1964, NCWC Press Department Files, ACUA.

38. McCool to Meyer, April 25, 1964, Meyer Papers, AAC.

39. McCool to Meyer, June 14, 1964, Meyer Papers, AAC.

40. Cantwell to Meyer, March 17, 1964, Cantwell Papers, Box 8, Folder Meyer–1964, CHS. A copy of Tannenbaum's letter to Cantwell dated March 13, 1964 is found in the same location.

41. "Cardinal Meyer: Condemn Anti-Semitism, Race Bias" *New World*, October 2, 1964; see also Yzermans, pp. 588–599; O'Donnell interview.

42. Interview with Monsignor Porter White, October 15, 1981.

43. "Cardinal on Religious Roots of U.S.," *New World*, October 30, 1964.

44. Meyer to Byrne, November 16, 1964, Meyer Papers, AAC.

45. A perfect example of this fanciful writing is found in Aloysius Wycislo's amusing memoirs, *Vatican II Revisited: Reflections by One Who Was There* (New York: Alba House, 1987). On pages 132–134, Wycislo repeats a very dramatic story from a supposed eye-witness view. However, correspondence indicates that Bishop Wycislo was safe and sound back in Chicago on November 12, 1964 and the incident happened a week later. See Wycislo to Meyer, November 12, 1964, Meyer Papers, AAC. Wycislo borrowed a lot of details from Xavier Rynne's *The Third Session* (New York: Farrar, Strauss, and Giroux, 1965), p. 257.

46. Letter of Bishop Francis Reh to author, January 21, 1982.

47. Letter of Cardinal Paul Emile Leger to author, July 10, 1983.

48. His friend Bishop John Grellinger spoke of visiting with Meyer on the evening of the confrontation and finding the cardinal dejected and depressed. Interview with Bishop John B. Grellinger, November 29, 1980.

49. "Cardinal Meyer 'Disappointed' on Liberty Issue," November 24, 1964, NCWC Press Files, ACUA.

50. Interview with Monsignor William Groessel, May 26, 1980.

51. Meyer to Ahern, February 16, 1965, Meyer Papers, AAC.

52. John Leo, "Cody in Chicago," *Commonweal* 74 (June 10, 1966): 334–336.

53. George Shuster, "Albert Cardinal Meyer: Council Father," Twelve Council Fathers Series (Notre Dame, Ind.: University of Notre Dame Press, 1964).

Index

Gleason, John R., 90, 214
Godfrey, Edmund, 228
Gonella, Guido, 58
Gorman, William, 214, 217–218, 220, 230, 266
Grail, Ladies of the, 128, 171, 159
Graney, William F., 231, 301, 331–332
Greeley, Andrew, 81–82, 164, 184, 236
Green, Dwight, 194, 197
Grellinger, John, 14, 398 n.48
Griffin, Domitilla, R.S.M., 199, 200
Griffin, James, 103, 134, 199, 272
Groessel, William, 342–343

Haas, Francis, 37, 126, 175, 180
Hackett, Edwin R., 178
Hales Franciscan High School, 304
Hannegan, Robert, 60
Hardiman, James, 7, 10–11, 18, 97, 103, 106
Harrigan, Ann, 297
Hartnett, Robert, S.J., 85
Hassett, William D., 58
Haston, Scotty, 129, 134, 369 n.46
Hayes, John, 5, 36–39, 117, 163, 175, 306
Hayes, Patrick, 6, 12
Heineman, Ben, 232
Hellreigel, Martin, 35
Herr, Dan, 6
Hesburgh, Theodore, C.S.C., 237, 300
Heschel, Abraham, 314, 338
Heywood, Robert, 261, 264, 372 n.17
Higgins, George G., 33, 67, 147, 158, 163
Hillenbrand, Frederick, 30
Hillenbrand, George, 30
Hillenbrand Reynold H., 22, 91–92, 117–118, 149, 174, 177, 179, 180, 183, 185, 283; and Christian Family Movement, 171–173; and Catholic Labor Alliance, 175; disagreement with Egan, 165, 231; dismissal from seminary, 158–163, 178; early life and career, 30–35, 186; and impact on Chicago Catholicism, 4; and liturgy, 151–153, 336; and post-seminary career, 164–167, 345; and racial issues, 253; as rector, 35–37, 157–158, 284; and social action, 37–39; and Specialized

Catholic Action, 39–42, 153–157; and racial issues, 253
Hillinger, Raymond, 100, 103, 106
Hishen, James D., 168
Hoban, Edward, 23
Hochwalt, Frederick, 92–93
Hoffman, Robert, 107
Holy Angels parish, 254–255, 260–261, 286–287, 321
Holy Cross parish, 224, 243, 259
Holy Family parish, 253, 258, 284
Holy Guardian Angels parish, 216, 218
Holy Innocents parish, 241
Holy Name Aeronautical/Flying School (Lockport), 24, 26
Holy Name Cathedral, 15, 22–23, 152, 154, 176, 180, 291, 293
Holy Name of Mary parish, 277
Holy Name Societies, Archdiocesan Union, 50
Holy Name Society, 23, 83, 103, 112, 154, 214, 217–218, 287
Holy Name Technical School (Lockport), 111
Holy Redeemer parish (Evergreen Park), 51
Holy Rosary parish, 241
Holy Trinity parish, 218
Hoover, J. Edgar, 61–63, 275
Hopkins, Harry, 24
Horne, Lena, 136
Horwitt, Sanford, 145
Hosty, Thomas, 210
Houtart, Francois, 235–236
Howard, Mr. and Mrs. Donald, 269–270
Howard, Martin, 158
Hunt, Lester, 224–225
Hurley, Joseph, 281
Hurley, Neil, S.J., 82
Hutchins, Robert Maynard, 228
Hyde Park, 227, 228, 231–233
Hyde Park-Kenwood Project, 165, 227–231, 234, 244, 245, 383 n.27
Hyland, Francis, 273–274

Ickes, Harold, 28–29, 44, 195, 269
Ihlder, John, 175
Illinois Institute of Technology (IIT), 197–200, 203